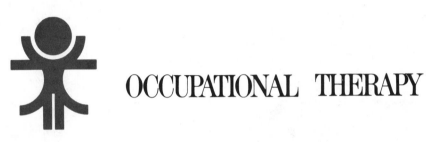

OCCUPATIONAL THERAPY

Contributing Authors

Gilfoyle, Elnora M., B.S., O.T.R.
Formerly Instructor, Department of Physical Medicine and Rehabilitation; Research Associate, John F. Kennedy Child Development Center, University of Colorado Medical Center, Denver, Colorado

Gillette, Nedra P., B.S., O.T.R.
Special Lecturer in Occupational Therapy, College of Physicians and Surgeons, Columbia University, New York, New York

Gleave, G. Margaret, O.T.R.
Executive Director, The Curative Workshop of Racine, Racine, Wisconsin

Grady, Ann P., B.S., O.T.R.
Director, Occupational Therapy Department, The Children's Hospital, Denver, Colorado

Hamant, Celestine, B.A., O.T.R.
Supervisor, Occupational Therapy Department, James Whitcomb Riley Hospital for Children, Indiana University Medical Center, Indianapolis, Indiana

Hopkins, Helen L., M.A., O.T.R.
Assistant Professor of Occupational Therapy, College of Allied Health Professions, Temple University, Philadelphia, Pennsylvania

Huss, A. Joy, M.S., O.T.R., R.P.T.
Assistant Professor, Occupational Therapy and Physical Therapy, Indiana University Medical Center, Indianapolis, Indiana

Hutchinson, Elizabeth L., O.T.R.
Formerly Vice-President, Division for the Blind, The Seeing Eye, Inc., Morristown, New Jersey

Mellinger, M. Arlene, M.A., O.T.R.
Senior Consultant, Occupational Therapists, Office of Rehabilitation Therapists, Division of Hospital Affairs, New York State Department of Health, Albany, New York

Slominski, Anita, B.A., O.T.R.
Coordinator, Cerebral Palsy Clinic, Indiana University Medical Center, Indianapolis, Indiana

Spackman, Clare S., M.S., O.T.R.
Associate Professor Emeritus, School of Allied Medical Professions, University of Pennsylvania, Philadelphia, Pennsylvania

Spencer, Elinor Anne, B.A., O.T.R.
Chief Occupational Therapist, Hospital of the University of Pennsylvania, Philadelphia, Pennsylvania

Wagner, Elizabeth M., O.T.R.
Formerly Specialist, Services for Deaf-Blind Children, American Foundation for the Blind, New York, New York

Walker, Alberta D., Ph.D., O.T.R.
Consultant in Homes for the Aged, Los Angeles Area, California

Zimmerman, Muriel E., M.S., O.T.R.
Assistant Professor, Clinical Rehabilitation Medicine, New York University Medical Center, Institute of Rehabilitation Medicine, New York, New York

OCCUPATIONAL
THERAPY FOURTH EDITION

EDITED BY

Helen S. Willard, B.A., O.T.R.

Professor Emeritus of Occupational Therapy, University of Pennsylvania, School of Allied Medical Professions

and

Clare S. Spackman, B.S., M.S. (ED.), O.T.R.

Associate Professor Emeritus of Occupational Therapy, University of Pennsylvania, School of Allied Medical Professions

J. B. LIPPINCOTT COMPANY

PHILADELPHIA • TORONTO

Distributed in Great Britain by
Blackwell Scientific Publications, Oxford and Edinburgh

ISBN-0-397-54118-X

Library of Congress Catalog Card Number 74-143334

Printed in The United States of America

9   8   7   6

Preface

This fourth edition of *Occupational Therapy* mirrors many of the changes which have taken place during the decade of the sixties. Much active research has been done and many investigative projects are now in process. Many occupational therapists have achieved Master's degrees and a considerable number have now attained or are in the process of attaining Ph.D's. or Ed.D's. The result is that there is now amassed a respectable amount of research literature which testifies to the professional caliber of occupational therapy.

The initial chapters of this volume dealing primarily with the status of occupational therapy and the principles of organization and administration have been relatively little changed. The subsequent chapters, written in part by previous authors who have expanded their material and by nine new authors, are direct evidence of the development of trends which were only beginning in the period covered by the third edition.

Such developments as the use in occupational therapy of technics to test and develop cognitive perceptual motor skills in persons with either psychosocial or physical dysfunction have brought the two areas closer together. Finally the highly specialized therapist in each field is recognizing that the patient cannot really be classified as suffering from only one type of dysfunction.

The occupational therapist has always dealt with the whole man and his development, but increasing emphasis is being placed upon knowledge of both physical and psychological human development and upon abnormalities which occur at all ages from childhood to old age. Occupational therapy has much to offer in the treatment of children. With the increasing number of neurological injuries from war and from automobile and sports accidents, knowledge and understanding of the character and degree of the injury present a challenge to refine methods of treatment and to devise ways of assisting the patient to adapt to his handicap. ADL, the activities of daily living, have become common parlance and have led to a general consciousness of the value of household arrangements and procedures which minimize effort and increase efficiency.

So this edition presents dramatic evidence of change in the profession of occupational therapy and of its readiness to meet the problems and the challenges of the seventies.

Community medicine and preventive measures for maintaining health are gaining greater attention and are involving the skills of the occupational therapist. Problems of drug abuse and many social and community problems are demanding the attention of medically trained persons among whom the occupational therapist is recognized as a valuable member of the team.

Convalescent and nursing homes are rapidly increasing and are demanding large numbers of personnel. In geriatric problems, certified occupational therapy assistants, who are also used in many other fields, are working under occupational therapists who serve as supervisors or consultants.

The contributors to this edition are all experts who have rendered outstanding service in the particular areas of occupational therapy in which they are or have been employed. They have prepared their chapters in their "spare time" without freedom from their regular jobs and without financial assistance of any sort. They have amply demonstrated their dedication to their chosen profession.

The editors wish to express their heartfelt thanks to all of the writers, past and present, who have contributed to the four editions of *Occupational Therapy*. Their interest and cooperation has been outstanding in making these publications of value to the oncoming members of our profession and are strong evidence of the character and spirit of occupational therapists.

The editors are aware of shortcomings and of possible omissions in this edition. We present it with great pride in the past and confidence in the future of the profession.

As this edition goes to press we know of others who are planning and writing books on specific areas. This is what was envisioned in 1947 and is a development most heartily welcomed. Some of the subjects omitted in this edition we hope will soon be covered with the breadth that they deserve.

Helen S. Willard
Clare S. Spackman

Contents

PART II

OCCUPATIONAL THERAPY

Occupational Therapy— Its Relation to Allied Medical Services

CLARE S. SPACKMAN, M.S., O.T.R.

> "Occupational Therapy is the art and science of directing man's response to selected activity to promote and maintain health, to prevent disability, to evaluate behavior and to treat or train patients with physical or psychosocial dysfunction."
>
> American Occupational Therapy Association, 1968

Occupational therapy contributes much to the treatment of the patient. It may be used with all types of patients after the most acute phase of illness has passed.

The unique contribution of occupational therapy is that it uses a program of normal activity to aid in the psychosocial adjustment of the patient, as specific treatment or as a simulated work situation. Thus it relates to the patient's everyday life and provides the link between hospitalization and return to the community. Its modalities are manifold, depending upon the needs of the patient, his physician's orders, the specified precautions, the ingenuity of the occupational therapist and the space and the funds available. The wide variety of activities which may be used provides an endless challenge to the therapist. The physician refers the patient for occupational therapy to achieve specified goals within his limitations. The occupational therapist selects occupations which are appropriate to the patient's physical and psychological condition and will aid in obtaining the desired results. Once the patient has reached a certain stage of convalescence, he should participate freely in normal activities—school, work or care of the home and recreation.

FUNCTIONS OF OCCUPATIONAL THERAPY*

Occupational therapy is a medically directed treatment of the physically and/or mentally disabled by means of constructive activities — such activities designed and adapted by a professionally qualified occupational therapist to promote the restoration of useful function.

The patient may be referred for occupational therapy by his physician for one or more of the following purposes:

1. As specific treatment for psychiatric patients — to structure opportunities for the development of more satisfying relationships, to assist in releasing or sublimating emotional drives, to aid as a diagnostic tool.
2. As specific treatment for restoration of physical function, to increase joint motion, muscle strength and coordination.
3. To teach self-help activities, those of daily living such as eating, dressing, writing, the use of adapted equipment and prostheses.
4. To help the disabled homemaker readjust to home routines with advice and instruction as to the adaptation of household equipment and work simplification.
5. To develop work tolerance and maintenance of special skills as required by the patient's job.
6. To provide prevocational exploration — to determine the patient's physical and mental capacities, social adjustment, interests, work habits, skills and potential employability.
7. As a supportive measure — to help the patient to accept and utilize constructively a prolonged period of hospitalization and convalescence.
8. For redirection of recreational and avocational interests.

Occupational therapy programs are a part of the medical services in such facilities as the following — general and special hospitals, rehabilitation centers, geriatric institutions, home care programs, reform institutions, special schools, clinics and any other organization which provides rehabilitation services for the disabled. The occupational therapist contributes to the total rehabilitation of the patient in conjunction with the doctor, nurse, physiotherapist, speech therapist, social worker, psychologist, vocational counsellor and other specialists, to return the patient to the greatest possible independence.

DEVELOPMENT OF OCCUPATIONAL THERAPY†

Occupational therapy, which developed as a profession during World War I (1914-18), grew rapidly in English-speaking countries with the

*Officially adopted by the World Federation of Occupational Therapists. — Revised October, 1962.
†See bibliography for source material on history and development of occupational therapy.

recognition of the need to rehabilitate the civilian patient as well as the disabled soldier. From earliest times the value of occupation for the mentally ill has been recognized. Its application as specific treatment for all types of patients has been accepted only since 1918. World War II (1939-45) did much to crystallize concepts of treatment. Since that time, with the increasing acceptance of rehabilitation as a medical responsibility, this type of treatment has developed in many countries.

In 1952 the World Federation of Occupational Therapists was founded. This organization has done much to develop educational programs which meet the minimum standards of education of occupational therapists throughout the world. Occupational therapy is well established in 25 countries and is growing rapidly in many others.

The education of the occupational therapist is divided into three phases: (1) The medical phase, which includes knowledge of the basic medical sciences, the conditions treated and the application of the theory of occupational therapy; (2) the study of the skills or activities used for treatment; (3) clinical practice or internship during which the student treats different types of patients under the supervision of a qualified therapist.

The profession is fortunate in that the educational standards are sufficiently similar throughout the world, so that it is possible for a therapist qualified in any member country of the World Federation of Occupational Therapists to work in any other country, provided that language and immigration requirements can be met.

CONCEPTS OF REHABILITATION

The rehabilitation of the patient is the responsibility of all medical personnel: the physician, the nurse, the social worker, the physical therapist, the occupational therapist and other closely related persons, such as the family, the teacher, the psychologist, the vocational counselor and the clergyman.

Essentially all types of medical treatment are rehabilitative procedures. Thus, rehabilitation is not a procedure per se but a philosophy, which postulates that, in order that the patient may attain maximum recovery regardless of the cause of his condition, not only the medical aspects but also the psychosocial and the vocational aspects must be considered.

Rehabilitation often is cited as the specific function of physical medicine. The physiatrist has specialized in methods of treatment which promote rehabilitation, especially for the physically disabled. However, it is the responsibility of all physicians to refer their patients for appropriate medical, educational, psychosocial and/or vocational services. If a physician is not aware of and does not utilize these services, his patients will not receive the full assistance that is available. In most instances in fields such as psychiatry, cardiology and ophthalmology, the referral for services which assist in achieving the rehabilitation of a patient may be entirely the responsibility of the physician in charge of the case.

Many services are needed in a community to provide for the total rehabilitation of a physically and/or mentally disabled person. Some of these are available in hospitals and outpatient clinics or through home services; others, in rehabilitation centers, in sheltered workshops or by the adaptation of the normal services, such as school, which are provided for all persons. It is only through the work of many agencies and many professions that the needs of all types of patients may be met.

REHABILITATION SERVICES NEEDED IN A COMMUNITY*

1. Services of specialists in the various medical areas.
2. Dental services which contribute to improved nutrition and the prevention of infection, to care for cosmetic defects and related problems of cleft palate and congenital anomalies of the mouth.
3. Nursing service in the hospital, in convalescent nursing homes and the patient's home.
4. Social casework which helps the patient and his family to accept and to adjust to the problems resulting from his disability.
5. Physical therapy services for the evaluation of physical abilities and disabilities and for treatment utilizing therapeutic exercise, physical agents, massage, and assistive devices.
6. Occupational therapy services for the evaluation of physical, psychosocial and vocational adjustment and treatment by the utilization of simulated home, social, recreational and work situations.
7. Speech and hearing therapy for the evaluation and the treatment of abnormalities in voice, speech and the hearing mechanisms.
8. Education, adapted to meet the needs of the handicapped individual, through special schools or hospital classes and/or tutoring in the hospital or home.
9. Psychological services to provide information concerning the patient's mental abilities, emotional adjustment, interests and vocational aptitudes.
10. Counseling which will enable the physically and/or mentally handicapped student to choose appropriate courses in school leading to a vocation by which he should be capable of earning a living.

*Chart 1—1 indicates the relationships of the above services.

CHART 1-1. PROCESS OF REHABILITATION

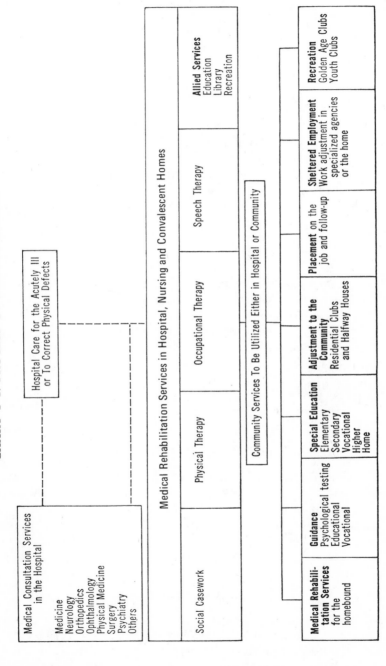

Medical Consultation Services in the Hospital

Medicine
Neurology
Orthopedics
Ophthalmology
Physical Medicine
Surgery
Psychiatry
Others

Hospital Care for the Acutely Ill or To Correct Physical Defects

Medical Rehabilitation Services in Hospital, Nursing and Convalescent Homes

Social Casework

Physical Therapy

Occupational Therapy

Speech Therapy

Allied Services
Education
Library
Recreation

Community Services To Be Utilized Either in Hospital or Community

Medical Rehabilitation Services for the homebound

Guidance
Psychological testing
Educational
Vocational

Special Education
Elementary
Secondary
Vocational
Higher
Home

Adjustment to the Community
Residential Clubs and Halfway Houses

Placement on the job and follow-up

Sheltered Employment
Work adjustment in specialized agencies or the home

Recreation
Golden Age Clubs
Youth Clubs

11. Vocational counseling services to provide guidance as to appropriate occupations in which handicapped clients may find employment; to suggest appropriate training facilities and to help the client to adjust to the working situation.
12. Selected placement for handicapped clients and follow-up in employment to assure adequate performance.
13. Residential clubs which help the patient to adjust to living outside of an institution while training or working.
14. Halfway Houses which aid in the readjustment of the psychiatric patient to the community.
15. Remunerative sheltered employment for those unable to function in competitive employment, where work can be adapted to the individual's capabilities and work adjustment and/or special training can be obtained.
16. Remunerative employment of homebound handicapped persons who can be made partially or wholly self-supporting.
17. Recreational programs in the community for the handicapped.

Team Approach

With the concept of rehabilitation there has been increasing emphasis on the importance of the team approach. Regular scheduled meetings are held at which all the professional members of the staff and the consultants meet to discuss new admissions, to plan treatment goals, to evaluate progress and to recommend further treatment or discharge. Thus realistic goals may be established for the patient, and the means of helping him to achieve them may be determined.

For team conferences to be successful all members must contribute to the discussion and the planning.

RELATION TO OTHER SERVICES

If the treatment is truly patient-centered, geared to achieve the patient's goal, then coordination occurs almost automatically, as each service considers the patient's needs rather than its own prestige. No one profession can state truthfully that it alone was responsible for the rehabilitation of the patient. Rather each must state that it provided certain services, treatment, guidance or support which contributed to the total result.

Medical Referral and Supervision

The occupational therapist may accept patients for treatment upon a written referral from a physician. The physician in referring a patient should state the diagnosis, if known, the present condition of the patient, the limitations or the precautions to be observed, the prognosis, the results to be achieved and the frequency and the length of treatment. It is the occupational therapist's responsibility to select suitable activities which should serve to attain the physician's treatment objectives.

The occupational therapist must be alert to changes in the patient's condition and should report these to the physician. The physician is responsible for changing the orders for occupational therapy when indicated. Reports should be made in writing or in conference relative to the patient's reaction to or progress in treatment.

In all matters relating to the patient's treatment the occupational therapist is directly responsible to the referring physician. Administratively, the director of the occupational therapy department is responsible to the director of the hospital or agency, or to whomsoever he may designate from the administrative staff.

Nursing

The nurse is responsible for all patients under her care. This includes not only specific nursing care but also seeing that, if necessary, the patient is transported to different clinics for treatment or diagnostic tests. It is the nurse's responsibility to account for the patient, and to give permission (with the physician's approval) for him to leave the ward. If occupational therapy is given at the patient's bedside or if he is to carry out certain activities in the ward, the nurse's understanding and cooperation is of vital importance. Praise and encouragement by the nurse in the absence of the therapist is invaluable.

If the patient's program includes activities of daily living, such as ambulation, eating, dressing or writing, the closest coordination must be maintained between nursing, physical and occupational therapy, as each is responsible in part for the instruction of the patient. When the patient is on the ward the nursing staff should supervise and encourage the use of activities of daily living learned in physical and occupational therapy. It is the therapist's responsibility to keep the nurse informed as to the activities which the patient should be able to perform.

The patient receiving occupational therapy makes considerably fewer demands on the nursing service. A physically handicapped patient, as he regains the ability to care for himself, relieves the nurse by caring for his own personal needs.

Social Service

The occupational therapist may obtain much valuable information from the social worker concerning the patient's background, his family and his financial problems, his reaction to his condition and to treatment. This is important in all types of hospitals.

In some instances it is only from the social worker that information concerning the patient's living conditions at home can be obtained. This is especially important for psychiatric patients about to be discharged, or when working out adaptations in the home for the severely disabled homemaker, or in planning a treatment program for convalescents to be continued at home.

The social worker is in most instances responsible for the referral of patients to other agencies upon discharge. The occupational therapist, having information concerning the patient which would be of value to other agencies at a later date, should give the social worker a report on the patient in duplicate so that this may be transmitted easily.

The occupational therapist should tell the social worker of pertinent reactions of the patient observed during treatment and/or comments made by him. This enables the social worker in doing casework with the patient to help him achieve a feasible goal.

Physical Therapy

In the treatment of physical disabilities occupational and physical therapy have a similar ultimate goal, namely, to contribute to the restoration of the physical function of the patient.

Personnel from these fields must work together closely and must have a mutual understanding of the goals and the treatment methods employed by each. Their work often supplements or complements the other in the treatment of the individual patient. For example, for the patient who is able to use an injured part voluntarily but does not do so because of pain, the objective of the treatment given by the physical therapist may be solely to relieve pain and precedes the treatment given by the occupational therapist which encourages voluntary motion and works to maintain power and endurance. In another instance the patient may be receiving treatment in physical therapy aimed to improve muscle strength and coordination through use of specific individualized exercise procedures, while simultaneously in occupational therapy the patient may be receiving a treatment which translates specific movements into useful, purposeful activities.

The physical therapist also administers various tests and measurements, the results of which, when interpreted in the light of the objectives of occupational therapy, may give a more realistic basis for formulation of treatment methods.

Speech Therapy

The speech therapist may provide the occupational therapist with information about the aphasic patient's comprehension of the spoken or written word. Aphasic patients vary greatly in their degree of comprehension. This defect affects the occupational therapist's approach to the patient and the type of activity suitable for the patient.

The occupational therapist, if fully aware of the patient's progress in speech therapy, can help to re-enforce this by encouraging him to use such words as he can and to name the simple objects used in treatment.

Education

Educational services are found in many types of hospitals. There should be close coordination between this program or special tutoring for individual patients and occupational therapy.

If the child has developed a physical handicap prior to school age, occupational therapy may be utilized to develop the hand skill and co-ordination needed to learn to write or to type.

The importance of providing adequate education for the handi-capped child cannot be overstressed. Too often a child with a physical handicap may, for lack of opportunity, develop a second handicap of inadequate education. Adults who lack education also profit by an op-portunity for further study during prolonged hospitalization.

Library Service

Library service is available in many types of hospitals, especially in large cities where it is usually an extension of the public library. Many of these provide page turners for persons unable to use their hands or prism glasses for patients who must lie flat in bed. Talking Book Rec-ords may also be obtained for patients with eye or other conditions which prevent them from being able to read.

Patients interested in special hobbies may request pertinent books. Persons unable to read English may get books in their own language.

Recreation

Recreation plays an important part in everyone's life. For hospitalized and handicapped persons it is often necessary to provide special facil-ities. Recreation has always been used as one of the modalities of occu-pational therapy. In some cases, however, a separate department is es-tablished. When this is the case every effort should be made to ensure coordination.

Vocational Counseling

Vocational counseling services are found increasingly in many types of hospitals. There should be close coordination between the occupa-tional therapist and the vocational counselor. When vocational train-ing or specialized placement is indicated, a report from the occupa-tional therapist on the patient's vocational potentialities as well as his physical abilities and adjustment should be presented.

Many occupational therapy departments have available a prevoca-tional evaluation service. The counselor desiring more specific infor-mation about the patient may request such an evaluation.

Extension of the Occupational Therapy Services

The shortage of qualified occupational therapists and the need for diversional activities for medically unrestricted patients with long-term or chronic illnesses, especially in the fields of psychiatry and geriatrics, has placed increasing emphasis on the valuable contribution which may be made by the members of the family and by volunteers. In many instances a wise mother, a friend or a volunteer can provide diversion for a convalescent patient whose condition is not such that medical guidance and/or specialized training are required.

A clear distinction should be made between occupational therapy and this worthwhile and valuable utilization of diversion and recreation.

To supplement further the services of the occupational therapist and to care for the many chronically ill institutionalized patients, certified occupational therapy assistants and instructors have been prepared through training courses to work under the supervision of registered occupational therapists.

Summary

This chapter has presented briefly the functions of occupational therapy irrespective of diagnostic category, the concept of rehabilitation and the coordination of occupational therapy with other services, and the team approach. Subsequent chapters in this book will deal specifically with the use of occupational therapy with certain types of patients.

BIBLIOGRAPHY

Dunton, W. R., Jr., and Licht, S.: Occupational Therapy, Principles and Practices. Springfield, Illinois, Charles C. Thomas, 1957.

Hirschberg, L. R.: Rehabilitation: A Manual for the Care of the Disabled and Elderly. Philadelphia, J. B. Lippincott, 1964.

Licht, S.: Occupational Therapy Source Book. Baltimore, Williams & Wilkins, 1948.

MacDonald, E. M., MacCaul, G., and Mirrey, L.: Occupational Therapy in Rehabilitation. ed. 3, Baltimore, Williams & Wilkins, 1970.

Pattison, H. A.: The Handicapped and Their Rehabilitation. Springfield, Illinois, Charles C. Thomas, 1957.

Viscardi, H.: Give Us the Tools. New York, Ericson & Taplinger, 1958.

Journals

Barton, W. E., Medical supervision in occupational therapy. Am. J. Occup. Therapy, 9:53, 1955.

Bennett, R. L., and Driver, M. F.: Role of occupational therapy in the rehabilitation of the physically handicapped. Arch. Phys. Med., 36:1699, 1955.

Clements, A. M.: Co-ordination of occupational therapy and the nursing service in treatment. Am. J. Occup. Therapy, 9:250, 1955.

Fox, J., Van D., and Orzack, L. H.: The contemporary meaning of work. Am. J. Occup. Therapy, 21:29, 1967.

Greer, I. G.: Motivation of the brain damaged patient. Am. J. Occup. Therapy, 9:156, 1955.

Johnson, J., and Smith, M.: Changing concepts of occupational therapy in a community rehabilitation center. Am. J. Occup. Therapy, 20:267, 1966.

Leopold, R. L.: Contributing therapists. Am. J. Occup. Therapy, 9:239, 1955.

Sokolov, J.: Working as a team. Am. J. Occup. Therapy, 9:270, 1955.

Spackman, C. S.: The world federation of occupational therapists. Am. J. Occup. Therapy, 21:301, 1967.

Stull, R. J.: Interdepartmental relations of ancillary medical services. Phys. Therapy Rev., 22:402, 1949.

Yerxa, E. J.: Authentic occupational therapy. Am. J. Occup. Therapy, 21:10, 1967.

2

Organization and Administration of Occupational Therapy Departments

G. MARGARET GLEAVE, O.T.R.

Organization and administration can be described very simply as the tools that turn visions into reality. One can see the need for expansion of a program, a new service in an institution, or even the need for a particular type of institution in a community. Until an organized way is developed to fulfill this need the vision remains no more than a dream, a wish, or a hope.

The same philosophy may be applied to existing departments and institutions. Improvement of services and operational technics can be accomplished only if a very realistic approach is taken to evaluate and analyze existing conditions.

Organization and administration need not be thought of as formidable. They form the basic pattern established for a program, the systems and the operational procedures to integrate the program, and the performance of duties to fulfill the obligations. In truth, they constitute management, integration and operation. They include all employees of the institution and apply equally to all departments as well as to the institution as a whole.

Organizational structure and administrative functions can be evaluated as good only when there is:

1. Balance between the overall structural design and the application of duties.
2. A well-established two-way flow of directions and results of operations between the executive and staff levels.

3. Flexibility to allow changes to be considered if they will produce a more satisfactory working relation.
4. Consideration for the administrative capacities and special interests of key personnel.
5. Evidence that the functions of the institutions are conducted in an orderly manner.

> The problems of organization and administration are closely integrated, frequently overlapping, and separable only by the fact that organizational considerations precede administrative matters.[5]

PRINCIPLES OF ORGANIZATION

We shall consider first the principles of organization from the institutional level. As these principles apply to the institution, so should they apply to each department within it.

MacEachern describes a hospital as follows:

> The departments of the hospital, including both in- and outpatient services, group themselves into two main divisions, those having to do with the professional care of patients, and those concerned with the business management.
>
> That section of the organization which has to do with the professional care of patients may be divided into four subgroups, viz.: (1) the medico-administration group, comprising medical social service, admission and discharge, and medical records; (2) the medical services, including the attending and resident staffs and the adjunct diagnostic and therapeutic departments; (3) the nursing service; and (4) the dietary service.
>
> Under the business section is included the organization for accounting, purchase and supply, mechanical, maintenance, housekeeping, and laundry.[2]

Among the essential considerations in an analysis of the organization of an institution, the following basic principles are generally accepted:

1. Central control, such as executive or management responsibility, should be established. This will provide a check on effectiveness of operations and propriety in the use of delegated authority.
2. Supervisory and executive relationships should be defined clearly to ensure lines of authority.
3. Responsibility and equivalent authority should be decentralized to the units or departments actually performing a function, without loss of overall control.
4. Functions should be assigned properly to ensure performance of essential tasks, prevention of confusion and duplication of effort.
5. A pattern of organization should prevail at each level. This will

ensure standardization as to functions, terminology and integration of policies.

6. Provision should be made for cooperative planning and performance through committees, councils and group meetings.

ORGANIZATIONAL STRUCTURES

Organizational structures can be of several different types. The three most common ones are known as line, staff, and functional. A line organization pattern is traditionally military and today refers directly to those elements which perform operations. A staff organization pattern refers to those elements which contribute indirectly to the performance of operations. A functional organization pattern is the most commonly used and is a combination of the line and staff patterns. It is more frequently referred to as the line and staff organization pattern. A line and staff chart illustrating the organization of a typical hospital is shown in Charts 2-1 and 2-2. A line and staff organization chart of a small rehabilitation center is shown in Chart 2-3.

PRINCIPLES OF ADMINISTRATION

Effective administration is a means of getting things done through people and of making the institution a good place in which to work. Basic to the accomplishment of effective administration are the following principles:

1. *Central Authority*. Investment of overall administration in one person provides control of operation.

2. *Proper Personnel*. Choice of properly trained and experienced persons in key positions assures effective operation.

3. *Indoctrinated Personnel*. All personnel should be acquainted with the organizational pattern of the institution and its departments.

4. *Delegated Authority*. Assignment of responsibilities with the power of decision is necessary to spread the work load efficiently.

5. *Communication*. Orders and directives to all personnel should be clear and concise, and reports of operation channeled back to central authority should be factual and succinct.

6. *Evaluation*. Through observation and study of reports on operation, effectiveness of programs of departments as well as of the total institution can be determined.

Since effective administration is the means of getting things done through people, an alert, effective and responsible staff is necessary. There are many practical ideas on how to build these qualities into a staff. Three basic ones are set forth here:

1. *Set a high standard of work habits*. If you are careless in your work habits, late for appointments, fuzzy in expressing yourself, care-

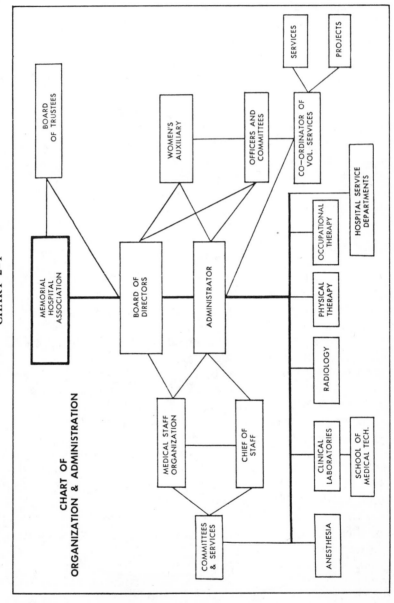

CHART 2-1

CHART OF
ORGANIZATION & ADMINISTRATION

CHART 2-2

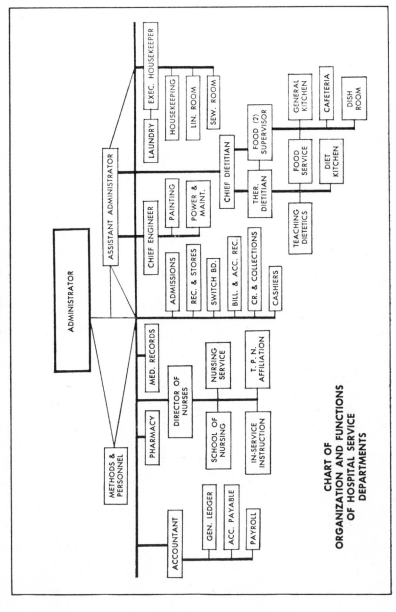

CHART OF
ORGANIZATION AND FUNCTIONS
OF HOSPITAL SERVICE
DEPARTMENTS

CHART 2–3. CURATIVE WORKSHOP – ORGANIZATION CHART

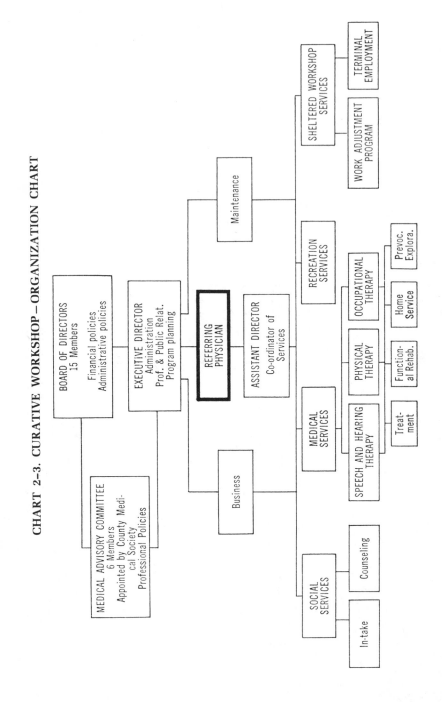

less about facts, bored in attitude, your subordinates probably will be too.

2. *Know the people who work for you.* What are their motives and attitudes? Do they respond best to praise, constructive criticism or other types of approval? Can they work effectively under pressure?

3. *Keep your subordinates informed.* Hold staff meetings regularly. Structure them to cover specific points. Allow time for discussion and questions. When necessary, use written communications between meetings.

West has aptly stated:

> One often hears of the envied "born" organizer or administrator, but the abilities generally deemed essential to success in this type of work are not necessarily inherited. They can be "made" or developed in the person who is conscientiously engaged in the executive phases of any effort. As in any undertaking, the prime requisites seem to be sincere interest, knowledge of the basic principles of the particular field and a devotion to the applications of these principles to both the *details* and the general plan of the total job.[6]

STARTING A NEW DEPARTMENT

Frequently, occupational therapists are called on to establish new departments of occupational therapy in institutions. One may be called in on a consultant basis or hired to organize and then to operate the department. There are definite procedures and guidelines that are applicable to both situations.

The procedures should include three steps: namely, the survey, the interviews and the planning. Sufficient time should be allotted to the survey so that it may be done thoroughly, covering every aspect, in order to get the truest possible picture of all circumstances. To supplement the survey, interviews should be held with key personnel of the institution such as the administrator, the medical director, the staff physicians, and the heads of departments with which the members of the occupational therapy department will be working. These interviews will be the principal way in which to determine the nature and the extent of the program desired.

Time and study should then be given to the information gathered through these two methods to evaluate it and to develop it into a workable plan for operation of the department. Careful planning cannot be overemphasized. It is essential in order to ensure a successful operation.

Guidelines to use in these procedures are presented in this section under seven topics: type of institution, size of institution, personnel, physical plant, supplies and equipment, budget and policies. The subject of Administrative Records and Reports is covered in another section of that title later in this chapter.

Type of Institution

Consideration should be given to the type of institution in which the department is being established. Is it a governmental or tax-supported (city, county, state, or federal) or a private voluntary institution? The American way of life demands of voluntary hospitals today the latest and best in facilities and services, both diagnostic and therapeutic. The choice of private care, semi-private care and ward care in voluntary hospitals and institutions requires a very different type of program in all of the diagnostic and therapeutic areas from that in a governmental type institution.

Does the institution serve all ages or is it limited to certain age groups? Does it handle outpatients only or both inpatients and outpatients? Is it a hospital, a rehabilitation center, a nursing home, a school, or another type? Is it a single diagnostic or a multidiagnostic center? All of these factors relate to the general philosophy of the institution's overall program and will have bearing on the type of occupational therapy to be offered.

Size of Institution

The size of the institution should be considered from the viewpoints of both the plant and the case load. Is the physical plant small and compact, or is it a large institution with scattered and widespread units? How many inpatients? How many outpatients? How many are bedridden and how many ambulatory? What is the rate of turnover in the census, if it is a hospital? What percentage of these patients will be referred to the occupational therapy department? What will be the frequency of their visits to the department?

Personnel

When the approximate case load requirements for the occupational therapy department have been determined, consideration can then be given to the number of therapists needed.

Experience has dictated that 10 treatments per day can be administered adequately by an occupational therapist handling very severe or involved cases. These types of cases will include amputees, cerebral palsied, selected orthopedic complications, selected neurologic conditions, tuberculosis or cardiac conditions, acute and severe psychiatric disturbances.

For those patients who can be handled in a group it has been found that a case load of 10 to 20 per group can be managed at one time by one occupational therapist.

To reach a decision relative to a realistic number of patients for one therapist to handle in a department which is being developed, there are several factors to consider. (1) Adequate time should be allowed for rounds, records and reports, preparation of therapeutic activities and the initial and ongoing planning of patient programs. Two hours a day is considered average. The dictates of a case load made up of severe and involved disabilities in all probability require more time. (2) It should be determined whether groups will be brought to the clinic or treated in designated space on the wards or in neighboring areas. (3) It should be determined also whether individual cases will be treated in the clinic or on the wards and whether outpatients are to be included. (4) Consideration should be given to scheduling occupational therapy with respect for other treatment and diagnostic needs of the patients. In many hospitals, groups in occupational therapy can be handled only in the afternoon; therefore, this type of service may be limited to one group per day.

Consideration should be given to use of certified occupational therapy assistants and non-professional aides to allow maximum use of the professional's time and expertise.

The final determination of the size of the staff needed will have to be governed necessarily by analysis of all factors under this section on Starting a New Department.

Physical Plant

There are three factors to be considered in regard to the physical plant of an occupational therapy department. They are location, size and layout.

1. **Location.** The occupational therapy department should be located comparatively near the patients' area of the hospital. This will allow for easy transportation of patients to the clinic. In those types of institutions where a physical therapy department exists, the occupational therapy department should be located close to it, as many patients will receive both treatments. This will allow for better coordination of the programs.

2. **Size.** In addition to the number of patients to be treated each day, or at one time, there are other factors that enter into determining the size of an occupational therapy department. Important ones are the type of disability field, the degree of involvement of the patients and the number of specific technics needed in treating them.

If the dictates of the institution limit the floor space of the department, one should give particular care to selection of activities. Woodwork, metal work, printing and minor crafts can be utilized effectively by many patients and do not tie up valuable floor space. Looms, particularly floor looms, may have to be minimal in number, especially if one is assigned to a single patient until the project is completed.

Where designated space is no problem, activities should be selected on results of a study of patient needs.

The work space for patients can be based on industrial standards plus room for supervision and for appliances such as carts, wheel chairs, beds, crutches and adaptations. Industry allows 16½ square feet per person for normal bench type operations aside from equipment space. It is safe, then, to assume that at least twice this amount, about 33 square feet per person, should be considered for patients in an occupational therapy department.

3. **Layout.** Because the occupational therapist will be supervising treatment of several patients at one time, the clinic area should be open so as to allow for easy visual and physical access to each individual patient. Where separate rooms are used for different technics, more therapists are needed to cover the area.

Office space should be private but with window vision to the clinic. Privacy is needed for three purposes: (1) to allow for interview and consultation with patients and students; (2) to keep confidential records of patients safely; and (3) to allow for telephone conversations with physicians and other professional staff relating to patient care.

General storage space should be located centrally to the clinic as a whole. Each treatment area should have accessible cupboards, drawers and storage bins. Safeguarding of tools should be provided for where any question of harmful use may be present.

Supplies and Equipment

The character of the disabilities to be treated will dictate to some degree the activities that will be used in the occupational therapy department. However, it has been found that certain activities lend themselves to all conditions treated by occupational therapists. Until a definite need is shown for the more unusual activities, initial planning should be around the basic ones.

The initial purchase of supplies and equipment should be governed by the evaluation made of possible case load and general needs in treatment procedures. Extensive lists of equipment and supplies may be found in the *Manual on Organization and Administration* published by the American Occupational Therapy Association.[1]

The initial expense for equipment and furniture (nonexpendables) will of course be the greatest. Ongoing equipment expense will occur only as demand is justified by either increase in the case load or addition in activities to reflect new trends in treatment procedures.

The initial expense for supplies (expendables) also will be greater than the ongoing purchases during operation. In a department to be operated on a limited budget, the therapist will have to be selective in the choice of activities and the type of supplies to be used with them.

There are always sources in a community where salvaged material can be obtained that will enable one to keep the supply item of the budget down. Managers of sheet metal works or lumber yards, and garment manufacturers are among those persons who are usually more than willing to save cuttings and scraps of usable size for occupational therapists.

Budgets

The fundamental purpose of budgeting is to find the most economical course through which the efforts of the department or the organization may be directed and to aid the management in holding to that course. Mott uses this definition:

> A budget is an administrative device useful . . . in relating financial resources to program goals . . . a means of ensuring that financial resources are available to meet program objectives and that program objectives are formulated with financial realities in mind.[3]

An occupational therapy department budget should be composed of two divisions. One should be capital assets having to do with equipment, tools and furnishings (nonexpendables). The other should be the operational items, such as salaries, supplies (expendables), maintenance and administration costs.

In both the capital and the operational divisions of a budget consideration should be given to income and expense. Income for equipment items may be fixed by allotment at the administrative level of the institution. Thus the therapist will know within a given period of time the degree to which additions may be made in new equipment.

Fees for Service

One of the major sources of income for operation for most institutions is fees for service. There is a growing trend, in institutions where fees are charged, to use a flat fee per visit and to include the cost of materials used in projects made during treatment. Problems can result when salvaged material is used with one patient, and costly materials with another. However, bookkeeping processes are simpler if the flat fee can be used. There are times when, if costly materials are used, an additional charge may be in order.

Policies differ among institutions charging fees. Some base their fees on actual cost, and others on a percentage of actual cost. For discussion here let us use actual cost for our basis. A fee can be estimated for a new department by projecting the volume of business and the necessary expense of operating the department.

Volume should be determined on a standard basis. This is generally considered in good business practices to be not more than 80 per cent of maximum capacity. Assume that capacity in volume for one therapist is 30 treatments per day. This includes a group of patients as well as individual treatments. In a month the total will be 600 treatments. Eighty per cent of 600 will be 480 treatments, which is considered to be standard volume.

Capacity figures are used to determine peak months of operation, when to expand facilities, and when to add more staff. Standard volume represents normal expectancy over a protracted term of time.

Monthly expenses for a department having one occupational therapist could be estimated as follows:

Salary	$ 725
Social Security	35
Retirement	40
Supplies	50
Percentage of Maintenance	200
Percentage of Administration	350
Total	$1,400

Thus, dividing the $1,400 of expenses by 480 treatments, the cost per treatment would be approximately $2.91. A base fee of $3.00 is, therefore acceptable.

There are institutions which prefer an hourly breakdown. This hourly based fee should cover expenses in a like manner. To determine the hourly fee as opposed to calculations made per visit, total treatment hours of all the patients involved in one typical day should be used instead of visits.

An example would be as follows: If 30 patients are treated in one day; 10 for 1 hour each, 10 for 2 hours each, and 10 for 3 hours each, a total of 60 treatment hours are given per day. This would be a capacity volume of 1,200 hours per month. Eighty per cent, or the standard volume, would be 960 treatment hours. Dividing the $1,400 of expenses by 960 hours will give an hourly fee of approximately $1.45 or an acceptable fee of $1.50.

Mott also has stated:

> A philosophy of fees . . . has been gaining widespread acceptance among rehabilitation centers . . . to recover as much of the cost of services as patients and third party sponsors can afford to pay. It combines the concept of charging for services with charity to the patient who cannot afford to pay. But charity is dispensed only in the degree to which it is thought to be needed, and patients of limited means are urged to pay for some portion of their services if possible.[4]

This simply means that those who can pay and third-party purchasers (such as medical insurance plans) pay their own way. Others pay according to their ability. If the policy of the hospital or the institution is to adjust fees for the medically indigent, the deficit created is a just one. It is appropriate for a Board of Directors to raise funds to cover this deficit.

After a department has been in operation for a few months a cost study should be made to reconcile the initial estimate. Consideration must be given to the capacity at which the department is operating at the time that the study is made.

At the end of the year when budgets must be prepared, it will be easier to forecast needs for the coming year from facts and figures kept in an orderly fashion.

Policies

Every organization should have policies under which it operates. Institutions should have policies set forth in one or more forms, such as personnel policies, professional policies and administrative policies. It is essential that these policies be clearly understood when a new department is to be established. It is also wise to develop policies for the department to ensure a good working relationship with the entire organization.

In addition to the existing policies of the institution, the vital information collected through the survey and interview procedures will provide the foundation for the development of departmental policies. There are a number of major areas that require the determination of policies.

1. **Scope of Case Load.** If the department is to be started on a demonstration basis, it may be necessary to establish a policy to limit the service of occupational therapy to a selected area, to a specific type of disability, to an extent of disability such as the degree of involvement, progressive type, ambulatory and/or to an age group.

2. **Scope of Services To Be Provided.** A demonstration basis may again be the reason for limited services. Availability of personnel or limitation of space may also be reasons. Specific policy should be established to cover the aims of occupational therapy. A few of the more basic aims are listed here:

Functional Restoration	Evaluations:
Social Adjustment	Activities of Daily Living
Stimulative Activity	Prevocational Exploration
Sedentary Activity	Functional Capacities
	Training:
Psychological Adjustment	Activities of Daily Living
Work Adjustment	Amputee
Supportive Activity	Handedness

3. **Medical Direction.** Relationships with referring physicians, institution affiliations and medical control should be understood and stated clearly.

4. **Administrative Direction.** Relationships with the administrator and with the business office on purchases and charges and with the nursing personnel on scheduling of patients should be determined clearly.

5. **Qualifications of Personnel.** Four areas of personnel should be considered: registered occupational therapists, certified occupational therapy assistants, aides and volunteers. A provision for selection of personnel for aides should be considered and a training period to have them become proficient in the less skilled and non-skilled duties of the department should be established. Volunteers should be selected and trained to be of the most help.

6. **Student Affiliations.** If occupational therapy students are to be accepted on affiliation an outline of the clinical affiliation program should be developed. It must be understood and stated very clearly in the policies that students *do not* relieve staff therapists of duties but rather add to them.

7. **Personnel Policies.** A clear understanding of the institutional personnel policies should be reached to provide for salary schedule, hours of work, vacation, holidays, sick-leave, employee benefits and professional and educational leave.

IMPROVING EXISTING DEPARTMENTS

Organizational structure and administrative functions of existing departments should be reviewed at regular intervals. Nothing ever stands still. It goes either forward or backward, and a rut only grows deeper.

The guide lines presented in the previous section of this chapter can well be applied to existing departments in any type of institution in order to keep them on an upward and forward growth pattern.

Periodic reviews and evaluations should be made of the professional relationship of the occupational therapy department to administration, to medical direction and to other departments with which it works such as physical therapy, social service, speech therapy and nursing. The use of and the results of the services that the department renders should be evaluated also in relation to the total function of the institution.

Only through an honest approach, involving again the procedures of surveying, interviewing and planning, can these evaluations become meaningful and be utilized positively.

ADMINISTRATIVE RECORDS AND REPORTS

One of the prime requisites of good administration is effective communication. Reports from each department give pertinent accounting of its activities to the central control. An administrator of an institution is able to keep his finger on the pulse of operations through study and evaluation of these reports.

To provide administration with these facts a system of reporting will have to be developed in accordance with the institutional needs. In most instances these systems originate at the administrative or business management level. Facts to be reported include the general categories of case load, staff, supplies, equipment, finances, maintenance and repair, accidents and emergencies.

Case Load. Census or total number of patients under care in the department will be requested at regular intervals. This might include admissions, re-admissions, patients pending treatment, active patients, patients awaiting discharge, and discharges.

Services rendered to this case load for purposes of charges will have to be reported daily. This may be done on individual charge slips or by means of a daily report of individuals treated.

Activity of the department may be requested through a breakdown of the services into diagnostic areas, treatment technics, inpatients, outpatients, ward and clinic visits. If these facts are not requested by the administration, it is advisable for the department to keep them for its own use in studying changing trends of case loads.

Staff. Administration requirements will include days worked, absences and reasons therefor, work load and in many instances efficiency reports. Similar information may be required of students as potential staff personnel. Such records should be kept on all volunteers assisting in the department.

Supplies. Supplies are requisitioned in accordance with need through the established method of the institution. Budgetary limits of the department should be considered. Should the case load go beyond the estimate used for planning a budget, purchase of supplies also may have to go beyond the budgetary limits. A running inventory, where large quantities of any one item are used, will permit efficient handling of this procedure.

Equipment. Purchases of equipment also will be requisitioned through the established method of the institution. The need for new or additional equipment should be substantiated through records of use, repairs, and through the projected estimate of use of new equipment.

Finances. In institutions where charges are made for services, again the procedure established by the institution will be followed. This may be done through individual charge slips for each patient or through daily reports of total business. Budgetary needs will be requested or budgets submitted for comment and/or approval, based on the trends of the past year.

Maintenance and Repair. Consideration should be given first to safety factors and then to appearance with respect to maintenance and repairs of equipment, furnishings, lights and building. Injuries from tripping over a break in the floor or from the collapsing of a weakened chair can be serious.

Maintenance of equipment, such as oiling bearings and tightening bolts, should be done regularly. To ensure regularity a record should be kept of the dates on which this maintenance was performed.

Accidents and Emergencies. Accidents or emergencies occurring to patients, staff, or any others while in the department should be reported to proper authorities immediately for first aid care and to ensure coverage by existing insurance policies, such as workmen's compensation and liability.

Another of the prime requisites of good administration is to provide central control with information from which an evaluation can be made of the program in relation to staff, to plant, to community needs and to long-range planning.

Relation to Staff. Analysis of the trends of the case load and of the number of treatments given is one of the major bases for determining when staff needs to be added and to what degree. It also serves as a means of determining acceptance of the program and the efficiency of staff performance.

Relation to Plant. Analysis of these reports will also provide information for deciding on reallocation of space for more effective use or planning for additional space.

Relation to Community Needs. The administrator of the institution, because of participation in community groups such as the Welfare Council, will undoubtedly be the first to hear of new needs within the health field of his community. With a realistic understanding of his institution and his staff he may be able to answer some of these needs through changes or additions to his program.

Relation to Long-Range Planning. Long-range planning is the projection of the program into the future. It is necessary in relation to staff, plant and needs in order to provide for growth and program development. Only through substantial data received from all departments can the administrator provide evidence to his Board of Directors for consideration and action.

PUBLIC RELATIONS

It must be remembered that at one time or another the occupational therapy department is directly or indirectly related to the community of which the institution is a vital part. Public relations is a major part of organization and administration. Interpretation of medical services is constantly being done through personal contacts, informal or formal talks to groups, tours of visitors through the hospital, and press releases. The occupational therapist is not exempted from the performance of these duties. Every occupational therapist should contribute through community relationships to a better understanding of the institution and the profession of occupational therapy. Vital to the future of occupational therapy is the recruitment of students into the field. This should be a major responsibility of each occupational therapist today.

BOOK REFERENCES

1. Am. Occup. Therapy Assoc.: Manual on Organization and Administration. New York, 1951.
2. ———: Occupational Therapy: Manual on Administration. New York, 1965.
3. MacEachern, M. T.: Hospital Organization and Management. ed. 2, p. 74, Chicago, Physicians' Record Co., 1946.
4. Mott, B. J. F., Kovener, R. R., and Mergie, M. A.: Cost Accounting, Budgeting and Statistical Procedures for Rehabilitation Centers and Facilities. p. 23, Chicago, National Society of Crippled Children and Adults, Inc., 1960.
5. ———: Cost Accounting, Budgeting and Statistical Procedures, for Rehabilitation Centers and Facilities. p. 16, Chicago, National Society for Crippled Children and Adults, Inc., 1960.
6. Willard, H. S., and Spackman, C. S.: Principles of Occupational Therapy. ed. 2, p. 63, Philadelphia, Lippincott, 1954.
7. ———: Principles of Occupational Therapy. ed. 2, p. 61, Philadelphia, Lippincott, 1954.

3

Medical Records and Reports

G. MARGARET GLEAVE, O.T.R.

Communication poses more problems than anything else man does, yet it marks man's superior intelligence over other living creatures. It is a part of human culture that was first initiated in written form some 5,000 to 6,000 years ago. Through communication, three bases of living are attained:

1. Wisdom (through reading what others have learned)
2. Expression (through writing what we know)
3. Socialization (through the exchange of thoughts and ideas with others)

In oral communication there is usually the opportunity to pursue the conversation until a maximum degree of mutual understanding is reached. In written communication one not only loses the chance to develop the message through exchange of ideas on the spot, but also one does not have the advantages of interpretation through gestures, facial expressions or tone of voice. The thoughts, the observations and the ideas that one puts into writing must be complete, clear, factual and readily understood.

In the medical field, and in all of its health related disciplines, more and more emphasis is being placed on communication through records—medical, social and administrative. Throughout the history of hospital standardization considerable emphasis has been placed on the maintenance of good medical records in accreditation. Its importance carries over into other types of institutions. An example is the Commission on Accreditation of Rehabilitation Facilities.

There are four basic reasons for records and reports in the medical field and its health related services:

1. To provide administrative control.
2. To assist in the treatment of the patient.

3. To aid in the advancement of the science of medicine.
4. To comply with the law and to aid in defense of a claim.

DIFFERENTIATION BETWEEN RECORDS AND REPORTS

It is important that we understand the difference between a record and a report. A *record* is a statement set down in writing or otherwise recorded for the purpose of preserving memory, or presenting authentic evidence of facts and events. Example:

> 7-17-70 Patient reported to the occupational therapy clinic but sat quietly removed from the group. No acknowledgment of therapist or other patients was evident.
> 7-18-70 Patient assumed same position in clinic. No notice was taken of other patients, but the patient when spoken to looked at the therapist twice during the hour.
> 7-19-70 No change from yesterday.
> 7-20-70 During the hour the patient moved from the chair apart from the group and voluntarily sat at a table with four other patients. Head was bowed when other patients or therapist spoke to her.
> 7-21-70 On entering clinic patient went immediately to table with other patients. She stared at embroidery being done by the patient next to her. On second attempt to show her the work this patient took it and clutched it in her lap staring straight ahead.

A *report* is a formal statement of the result of an investigation or an account of occurrences for the purpose of circulating related facts. Example:

> During the week of July 17 through 21 this patient has progressed from sitting removed from the group of patients to sitting voluntarily at a table with four others. When shown embroidery being done by the patient next to her, she took it and clutched it in her lap.

Records and reports need not be a chore to the occupational therapist. They should be tools which verify and augment the activities of the profession. It is not an overstatement to say that records are equally as important as the treatment given. In this age of specialization which produces a team of medical personnel working with an individual patient, communication becomes a tool as essential as the treatment itself.

We have reached a point in medical care where no one professional individual, regardless of his medical specialty, can be all things to all people. This may be applied to every branch of the science of medicine. The physicians were the first among us to develop well-defined specialties. In addition to calling in consultants from among their own colleagues, they are using the health related services more and more to assist them in the treatment of their patients.

Occupational therapy holds a rightful and necessary place among these health related services. Therefore, it becomes necessary for occupational therapists to be able to impart their contributions to the treatment program of a patient verbally and by the written word in relation to all other medical disciplines.

DUTIES OF THE OCCUPATIONAL THERAPIST

A definition of occupational therapy is submitted here for your consideration:

> Occupational therapy is ordered by physicians and administered by registered occupational therapists using work processes and purposeful activities to assist in the improvement, the development and/or the maintenance of mental, social or physical abilities which have been impaired by disease or injury.

Essential to the fulfillment of this definition, the duties of the occupational therapist may be listed as follows:

1. Interpretation of the aims of the referral in relation to the needs of the patient.
2. Establishment of rapport with the patient.
3. Selection of the proper activities to accomplish the aims of the treatment.
4. Direction of the patient while engaged in these activities to obtain the best possible results.
5. Awareness of the patient's degree of progress.
6. Awareness of the patient as a total person, psychologically as well as physically.
7. Recording and reporting the results to the persons concerned.

Through an intelligent straightforward approach to these duties a good working relationship is developed with other health related services and with the medical profession.

LEGAL ASPECTS

Information set forth in this section is given with the intent of emphasizing the importance of the legal aspects of medical records. There are certain incontrovertible facts that should be recognized by all practicing occupational therapists. These will be cited and discussed briefly. Beyond this, the occupational therapist should consult with the administrator and/or the medical director for guidance as to the use of, the release of and the disposition of such records as are produced in the occupational therapy department.

Legal complications often develop because of a lack of knowledge of what constitutes the "patient's record." It is generally accepted that patients' records may include three sections: an administrative record, a clinical record and a social service record. The clinical or medical record is the one to which is attached the importance of legal aspects. Hayt, Hayt and Groeschel state:

> The medical record is the property of the hospital, but is kept for the benefit of the patient, the physician, and the hospital. It serves as a tool for the physicians, the nurses, and the other professional personnel, enabling them to have a detailed and current record of the patient's condition or progress.[2]

It should be emphasized that the term "hospital" in the above paragraph may be applied to any type of institution where medical services are administered, such as rehabilitation centers, nursing homes and orthopedic schools.

The institution, as owner of these records, is obligated legally and ethically to protect them. The Code of Hospital Ethics adopted by The American Hospital Association and the American College of Surgeons stipulates:

> . . . it is the responsibility of the hospital and its personnel to safeguard the clinical records of the patients and to see that such records are available only to properly authorized individuals or bodies.[3]

Information in medical records falls into two categories: nonprivileged and privileged. Nonprivileged information is unrelated to the treatment of the patient. Privileged information is related to the treatment, the condition and the progress of the patient. Hayt, Hayt and Groeschel state:

> No authorization from a patient is necessary to disclose ordinary facts unrelated to treatment, such as the number of times and the dates on which the physician attended a patient, that the patient was ill and was operated upon, the complete name of the patient, address at the time of admission, verification of his hospital admission and discharge dates, name of relative or friend given on admission. However, discretion should be used and care taken to make certain that the inquiry is a proper one.
>
> Any other information, including age, address on discharge, if to a sanitarium or state hospital, the service on which the patient was hospitalized and all professional information, particularly the diagnosis, should not be disclosed without proper authorization.[3]

Proper authorization is written consent of the patient or guardian. The consent of the physician is unnecessary legally but may be obtained as a professional courtesy.

Press releases for promotional purposes may be allowed if the identity of the patient is withheld, and the physician's name omitted. It is still wise to have the permission of the patient for the use of the material. Hayt, Hayt and Groeschel are cited again as follows:

> The hospital should not release information regarding a patient to the press or permit photographers to take pictures of patients without the written authorization of the patient, and the attending doctor. Final consent rests with the patient, whose consent is sufficient, unless his condition is such as to preclude interviews or pictures without the approval of the attending doctor. It must be emphasized that good administration and the best interests of the patient may sometimes bar pictures even when permission of the patient has been obtained. Sound judgment must govern such exceptions.[4]

The preservation of medical records will differ according to the law in different states. The length of time records should be kept will vary from 10 years to indefinitely. For the purposes of possible readmissions, medical studies and research most institutions keep the medical records indefinitely. In this respect little has been written specifically about occupational therapy progress notes and reports. The American Hospital Association states in relation to Special Therapy Departments (Occupational and Physical):

> After the department's monthly and annual reports have been made the files should be destroyed since the report of treatments and results observed by the technicians are placed on proper record in the patient's hospital record folder. These departments may retain a copy for special studies.[1]

Emphasis should be given to the legal implications of every entry made in a medical record, since it is essential that it be accurate, objective and complete. Any omissions or mistakes, from the intake procedures through to the discharge procedures, may undermine confidence in the record as a whole. Doubt could be created as to whether or not other information has been reported, or whether or not it is accurate.

REASONS FOR KEEPING GOOD RECORDS

Keeping records of the patients treated in occupational therapy departments is a matter of serious importance. Like anything else that is done for the benefit of patients, records and the procedures involved in keeping them should always be checked for ways of improvement. Integration of the departmental records with the general medical records will be governed by the policies of the hospital. However, if a physician prescribes any specific therapy for his patient it should be accepted that he wishes progress reports. The *Journal of the American Medical Association* has stated:

Progress notes reflect the patient's response to or failure of particular therapy. Thus a collection of many facts in an orderly manner
in one place and for one person enables the doctor to "keep on top"
of each case he treats within the hospital. Additionally they can be
of inestimable value to any other physician who may be called upon
to aid or to replace the original attending physician.[5]

In the preceding section and in the latter paragraph two reasons for
keeping good records have been discussed. A list of all reasons follows:

1. To comply with the law or to substantiate a claim.
2. To communicate information as to progress to the attending
   physician and to other disciplines working with the patient.
3. To interpret the treatment program to the patient, to his family, to
   the public and to professional groups.
4. To facilitate efficient operation of a department when staff
   changes occur due to illness, vacations, or new personnel.
5. To aid in in-service training and student training programs.
6. To evaluate the effectiveness of the department's program.
7. To aid in special studies and research.

With respect to this last point it should be noted that a real opportunity and a challenge exist with the tremendous impetus toward research in all fields of medicine through the availability of public
funds for research.

RECORDING

Recording in medical records covers four major areas. They are discussed here in relation to occupational therapy.

1. **Identification Information.** This consists of the patient's name,
address, age, family status, educational background and work experience. This type of information is obtained most frequently by the ad-
mitting officer of the institution. If routine information so obtained in
your institution does not provide you with all the background that you
need, additional information should be obtained on the patient's first
visit. This can be done through formal interview procedure or informal
conversation, whichever lends itself better to your situation. However,
respect must be shown for the confidential character of the information
and for the way that it is obtained from the patient.

2. **Condition on Admission.** (A description of the physical and/or
mental status of the patient at the time the treatment is started in the department.) The information in the patient's medical record may be
complete and current and usable for your need. If not, an evaluation of
the patient's abilities should be made in your department and recorded

systematically. This information will serve as the basis from which changes in the condition of the patient can be measured as the treatment progresses.

3. **Progress Notes.** (Recording observations of the patient's response to treatment.) This is the most important item of recording in the medical area and will be discussed in greater detail later.

4. **Supplementary Information.** (Recording observations of the patient not related to occupational therapy.) These facts should not appear in the progress notes but should be recorded separately and forwarded to the other disciplines concerned. For example, if a patient should tell you of a problem regarding another member of his family that was worrying him, this should be recorded as told to you and then should be reported to the attending physician and to the social service department.

REPORTING

Reporting is an abstract of the facts of the records. In many instances this will be the information requested most often by the attending physician. This information, too, probably will be the information filed with the patient's medical record. Four major areas should be considered.

1. **Initial Evaluation of Condition.** A summary should be written of the condition on admission with an estimate of the patient's initial potentials to accept and to adjust to treatment.

2. **Treatment Plan.** A summary of the treatment program as initiated and interim summaries of changes instituted as it progresses.

3. **Progress During Treatment.** Summaries of the progress notes.

4. **Final Evaluation of Treatment.** Summary of the whole treatment program and results.

WHEN TO WRITE

One of the questions most frequently asked by occupational therapists and other professional personnel is, "How often should notes be written?" Because recording is a means of preserving memory, observations should be recorded at the time of occurrence, not a week later or a month later. Prompt recording is also essential in order to disseminate information to all others working with the patient.

Reporting should be timed with (1) results obtained in the treatment, (2) the physician's examination, and (3) the needs of other interested disciplines. We must be aware constantly that all results obtained will not be of a positive nature. Regressions, failures, plateaus reached are as important to report as progress.

HOW TO WRITE

The specific art of writing good records and reports needs to be developed and improved constantly in all fields of medicine. Essential to good writing is the ability to observe. To observe is to see or hear skillfully. This is a skill that is developed primarily through experience. Fundamental to the development of this ability is the knowledge that one must have of the disabilities, the diseases and the conditions of the patients observed, and the skills, the activities and the procedures used.

In relating observations three necessary qualities should be developed:

1. **Accuracy.** The ability to express exactly, precisely and correctly what has been seen.

2. **Honesty.** The ability to be fair, true and just in putting one's observations into words.

3. **Thoroughness.** The ability to give careful attention to all facts without being superficial or superfluous.

ESSENTIAL PARTS OF RECORDS AND REPORTS

Records and reports are composed of three essential parts: the aim of treatment, the treatment procedure and the patient's response.

1. **Aim of Treatment.** Physicians give medical direction to the occupational therapist by checking statements on referral blanks or by writing directions in a narrative form. These medical directions include such statements as "increase muscle strength," "develop physical tolerance," "train in daily skills," "stimulate," "maintain morale," "alleviate guilt," "develop interest in group activities." These aims should be defined in the record by the occupational therapist in relation to the needs of each individual patient.

2. **Treatment Procedure.** A description of how the aim is being accomplished should be entered on the record. This should include procedures used such as: positioning necessary, adaptation used, types of groups initiated, use of colors, methods of socialization.

3. **Patient's Response.** Observations such as the patient's progress, regression, attitude, co-operation, should be recorded as they occur.

An example of how these three steps may be incorporated into a record is as follows:

Date   Progress Notes
4-1-70 AIM of treatment is to strengthen musculature of both upper and lower extremities on right side and to encourage use of right hand.

    1. Patient started small wood project, using bicycle saw to cut out pieces. Filing and sanding at work bench, seated, to

encourage reaching to shoulder height, and to use bilateral hand tools. Patient also rode toy tractor, and played with hammering toys, using right hand to hold hammer.

2. Patient is very friendly and co-operative. Had some difficulty following lines while sawing due to visual defect in right eye. Some fatigue was evident at the end of first treatment.

                                                            Signed O.T.R.

Each dated entry should carry the therapist's signature. If notes are typed either by the therapist or a stenographer, the therapist's name may also be typed out but should be initialed after being read for accuracy.

In using a system of this type only that section of the three divisions involved need be written in continuing notes, using AIM or the numbers 1 or 2 as indicated. In this way it will be easy to check the times that the AIM or the procedures are changed, and to follow the patient's response to treatment. It will also facilitate writing summaries for reporting to the physician and others interested in the case.

In writing records and reports the command of language is important. It is not the easiest thing to put your thoughts on paper for another to read. Too often misinterpretation is the result. Through practice one can learn to describe aims, treatment procedures and observations so that they will tell the treatment story in logical sequence. There are a few rules to be followed in writing.

1. One should learn first to identify and then to exclude vernacular or jargon words, abbreviations and phrases. ADL means little to others than those working in rehabilitation. Activities of Daily Living means a bit more to others. There are those persons with whom occupational therapists work who may need to have this phrase broken down into feeding, dressing, communication and transportation. Technical vocabulary of a specific discipline is meaningless to others who read the record.
2. All writing should be done in the third person. "This," or "the patient" . . . not, "Mr. Brown." "It was observed" . . . not, "I saw."
3. Eliminate empty phrases. "Such as," "so that," "in case of," and other phrases like them make the record more difficult to read. Terseness in writing should be developed. Terseness is nothing more than being elegantly concise, short and to the point.
4. Flowery descriptive passages or overuse of scientific words should be avoided. Scientific words have their place in reports and records, but many times everyday language will describe thoughts better and will be understood more accurately.
5. Description of the patient's progress should be explicit. Until

such terms as "good," "moderate," "fair," "poor" are defined and marked into logical steps with meaningful interpretations, no more is done than to risk a guess at the results recorded about the patient.

Two notes on the same patient, taken at random from samples from the field are presented here for analysis and rewriting.

9-30-70 A man of constantly changing moods. Today he appreciates anything done for him and tomorrow the same action may agitate him. His unusual and varying personality makes him understood by some and disliked by others.

Signed (first) O.T.R.

10-29-70 Patient has been ill most of therapist's time with him. In last week or so, however, he has regained strength sufficiently to participate again in program. During this time, the therapist's comments concerning this patient are in agreement with the above.

Signed (second) O.T.R.

Comments are as follows about the note written 9-30-70:

This borders on being a flowery description. A question arises as to the things done for him that create this agitation. It is doubtful that one's "unusual and varying personality" makes one understood. Therefore, a question arises as to whether it is not the personality that is understood, not the patient. A suggested rewrite is as follows:

9-30-70 This patient displays constantly changing moods. A typical example was his acceptance of help to untangle a knot in his weaving on Monday, and on Wednesday becoming agitated over the same help and refusing it. This behavior has caused some of the other patients to resent him.

Comments on the note written on 10-29-70 are as follows:

Did the therapist cause the illness? If so, change therapists! It is indefinite as to when participation in the program was resumed. The word "however" belongs to the empty word category and can be eliminated. To whom is the therapist commenting during this time? A suggested rewrite is as follows:

10-29-70 This patient has been ill since this therapist was assigned to treat him on 10-12-70. During the past week improvement in his condition has enabled him to resume his treatment. No change in moodiness or in acceptance by other patients has been noted.

CHARTS AND GRAPHS

Another method of recording and reporting which should be developed is the use of charts and graphic records, especially in treating physical disabilities. Graphic records are easily read and simplify the recording process. An illustration is shown in Chart 3-1.

There is no limit to the refinement that can take place in recording and reporting. The development of good medical records is a continuing process of systematic re-evaluation. It is the medium through which the profession of occupational therapy communicates with the physicians about their patients and with other health related services working with these patients. When well done, it will command respect.

CHART 3-1

CURATIVE WORKSHOP

OCCUPATIONAL THERAPY MEASUREMENTS

Name_____ # _____   UPPER R____L____   LOWER R____L____

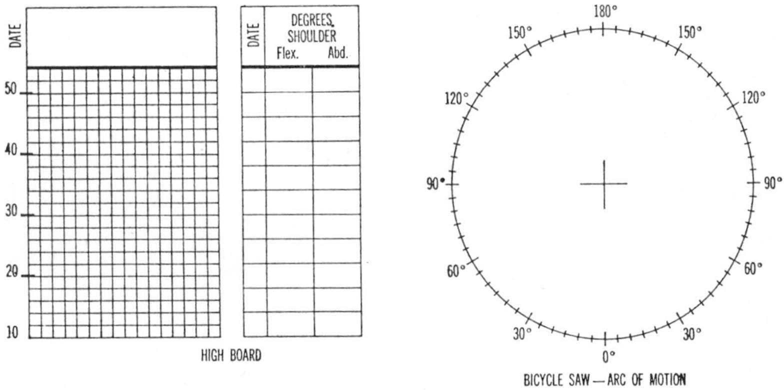

HIGH BOARD

BICYCLE SAW — ARC OF MOTION

BICYCLE SAW NO._____
USE STEP ON R____L____ TO MOUNT   BOOT ON R____L____
R____L____ LEG ONLY   BOOT DISCONTINUED_____

DATE: 19____																								
SEAT																								
PEDAL SHAFT																								
PEDAL LENGTH																								
FORWARD { Time																								
REVERSE { No.																								
LBS. RESISTANCE																								
DEGREES																								
HIP FLEXION																								
KNEE FLEXION																								
KNEE EXTENSION																								

ELEVATED SANDER									
DATE: 19____									
ANGLE NUMBER									
REACH									
LBS. RESISTANCE									

HANDLES								
19____								
SIZE	4″	3½	3″	2½	2″	1½	1″	½″

REFERENCES

1. American Hospital Association: Hospital Records Administration. p. 19, Chicago, A.H.A., 1949.
2. Hayt, Emanuel, Hayt, L. R., and Groeschel, A. H.: Law of Hospital, Physician and Patient. ed. 2, p. 652, New York, Hospital Textbook Co., 1952.
3. ———: Ibid., p. 654.
4. ———: Ibid., p. 662.
5. Medicine and the law. J.A.M.A. 166:7, 1958.
6. Welles, C.: The implications of liability: guidelines for professional practice. Am. J. Occup. Therapy 23:18, 1969.

4

Methods of Instruction

CLARE S. SPACKMAN, M.S., O.T.R.

For the successful application of occupational therapy it is necessary that proper instruction be given in the required activities. The therapist, confronted with the varying abilities and intelligence of his patients, needs to be well grounded in how to teach the processes of treatment so that the patient understands clearly what he is to do and requires the minimum of correction and supervision. If faulty methods are used and work is done incorrectly, it may result in actual harm in the patient's physical or psychological reaction. If the patient has difficulty in learning the processes he may become discouraged, lose confidence in the treatment and fail to get the proper exercise. Poor methods of instruction result in a waste of time and effort for all concerned.

The following suggestions for the instruction of patients have been adapted from a publication issued many years ago, the "Job Instructor Training Plan for War Production" developed by Training Within Industry, War Manpower Commission, Washington, D. C. This adaptation has been tried in different occupational therapy departments through the years and has been found to be helpful. Although not a new procedure it is a simplification and an application of basic rules of successful instruction.

DESCRIPTION AND DEMONSTRATION

A technical procedure may be taught by telling how to do it or by showing how to do it. The average person's memory span is too short for the use of verbal instructions of any length, so that if teaching is done by telling alone, numerous repetitions are necessary. With a person of dull mentality mere explanation of a process may result in complete failure to learn. Showing a person how an activity is done also may present difficulties. Unless the learner is in the correct position to see properly what is done, it is very difficult for him to form a correct visual image of what he is to do. The visual image in any case tends to be hazy, and repetitions of the demonstration are necessary. Both telling and showing are recognized methods of instruction, but neither when used alone is completely satisfactory.

The method of instruction combining both telling and showing gives excellent results. There are four basic steps in using this method: (1) the preparation of the patient, (2) the presentation of the activity, (3) the tryout performance and (4) the follow-up.

STEP 1. The Preparation of the Patient

A. *Put the patient at ease.* The person who is fearful and ill at ease is handicapped in learning an activity. An informal chat with the patient for a moment or two about familiar things in a friendly and cordial manner does much to put the patient at ease and to establish rapport. An understanding of the patient's psychological reactions to his disability also helps in this phase.

B. *Find out whether the patient knows how to do the activity.* It is annoying to be taught something that one already knows; therefore, it is important for the therapist to find out whether or not the patient can do the proposed project, and if so, how well he can do it.

C. *Get the patient's interest.* A basic maxim of occupational therapy is that the patient should be interested in the activity. Interest is also important for learning. In the treatment of patients with physical disabilities a patient may be given a piece of work requiring exercise of the correct type but in which he is totally uninterested. His interest may be increased if the reason for the particular activity given him is made clear.

D. *Place the patient in the correct position.* Through inexperience the error may be made of facing the patient while demonstrating the work to be done, and as a result the patient has a reversed mental image of the activity. Both the demonstrator and the patient should face in the same direction, with the patient to the side that permits him to see the process most easily. If an activity requiring use primarily of the right hand is being demonstrated, the patient should be on the left side so that the right hand does not hide the work.

STEP 2. Presentation of the Activity.

The therapist should tell and show the patient how to do the activity. In the verbal instruction the English used should be adapted to the patient's comprehension, and technical terms should be avoided or explained if used. The material to be learned should be presented slowly and patiently, avoiding any appearance of being hurried or impatient. Not more than one step at a time should be taught. Key points that are particularly helpful to know, such as knacks or hazards, should be stressed. It is poor instruction to give more at one time than can be mastered, therefore, a complicated activity should be broken down into smaller learning units.

STEP 3. Tryout Performance

A. *Have the patient do the activity.* After the patient has been shown how to do the work, he should do it himself. It is better to use the phrase "Now you try it," than, "Would you like to try it?" for the latter gives the patient an opening to reply, "No," or "I can't." After he has done the process once, he should be asked to repeat it and should be asked carefully worded questions as he works, queries that are based on the key points of the procedure, such as, "How long should the cord be cut?" or "Why is the cord placed on the right?" Questions that can be answered with "Yes" and "No" should not be asked but rather those beginning with "How," "Why," "What," "Where" and "When."

B. *Correct all errors as they occur.* Errors should be corrected at once; if possible, they should be anticipated and prevented. The patient never should be permitted to repeat an error, because repetition fixes the incorrect method in his mind. If necessary, the process should be demonstrated again.

C. *Repetition of the activity.* After the patient has done the activity a second time, he should be asked to repeat it a third time and to explain the process in his own words. These repetitions are necessary in order to be sure that the patient knows how to do the activity and that he has not done it right the first time merely by chance. He should not be asked if he understands; he should prove that he does.

STEP 4. Follow-up

A. *Put the patient on his own.* When the patient knows what to do and how to do it, he should work independently for the time indicated.

B. *Designate to whom the patient is to go for help.* It should be stressed that if the patient has difficulty in working on the assigned project he should wait until the therapist returns to show him what to do. It may be explained to the patient that others are busy on their own jobs and should not be interrupted and that help should be obtained only from the therapist or the person whom the therapist designates to help him.

C. *Check up on the patient frequently.* After the patient is put to work alone, his progress should be checked frequently to be sure that he can continue the work without further instruction. Of course, help should be given if errors occur.

D. *Taper off.* As the patient gains skill in doing the process, the check-ups need be less and less frequent.

METHODS OF PREPARATION

The successful use of the preceding outlined basic steps of instruction depends upon the preparation for instruction, which includes the following three procedures:

1. **Have Everything Ready.** The proper tools and the necessary material and equipment should be at hand for use.

2. **Have the Work Place Properly Arranged.** The arrangement of the work place is important. This should be set up in the way it is expected to be used. The posture of the patient must be considered in the choice of a workbench or a chair. If the treatment is being given in the ward, the patient's position in bed or wheel chair must be correct, for the importance of good posture while working on a project cannot be overstressed. Special adjustments of the equipment or the position of the patient may be necessary in order to obtain the desired type of exercise.

Safety precautions for the patient and others working in the clinic must be observed. This is particularly true when the patients are persons prone to have accidents or persons who have been injured previously because of poor safety habits. Safe work habits should be stressed constantly.

3. **The Breakdown of an Activity.** The analysis of the processes involved in a procedure is perhaps the most important of the steps in the preparation for instruction. It is impossible to instruct a patient in the performance of an activity unless the steps and the key points have been determined previously.

A breakdown for each of the activities frequently used should be made so that it will be available when needed. Only a few minutes are required to do this; and once done, it can be used indefinitely. In departments in which more than one person may work with the same patient, confusion is lessened if the breakdown is the composite work of the staff, all of whom then use the same technics.

A breakdown of the process to be taught is vital to good instruction, for it is a brief memorandum of the essential steps and the key points involved in the performance of the activity. A step may be defined as an important action that furthers the process. A key point emphasizes the "knack" of a performance or stresses the inherent hazards to be avoided. In analyzing an activity the process is done slowly, and note of each step is taken. Then the activity is repeated step by step, and each key point in the step is noted. The breakdown is checked by repeating the process to be sure that nothing has been omitted. Then it is tried out on another person.

Breakdown of an Activity

Activity: Typewriting   Process: Insertion of paper in typewriter

Important Steps	Key Points
1. Pick up paper	1. Left hand Thumb and first 2 fingers Lower left-hand corner
2. Insert paper	2. Back of platen against left side Bottom of paper touches feed-rollers Paper straight
3. Twirl platen knob	3. Right-hand platen knob Thumb and first 2 fingers Twirl with snap motion
4. Straighten paper (if necessary)	4. Use of paper-release lever

Units of Learning. Many of the activities used in occupational therapy include several units of learning, each of which should be taught separately, using the 4 steps of instruction for each unit. In many instances the second learning unit may involve parts of the first, thereby providing opportunity for valuable repetition and for checking on the facility gained in the previous unit.

"How Tight Is Tight?" One of the problems that frequently arises in occupational therapy is the use of such words as "tightly," "firmly," "loosely" or "hard." When a patient is instructed to screw a nut "tightly," how is he to know the degree of tightness? And if he is told to tighten a nut as much as he can, the results vary according to the individual's strength. The difficulty is solved best by the use of the sense of touch. The nut is screwed to the desired degree of tightness, and the patient is allowed to determine how tightly it has been twisted, after which he tries to duplicate the procedure. Then his efforts should be checked. The patient should recheck, repeating the process until there is no question of the interpretation of the term "tightly." This difficulty arises particularly in cord knotting, adjusting the warp on a loom or tightening the bolts on equipment.

SUMMARY

The 4 basic steps in good instruction are:

1. Preparation of the Patient:
   A. Put the patient at ease.
   B. Find out what he knows.

      C. Get the patient's interest.

      D. Place the patient in the correct position for observation of the demonstration.

  2. Presentation of the Activity:

      A. Show and tell how to do it.

      B. Teach step by step, stressing key points.

      C. Explain carefully and patiently.

      D. Teach no more than can be mastered at one time.

  3. Tryout Performance:

      A. Have the patient perform the activity.

      B. Ask questions and have the patient explain the process.

      C. Correct errors as they occur.

      D. Repeat until the patient knows it.

  4. Follow-up:

      A. Put the patient on his own.

      B. Designate the person to whom the patient is to go for help.

      C. Check frequently.

      D. Taper off.

The basic steps for preparation to instruct are:

  1. Have everything ready.

  2. Have the work place properly arranged.

  3. Make a breakdown of the activity.

     If the patient has not learned, the occupational therapist has not taught.

ADAPTATION OF TEACHING METHODS FOR DIFFERENT HANDICAPS

Visually Handicapped

The work area should be set up precisely as the patient is to work. The therapist should make a plan of it so that every time the patient comes to the clinic, or every time the occupation is given to him to do on the ward, each tool is in the same place.

    Before instructing a patient in any activity the therapist should endeavor to do it blindfolded and should make a breakdown accordingly. The breakdown used for sighted persons will not be adequate, especially for those patients unable to see because of a temporary condition which has necessitated the bandaging of their eyes.

    When the patient is introduced to the work area he should feel the position of each object. The therapist should tell him specifically where each tool is. For example: The pliers are on your right side 3" from the edge of the bench. The copper wire is 10" in front of you, lying in a coil.

The methods of instruction used, although basically the same, will depend on whether (1) the patient has complete loss of sight and has adjusted to his handicap; (2) the patient has a temporary (or perhaps permanent) handicap which prevents him from seeing and is of recent origin; or (3) the patient has lost his sight gradually. The first will learn quickly, often instructing the therapist. However, this type of patient is rarely referred to occupational therapy unless in a hospital for another reason. The second presents the greatest problem, as he is completely unaccustomed to doing anything without sight. Therefore, great care must be taken in instructing him so that failure will not occur. The third has gradually become accustomed to diminishing vision. This may help or hinder, depending on his acceptance of his condition.

Instruction is not dependent on telling alone, but the verbal instruction must be clearer and more specific than that given to sighted persons, for example, in stating the position of the hands, right or left. The patient should be encouraged to feel the different positions as instruction proceeds. Samples worked out step-by-step are of great value.

For the patient temporarily unable to see or for the recently and suddenly blinded the sensitivity of the hands affects the speed of learning, in that feeling must replace sight. The patient should be encouraged to develop his tactile sense. For the blind patient directions in Braille may be of assistance.

Among the visually handicapped are primarily persons somewhat over 45 years of age. Presbyopia, inability to see clearly at close range, begins to develop at this time. Patients who read habitually will have reading glasses. Any patient who has always worn glasses may have bifocals or trifocals. However, many patients will be unable to do close work such as embroidery, sawing a fine line or close assembly work. If there is no refractory error, the ordinary magnifying glasses which can be purchased at a variety store will be adequate until the patient can obtain proper ophthalmologic care. Patients with bifocals or trifocals must have their work placed at correct distances.

The Hard of Hearing

The hard of hearing also require adjustment in teaching methods. For those who read lips, the therapist should tell and show separately, not simultaneously. He should turn his head toward the patient when talking so that his lips can be seen. Before giving verbal instructions the therapist should attract the patient's attention.

Many patients who use hearing aids often turn them off in a noisy clinic because of the amplifying of certain sounds. If the therapist wishes to give instruction he should wait until the patient reconnects his hearing aid.

Non-English-Speaking Patients

It is common to have patients who speak little or no English. In such instances the following points will be helpful:

Do not shout at the patient. He is not deaf.
If you know even 2 or 3 words of the patient's language, try to use them so that he can laugh at you. Then he will not be ashamed to try his poor English.
Speak slowly and distinctly.
Avoid verbs.
Write numbers.
Use gestures or sign language.
Print out a word. Do not spell it orally.

Often interpreters may be found among the patient group.

Patients Able to Use Only One Hand

In demonstrating a process to a patient who can use only one hand, the therapist should demonstrate using only one hand. This requires that the therapist learn to do the activity one-handed, either right or left, before starting to teach the patient. The teaching method remains the same.

BIBLIOGRAPHY

Ey, J. A., Jr.: Techniques and psychology of instructing. Am. J. Occup. Therapy 9:248, 1955.
Hoberman, M., and Cicenia, E. F.: Teaching: a factor in functional training. Phys. Therapy Review 38:245, 1958.
Shaperman, J. W.: Learning techniques applied to prehension. Am. J. Occup. Therapy 14:70, 1960.
Walters, E. C.: The application of the overload principle to the learning of a motor skill. Am. J. Occup. Therapy 10:1, 1956.

5

Occupational Therapy And Mental Health

NEDRA P. GILLETTE, B.S., O.T.R.

A HISTORICAL PERSPECTIVE

The occupational therapist in the field of mental health must look both to the past and to the future. From the past, he gains a rationale for his being; from the future, he receives an invitation to apply his heritage, to collaborate in the development of a new society. For the field of mental health is not restricted to psychiatric problems, to failures in adaptation, or to dealing with medically described entities which imply illness and the need for externally applied treatment. The concept of mental health requires that we explore and understand those behaviors which portray the individual's life-style, which reflect his needs and the ways in which he attempts to find personal satisfaction while meeting social and economic standards. The individual's relationship to society, as revealed through his behavior patterns, his choice of leisure activities, his motivation for work and his ability to be productive—these are the concerns of the occupational therapist.

How has the past provided us with a rationale which so clearly contributes to the solution of current problems?

The first article in the first issue of the first publication devoted to occupational therapy, *The Archives of Occupational Therapy*, printed in 1922, was called, "The Philosophy of Occupational Therapy."[1] It was an address by Dr. Adolph Meyer, the leading remaining advocate of moral treatment in this country. Moral treatment had been the highly successful form of care for the psychiatric patient during the early nineteenth century. That it failed to survive is one of the tragedies in the history of the medical and social professions.

Patients were treated as peers of the staff, and were expected to respond in socially appropriate ways. The most important factor influencing recovery undoubtedly was the new concept Dr. Meyer described of mental problems as problems of living, and not merely diseases of a structural and toxic nature on the one hand, or of a final, lasting constitutional disorder on the other. His description of the moral treatment programs anticipated the coming of existential psychiatry when he wrote:*

> ... Direct experience and performance were everywhere acknowledged as the fullest type of life. Thought, reason and fancy were more and more recognized as merely a *step* to *action*, and mental life in general as the integrator of *time*, giving us the fullest sense of past, present and future, but after all the best type of reality and actuality only in real *performance* ... *performance* is its own judge and regulator and therefore the most dependable and influential part of life. ....[2]

Performance is a keystone in the foundations of occupational therapy.

The moral treatment programs of the early nineteenth century and those which were briefly revived again by Dr. Meyer and his colleagues in the 1920's were directed toward creating institutional standards of living and patterns of behavior which were synonymous with those the society at large could tolerate and accept. Through these methods differences between hospitalized persons or mentally ill persons and their fellow citizens and family members were significantly reduced, so that barriers between patients and society were largely unnecessary, since both groups shared the same values and regarded the same patterns of behavior as appropriate and desirable.

The programs of social recreation and therapeutic work which were in evidence during the periods of moral treatment were the prototypes of some of the best occupational therapy programs today. Occupational therapy speaks to the outer reality of man. Its concerns are with the quality of his daily routines, as seen through the skills he possesses: grooming himself, carrying out his domestic chores, handling the decisions required by the jobs and challenges confronting him, developing the strategies required in the competition of games, deriving satisfaction from the commonplace interactions involved with living among friends and relatives, participating in neighborhood affairs, and collaborating appropriately in economic endeavors. When these aspects of behavior have been balanced by means of the normal developmental process, it is believed that the mature function of work or occupation emerges. The methods of developing or modifying the desired occupational behaviors when they are either inadequate or inappropriate are imbedded in the prevailing culture, and therapeutic interventions are

* Meyer, A.: The philosophy of occupational therapy. Archives of Occupational Therapy, 1:5, 1922.

based on the practices and values which the society permits. Thus, the mandate for occupational therapy is derived.

Dr. Meyer went on to say:

> ... somehow I see in all this a profound importance extending far beyond our special field. Our efforts seem to me destined to be the soil for helps of much wider applicability. Present day humanity seems to suffer from a deluded craze for finding substitutes for actual work ... Our special work, which tries to do justice to special human needs, I feel is destined to serve again as the center of a great gain for the normal as well[3] [as those whom we have identified as being mentally ill].*

He therefore anticipated the role of occupational therapy in community health, with directed work and leisure time activities being used to prevent illness and to maintain good health. This humanitarian philosophy serves us well today as we move into a period in which more and more people appear to be distressed, to be unable to find meaningful ways to use their time. Not only our patients but our neighbors describe the lack of purpose in their lives: an inability to find gratification through the tasks they must routinely do. They fail even to recognize the basic human right to have creative experiences which are personally fulfilling, and which lead to the ability to extend oneself and to be concerned about the rights and well-being of others.

Several other facets of our heritage have been incorporated into the rationale of occupational therapy. The contributions of Eleanor Clarke Slagle, of Mr. Louis J. Haas, and the thoughtful writing of Dr. L. Cody Marsh regarding therapeutic work programs are integral parts of present-day practice. Each of them was a product of the school of moral treatment. Their work preceded the era of psychological psychiatry, and yet their foresight anticipated the development of the current social psychiatry movement.

Eleanor Clarke Slagle was the personification of the humanitarian of the 1920's. She was also at various times something of a militant, an aggressive and imaginative woman who got things done. She developed a training program for a group that she named *occupational therapeutists*. They were to be concerned with social rehabilitation, primarily of patients in the back wards of state hospitals.

> By social rehabilitation, I mean three distinct groups: one group that will, in all likelihood, remain in the hospital for the balance of their days; the second group that may be returned to community life and activity, and the third group who may profit by work directed with understanding in a pre-hospital work clinic with an idea and hope of preventing hospital experience.

* Meyer, A., p. 8.
** Slagle, E. C.: Training aides for Mental Patients. Archives of Occupational Therapy, 1:12, 1922.

She, too, foresaw the role of occupational therapy in community programs directed toward preventing illness and maintaining the stability of community life, as well as helping to insure the health of the citizens of that community. Her philosophy of rehabilitation was as follows: "For the most part, our lives are made up of habit reactions. Occupation, used remedially, serves to overcome some habits, to modify others, and to construct new ones, to the end that habit reaction will be favorable to the restoration and maintenance of health."[5] Much of her thinking probably would be supported by the operant conditioning principles in use today. Her technics, however, were more humanistically determined; they reflected concern for the interpersonal rights and the dignity of patients with whom she worked and belief in the value of organized, productive time.

Mrs. Slagle went to great lengths to describe the ideal personality of the *occupational therapeutist* who was to work with the back ward patients. Her description is, in fact, an excellent one for the ideal personality of the mother of a pre-school child: infinite kindness, gentleness and patience, imagination, the ability to slip into the fantasy world of another, and to lead him gently back to normal reality when such is desired. Pre-school years are, after all, that period of time when habits are most clearly formed, when the child learns what his home and community value, when he learns what kinds of behavior will be tolerated, and when he learns which things are punished and which ones are rewarded. This is the time when he develops his sense of autonomy: his ability to know what he can control and what he cannot control, and when he sets up a pattern of habits and behaviors which stand him in good stead as he faces the larger community outside his home. This is also the time when his self-concept is formed, when he sees himself as a lovable person or one who is not approved and loved, when he begins to value himself and to have self-respect which allows him to value and respect others. These were attributes which were needed by the back ward patients with whom Mrs. Slagle dealt, and while the concepts of developmental psychology were perhaps not immediately in her awareness, they were beautifully demonstrated in her description of therapeutic relationships.

If the development of habits represents the pre-school years in the resocialization of the chronically ill, the introduction of creative activities might be likened to the next period of learning. Mrs. Slagle said, "Kindergarten follows habit training; that is, grading the occupation from the simple to the complex. Passing from the known to the unknown, tasks must be of increasing interest and must require an increasing degree of concentration."[6] Following "kindergarten," her patients progressed to an occupational (therapy) center. Thus, they entered school, just as a child faces a new environment, meets new people from other backgrounds, and begins to test his ability to get along in a new setting. He refines the skills that were developed through the habit training period and through mastery of tasks that involved learning and coordination, and he begins to develop a picture of himself as an integrated person with certain abilities, some limitations, and some ideals.

Mrs. Slagle's patients next moved into a pre-industrial group. Jobs were found within the hospital structure which allowed both the patient and the staff to assess his ability to function in the economic world. Mrs. Slagle wrote that she would not presume to say that her *occupational therapeutists* did job training, but rather that they prepared persons to assume job responsibilities within the institution or the community, if discharged.

Eleanor Clarke Slagle, then, foresaw the development of occupational therapy on principles of work and play and human relations as they are experienced throughout the life cycle. She emphasized the needs of childhood in her programs.

Mr. Louis J. Haas provided some basic concepts relative to the adolescent period of life. Mr. Haas was a master craftsman, a teacher and a perfectionist. He developed problem-solving technics and presented them through crafts and work procedures, and he based his treatment programs on specific explorations of social, economic and family problems which the patient would face when he left the hospital. Discipline through structured activity was basic to his thinking, and he urged the patient toward more adequate control of himself and more appropriate response to his own reality. Standards for performance were exquisitely high and were never compromised, but Mr. Haas's sensitivity to the patient's current level of competency was also unique. He wrote, "The treatment program presents a controlled environment wherein the individual can be aided to face a modified reality with increasing success and assurance."[7] He gave explicit instructions for each activity and was alert to determine the means by which each patient learned best: visually, orally or kinesthetically. He ascribed to a lack of coordination many of the deficits in the patient's ability to master problems outside the hospital, surely an antecedent to the present-day interest in cognitive-perceptual-motor theories.

Exploratory interviews assessed the patient's interests, skills and unfulfilled wishes. The occupational therapy staff were skillful in using tools, media, and instructions to provide reality testing, a method of confrontation which helped the patient assess himself more easily. The professional responsibilities of interview, evaluation and critical appraisal of the patient's work were considered to be teaching methods which enabled the patient to grow to his own highest potential.

The primary challenge of adolescence is to develop a set of values consistent with those of the society at large, and which is congruent with the self-concept of the individual. The adolescent must also define for himself an economic role which is within his capabilities, and develop the personal identity which fulfills the sexual role society expects of him. In the Haas method of occupational therapy, such opportunities were provided through the disciplined use of crafts and work, supported by an identification with a masterful teacher who was comfortable both in his occupational behavior and in his sexual role in the social system.

The third pioneer whose work has enriched the occupational therapy rationale was a psychiatrist, Dr. L. Cody Marsh. In an address read at the Sixteenth Annual Meeting of the American Occupational Therapy Association, September, 1932, he described the industrial therapy program in the Worcester (Massachusetts) State Hospital, which employed nearly all of its 2,000 patients.[8]

A system of job analysis had been applied to every conceivable kind of job a hospital community might offer. A method of history-taking was devised which elicited the abilities, skills and potential of each patient admitted. The hospital was considered to be an independent community which could serve as a model of retraining and preparing patients to return to the community at large. Dr. Marsh felt that the hospital needed to be more responsive to society, to be more empathic with the kinds of life styles that society supported, and he challenged both psychiatry and occupational therapy to prepare patients to return to the community by teaching those values and work habits which society approved. He presented a mock psychiatric conference wherein the profession of psychiatry was reviewed as a patient. This delightful analogy demonstrates the fundamental difference between psychiatry and occupational therapy, and should be read by all who are presently concerned with the potential collaboration between the two disciplines.

Dr. Marsh spoke of the developmental period of adulthood—that stage in life when one is engaged in an economic role based on the occupations developed and rewarded by his society.

Successful adulthood is characterized by productivity and creativity. One's pursuits are in the direction of economic independence, and gratification is indirectly obtained, while most of the individual's efforts are directed toward the benefit of his family and of society as a whole. To Dr. Marsh it appeared that the apathetic and lonely persons sitting in the wards of the state hospital should be directed into activities relevant to their needs as self-respecting adults. Jobs provided training in skills and occupational roles, and were therefore gratifying as the patients contributed to the welfare of the community where they were temporarily residing.

Other Principles Derived from the Past

Certain other principles relative to present-day practice may be derived from the past. Each of these pioneers has placed special emphasis on function, on the need to provide the means by which an individual recognized and developed those skills and attitudes which, for him, led to improved adaptation and greater satisfaction. Assessment of the patient's level of function took into account the pathology evidenced as a means of understanding temporary or more permanent limitations. The occupational therapists and the psychiatrists with whom they worked apparently deemed the greatest value of therapeutic work to be the development of independent function, adaptive skills, useful habits, and satisfying behaviors. They were challenged[9] to develop evaluation technics for determining the nature and extent of the patient's deterioration, so as to have a base line from which to develop a therapeutic work program. Others saw the therapist as being a significant link in the communications between doctor and patient, sharing information as to accomplishments and behavioral changes demonstrated through the occupational therapy process.[10] But the implication seems to have been that these new skills and habits were superimposed upon the psychopathology, and the patient learned more satisfactory ways of engaging with the world. No thought apparently was given to the idea that the patient's personality structure or the pathological process itself were significantly touched by the activities provided through occupational therapy.

Another area of concern was with behavior and the social system. Moral treatment was based on the assumption that the patient had failed to reconcile his own behavior with that required by the community in which he lived. Today, social scientists point out that the community determines which of its members shall be free and which shall be restrained. The range of behaviors which the community will tolerate is clearly identified with, though seldom written into a legal code. The choice of restriction is between prison and mental hospital, and the nature of the deviant behavior, coupled with the degree of its deviance, determines which institution will receive the non-conformer. The mental hospitals of the moral treatment era attempted to demonstrate through the personal behavior of the staff that code of behavior which would readmit the patient to society. The patient was considered to be able to benefit from this kind of example, a technic now used by some behavioral therapists. Occupational therapists in such programs would have established the work norms which were congruent with those of the community to which the patient was to return. In a sense, occupational therapy was a training program, wherein the patient was conditioned, by rewards and approval, to adopt the standards of production and interpersonal responses which were considered appropriate. Insights as to why he had become deviant or had failed to develop the appropriate skills and attitudes were not expected to be necessary results of the therapeutic program.

As the movement of psychological psychiatry evolved, therapists began to question the scope of their work, and some began to feel the need to ally the profession with that group of psychotherapists who explored unconscious processes and attempted to intervene directly in psychopathology, with the objectives of correcting personality structure, modifying self-concept, and assisting the patient to re-integrate through cognitive and affective processes. The profession as a whole, however, continued to work on the assumptions of the past, and did not attempt to formulate a theoretical basis for its methods until much later.

Therapeutic Role Models

Another set of ideas which are important in today's practice also have historical antecedents. During the 1950's, the idea of "therapeutic use of self"[11, 12] became prominent. This, too, was related to the growing emphasis on the need to collaborate more closely with psychiatrists, relying more heavily on similar technics, and simultaneously devaluing the activities process. The pendulum seems to be swinging at the present time toward a position of balance between the meaning of work and activities and the necessary therapeutic interpersonal encounters. Some models for the "therapeutic use of self" had been developed by the early pioneers.

Mrs. Slagle portrayed the tolerant, loving, nurturing mother, a role too often lacking in the developmental experiences of the psychiatric patient. She gently urged the acquiring of habits which were socially acceptable, and gave love and warmth as rewards. She placed such high value on human dignity that she quietly refused to allow patients to live in degenerative conditions, slowly leading them into behavior patterns which brought forth self-esteem and the ability to recognize one's own worth in the work-a-day world. Such nurturing, accomplished through carefully and clearly established routines, is the essence of the good mother's role as the child's self-concept evolves and he begins to develop a sense of autonomy. We now know that the activities of daily living which represent grooming, feeding, sharing, communication, creative play and self-expression are all best carried out in the atmosphere created by the representative mother.

Mr. Haas provided the role model of teacher. As mentioned earlier, this is an important figure during the adolescent period of development. A common aspect of many psychiatric problems is an identity crisis, a period during which the individual struggles to define both sexual and vocational roles for himself. This is a normal crisis in adolescence; yet it has led certain writers to question if, in fact, adolescence itself is a state of normality! Certainly it is a difficult period for adolescent and parent alike. One of the necessary figures in the resolution of the adolescent crisis is a parent surrogate, an outsider who provides essentially the same moral values and standards as do the parents, but one whom the adolescent can accept and with whom it is safe and desirable to identify because he is not an actual member of the family, and is someone whom the adolescent himself chooses. A teacher, an athletic hero, a political figure, a movie star, a summer employer, or someone who is really "in" on the activist scene, may be taken as the significant figure.[13]

The occupational therapist, through the use of activities which represent the leisure time pursuits, the educational requirements, or the vocational choices with which the adolescent must deal, may serve as the parental ideal so badly needed if the identity crisis is to be resolved. High standards of workmanship, challenges provided through graded activity, supervised experiences with peer group members, and problem-solving with peers in task-oriented groups are the means by which the therapist in this role provides the essential experiences for this developmental period. Louis Haas was the prototype for this therapeutic model.

And finally, the therapist needs to be able to assume the role of supervisor and employer. He may, in fact, be a supervisor or employer, as well as a therapist, and these responsibilities have direct bearing on the quality of the mental health program which he serves.[14,15,16] As a therapeutic process, however, the role of supervisor/employer should be used with those persons who are attempting to develop appropriate adult occupational behaviors. Supervision is considered to be a process in growth and development, a collaborative relationship wherein two persons work toward the expanded capabilities of the supervisee. This differs from a therapeutic process in that only those behaviors relevant to the job are within the purview of the supervisor, while during therapy, the broader range of maladaptive behaviors must be explored, as they represent the self-concept of the individual and his capacity for integrating his own needs with those of his society. Nevertheless, many of the same technics of supervision apply, modified so as to be typical of employers, foremen or supervisors whom the patient is likely to encounter in a real work situation. Emphasis should be on production, upon meeting quotas and standards, and upon appropriate interpersonal responses to fellow workers. The hospital community, as L. Cody Marsh pointed out, represents the real society in miniature. The therapist must be carefully attuned to the workman's values and to the standards of the local housewife, if he is to represent fairly the community in which his clients must be prepared to function. With the movement toward fewer hospitalizations and more mental health programs operating in the community itself, this becomes a therapeutic role of increasing importance.

THEORETICAL BASIS FOR PRACTICE

Occupational therapy, as a discipline concerned with the self-directed, productive behavior of human beings, derives its primary rationale from the developmental processes which are fundamental to growth and creativity. The pioneers whose work led to the establishment of the profession have provided an introductory rationale on which to build a theoretical construct relevant to the needs of the practitioner of the present. This chapter cannot present a single unified theory of occupational therapy because none currently exists. Rather, the several partially validated theories which guide present practice are reviewed here so that methodologies may be presented through a theoretical framework.

Developmental Theory

Theories of human development ordinarily are concerned with four aspects of growth and change. First is the biogenetic core, which determines the biological dimensions of human development. It includes the phylogenetic predispositions through which unfolds the ontogenetic life unique to each individual. These are sometimes referred to as hereditary or constitutional factors and much remains unknown about their potential for change through educational or therapeutic intervention.

The second area concerns cognitive-perceptual-motor functioning. The assumptions made about this area of development are fully discussed in Chapter 14 of this book. Basically, this system provides the perceptual mechanism through which the inner biological sphere of the individual relates to the outer world of phenomena and events. It allows the individual to gain access to and knowledge of (cognition) those environmental encounters which he experiences.

The process of socialization is the third developmental function. It evolves from a series of interactions with other human beings, primarily family figures at first, and later expands to include peer groups and others in the community. This is considered to be an affective kind of development as differentiated from the cognitive or intellectual development of the previously mentioned phase.

And finally, there is the process of enculturation, the learning through and about the social system in which the individual resides. This learning is cognitive and task-oriented. It is concerned with the inanimate

CHART 5-1A PSYCHODYNAMIC DEVELOPMENT . . . FREUDIAN SCHOOL
Developed by N. Gillette for AOTA/SRS 123 Regional Institute 1968

Oral	Anal	Genital-Oedipal	Latency
Dependence	Attempts independence	Genital interest	Quiescence of primitive impulse struggles
Passivity	Resistance shown	Possessiveness to opposite parent	Interest in mastery of skills
Initial aggression	Negativism Self-assertiveness	Antagonism to same parent	Identification
Oral-erotic activity	Selfishness	Castration anxiety or disappointment	Tolerates competition
Incorporation	Narcissism		More accepting of reality principle
Projection	Magical thinking Anal preoccupation Ambivalence Sadistic means of control		Strong defenses develop

CHART 5-1B EIGHT AGES OF MAN . . . ERIK H. ERIKSON

The Developmental Problem	The Physical and Social Era	The Essential Strength of the Era
Basic trust vs. Basic mistrust	Oral-sensory	Drive and hope
Autonomy vs. Shame and Doubt	Muscular-anal	Self-control and will power
Initiative vs. Guilt	Locomotor-genital	Direction and purpose
Industry vs. Inferiority	Latency	Method and competence
Identity vs. Role confusion	Puberty and adolescence	Devotion and fidelity
Intimacy vs. Isolation	Young adulthood	Affiliation and love
Generativity vs. Stagnation	Adulthood	Production and care
Ego integrity vs. Despair	Maturity	Renunciation and wisdom

objects that the culture uses to deal with the processes of daily living. Jobs, tools and games are examples of the factors dealt with in the enculturation process.

Some developmental theorists have been concerned primarily with the experiences of childhood and adolescence. More recently, the developmental processes which are a part of the adult's experience have been recognized. Failure to attribute purposeful development to all phases of an individual's life results in devaluation of the later years and a decline in self-esteem of the older citizen. For the purpose of occupational therapy, therefore, it is essential that the entire life span be treated as a dynamically evolving process.

Chart 5–1 may assist in comparing the developmental theories most frequently used in relation to occupational therapy.[17,18,19,20]

Theories of Occupational Therapy

In 1966, the challenge was raised that no existing theoretical structure existed on which to develop methodologies or to predict the nature of the practice of the future.[21] The single existing text devoted to the psychiatric aspects of occupational therapy presented a series of methods and practical procedures for treatment, evaluation and meeting mental health needs, based on the interpersonal theory of psychiatry and the authors' extensive experience with psychiatric patients. Because the Fidler proposal* pre-supposed adequate knowledge of psychodynamics, object relations, and symbolic representation, it was not immediately usable by the majority of therapists whose educational backgrounds had not included these concepts. Therapists who had adequate preparation in these areas or who were able to find psychiatric supervision while they practiced the technics outlined, found the results to be both effective and gratifying. The level of psychiatric sophistication required, however, was not immediately available through the occupational therapy curricula of that period, and the methods and concepts set forth continue to pose a relatively untested challenge to the profession as a whole.

To some occupational therapists and psychiatrists, however, the essence of the occupational therapy process lies in the realm of productive, gratifying socioeconomic development of the individual. (A concept not at all argued by the Fidlers, but their emphasis on unconscious processes and psychopathology has been read by some as devaluing †

---

* This model is similar to the one proposed by another husband and wife team in Canada. The Azimas challenged the profession of occupational therapy to develop a rationale based on use of the media as a free projective mode of revealing and modifying thought processes and behavioral motivations. They outlined both treatment and evaluation procedures which they had demonstrated to be effective. Object relations, deliberate regression through selected activities, and gratification of primitive needs through appropriate object experiences were integral parts of the occupational therapy process they proposed.[22]

† Text continues on page 68.

CHART 5–1C DEVELOPMENTAL TASKS AND EDUCATION ... R. J. HAVIGHURST
Developed by N. Gillette for AOTA/SRS 123 Regional Institute 1968

Infancy and Early Childhood	Middle Childhood	Adolescence
1. Learning to walk	1. Learning physical skills necessary for ordinary games	1. Achieving new and more mature relations with age-mates of both sexes
2. Learning to take solid foods	2. Building wholesome attitudes toward oneself as a growing organism	2. Achieving a masculine or feminine social role
3. Learning to talk	3. Learning to get along with age-mates	3. Accepting one's physique and using the body effectively
4. Learning to control the elimination of body wastes	4. Learning an appropriate masculine or feminine social role	4. Achieving emotional independence of parents and other adults
5. Learning sex differences and sexual modesty	5. Developing fundamental skills in reading, writing and calculating	5. Achieving assurance of economic independence
6. Achieving physiological stability	6. Developing concepts necessary for everyday living	6. Selecting and preparing for an occupation
7. Forming simple concepts of social and physical reality	7. Developing conscience, morality, and a scale of values	7. Preparing for marriage and family life
8. Learning to relate oneself emotionally to parents, siblings, and other people	8. Achieving personal independence	8. Developing intellectual skills and concepts necessary for civic competence
9. Learning to distinguish right and wrong and developing a conscience	9. Developing attitudes toward social groups and institutions	9. Desiring and achieving socially responsible behavior
		10. Acquiring a set of values and an ethical system as a guide to behavior

CHART 5–1C (Continued)

Early Adulthood	Middle Age	Later Maturity
1. Selecting a mate	1. Achieving adult civic and social responsibility	1. Adjusting to decreasing physical strength and health
2. Learning to live with a marriage partner	2. Establishing and maintaining an economic standard of living	2. Adjustment to retirement and reduced income
3. Starting a family	3. Assisting teenage children to become responsible and happy adults	3. Adjusting to death of spouse
4. Rearing children	4. Developing adult leisure-time activities	4. Establishing an explicit affiliation with one's age group
5. Managing a home	5. Relating oneself to one's spouse as a person	5. Meeting social and civic obligations
6. Getting started in an occupation	6. Accept and adjust to the physiological changes of middle age	6. Establishing satisfactory physical living arrangements
7. Taking on civic responsibility	7. Adjusting to aging parents	
8. Finding a congenial social group		

CHART 5-1D DEVELOPMENTAL CONCEPTS ADAPTED FROM THE INTERPERSONAL THEORIES OF H. S. SULLIVAN

Infancy	Childhood	Juvenile Era
Necessary early physiological adjustments and adaptations: heat regulation respiration movement and pattern of GI functions sensitivity to touch, kinesthetic stimuli defenses against bacterial and viral invasions establishment of diurnal pattern maturity of nervous system	Development of speech	Learns to accommodate to values of those outside family circle
	Development of conscious need for playmates	Explores roles different from those played (allowed) at home
	Self-image initially formulated	Fear of ostracism is a dominant motive
	Adult's earliest memories usually from this period	Need for group relatedness is primary motivator
	Verbalization becomes major means of communication	Formal education allows for further mastery of physical world
	Overt consensual validations become possible, with speech	No serious concern for other person's needs, but value concepts such as fairness, justice, are developed
	Child becomes aware of ambivalent message: words vs. affect	
Identification of emotional experiences: Good Mother, Bad Mother leads to Good Me and Bad Me; self-image must incorporate both	Sees self as child in adult-dominated world	Words take on more importance as means of communication
	Concern with patterns of relationship to authority	Expansion of mastery of inanimate objects
Develops range of emotional responses, uses appropriately	Mastery of shapes, coordination, body image	
Mastery of gross motor responses	Integration of the positive function of parallel play	
Mastery of some concept of three-dimensional space	Peer relationships lack real continuity	
Beginning sense of body image	Importance of transitional objects	

CHART 5-1D (Continued)

Pre-Adolescence	Adolescence	Young Adult
Development of a chumship, where the other person's true needs are equal to one's own	Further development of one-to-one relatedness	Separation of self from home: parents, dependency, controls, values
This becomes basis for validating one's feeling of humanness	Developing capacity to love	moving out
Leads to development of compassion; can be extended in the abstract	Experience in integration of partnerships	financial independence
First expansion of sources other than parents to validate and affirm one's values, to attempt expansion of the self-system	Learns to live and to share with a contemporary	marriage
May be the highest point of humanness in the whole life span	Thus, opportunity for consensual validation and correction of perception for sharing of everyday experience	Children: declaration of equality with parents
	Need to reintegrate the disassociated experience of touch; produces anxiety	affirmation of continuity
	Must gain confidence re capacity to give and receive sexual gratification	impact on world
	Assumption of responsibility for one's own growth	

CHART 5–1D (Continued)

Middle Age Crises	Maturity	Old Age
Central problem shifts from how to survive to how to enjoy life	Defined as: "proportional to one's capacity to relate to his contemporaries, regardless of age, in the context of the process of extending love to include more and more people, and to find the common denominator with oneself in more apparently divergent people."	Strong cultural pressures to discourage growth, changes, adaptation; possibilities would be: hobbies, group relationships, friendships or productive work
Emotional responsibility for children has ended		Cultural conception that physical age involves emotional deterioration is false
Ability to continue to control and direct children greatly diminishes		Growth, with no limits ahead
Culture ridicules "growth" making it hard to make a healthy adjustment	Conceives of self as independent, free to choose own associates, to implement own decisions; sees self as integral factor in the chain of cause and effect	Access to widest range of emotional responses
Social prejudices restrict career changes, see them as foolish		
Decision to grow or to die is the real crisis of middle age		

this aspect of occupational therapy.) Thus, they would search for a model based on developmental processes as reflected through the very activities so familiar to therapist and patient alike: work and play. This group, whose leading spokesman is Reilly,[23] proposes that the major concern of occupational therapy is with the functional capacities of the individual, his ability to be self-determining in a social and economic capacity which for him is satisfying, and which in the eyes of society is necessary and respectable. By stressing work and play in the daily lives of people, this group tends to minimize the close allegiance with psychiatry which the Fidler model presupposes. The Fidlers conceive of occupational therapy as active intervention into pathological conditions, or a means of maintaining mental health in the face of potentially disorganizing forces. Reilly believes that the occupational therapy allegiance should be with health, with establishing a functional diagnosis based on an assessment of strengths; "treatment" then becomes improving innate skills or previously learned behaviors in order to solve problems of daily living more effectively.

In 1968, the American Occupational Therapy Association's Consultant in Psychiatric Rehabilitation invited therapists to submit their own working theories for publication, toward the effort to establish an integrated theory. Four theories were selected, and they appeared in the *American Journal of Occupational Therapy*, Vol. XXII, No. 5, 1968. The student is urged to study these in the original, and to develop his own comparisons of the four basic concepts. Two of these proposals were related to principles of learning theory and behavior modification.[24,25] A third was based on the concepts of life-style developed by Kurt Lewin.[26] The fourth [27] has been expanded into a comprehensive theory and published as a text, *Three Frames of Reference for Occupational Therapy and Mental Health*. Each of these proposals is related to, though not necessarily developed through, existing behavioral science correlates. Chart 5–2 illustrates some of these relationships by providing a cross-reference system, which may be used comparatively.

While it is not the purpose of this chapter to establish a single unified theory for the practice of occupational therapy in the field of mental health, the following components are believed to be essential in the formulation of a viable theory and for the development of appropriate and effective methodologies related to evaluation, treatment and consultation: (1) the processes of human development; (2) the neurophysiological aspects of maturation; (3) the psychosocial aspects of human behavior and learning. Such a theory would thereby encompass genetic and biological factors and their positive potential or limitations for the behavior and adaptation of the individual; knowledge of*

* Text continues on page 73.

CHART 5-2A PSYCHOANALYTICAL

Modified from tables developed by Kenneth Overly, OTR, for the AOTA Reference Handbook on Continuing Education, Kendall/Hunt, Dubuque, Iowa, 1969.

Theoretical References	Core Concepts	Focus of Practice	Clinical Treatment References

Freud, S.: Interpretation of Dreams. London, Hogarth Press, 1953.
 	
Psychotherapy of Everyday Life, in the Basic Writings of Sigmund Freud. New York, Modern Library, 1958.
 	
Jung, C. G.: Man and His Symbols. New York, Doubleday & Company, 1964.
 	
Brenner, C.: An Elementary Textbook of Psychoanalysis. New York, Doubleday & Company, 1957
 	
Freud, A.: The Ego and the Mechanisms of Defense. New York, International Universities Press, 1946.
	Basic Unit of Analysis
	individual psyche
	Bio-Genetic Determinism
	(structural)
	drive-object
	libidinal energies
	Unconscious
	Conscious
	Id
	Ego
	Superego
	Defense mechanisms
	Symbolization
	(dynamic)
	Psychosexual stages
	oral
	anal
	oedipal
	latent
	Object relations
	concept of introjection, object incorporated into intrapsychic reality
		Focus on individual
		Gaining access to and control of his intrapsychic process through:
		1. Free association
		  a) analytical art therapy
		  b) movement
		2. Transference in terms of primary process
		3. Anaclitic treatment
			Fidler, G. S., and Fidler, J. W.: Occupational Therapy: A Communication Process, pp. 122–127. Macmillan, New York, 1963.
			
			Naumberg, M.: Schizophrenic Art: Its Meaning in Psychotherapy. New York, Grune & Stratton, 1950.
			
			Pesso, A. I.: Psychomotor Therapy. In Press.
			
			Sechehaye, M.: Symbolic Realization. New York, International Universities Press, 1951.
			
			Green, H.: I Never Promised You A Rose Garden. New York, Holt, Rinehart & Winston, 1964.
			
			Azima, W., and Azima, L.: Object relations therapy in schizophrenic states. Am. J. Psychiat., Vol. 115, No. 1, 1958.

CHART 5-2B INTERPERSONAL

EXISTENTIAL PSYCHIATRY

Primary Reference: Sartre, J. P.: The Emotions. New York, The Phil. Library, 1948.
Treatment Reference: (1) VanDenberg, J. H.: The Phenomenological Approach to Psychiatry,
Springfield, C. C Thomas, 1955
(2) May, R., Angel, E., and Berger, E. (eds.):
Existence. New York, Basic Books, 1958.

Theoretical References	Core Concepts	Focus of Practice	Clinical Treatment References
Sullivan, H. S.: The Collected Works, Vol. I & II. New York, W. W. Norton & Co., 1956. Pearce, J., and Newton, S.: Conditions of Human Growth. New York, Citadel Press, 1963. Erikson, E.: Childhood and Society. New York, W. W. Norton & Co., 1963. Searles, H.: The Non-Human Environment. New York, International Universities Press, 1960.	Basic Unit of Focus: interpersonal dyad Anxiety occurs when needs for security or satisfaction are not met mechanisms for negative reductions and/or positive resolutions: tension selective inattention focal awareness Communication distortions in consensual validation Psychosocial stages of development—through total life span Behavior is product of self interacting with significant others Object relations	Examination of one's actions in an interpersonal setting Learning occupational therapy as a setting in which: object, action process, interpersonal relations occur Both individual and group treatment	Sullivan, H. S.: The Collected Works. Rogers, C. R.: Client-Centered Therapy. New York, Houghton-Mifflin Press, 1951. Haley, J.: Strategies of Psychotherapy. New York, Grune & Stratton, 1963. Parker, B.: My Language Is Me. New York, Basic Books, 1962. Ruesch, J., and Bateson, G.: Communication: The Social Matrix of Psychiatry. New York, W. W. Norton & Company, 1957. Fidler, G. S., and Fidler, J. W.: Occupational Therapy: A Communication Process in Psychiatry. New York, Macmillan Co., 1964. (see especially chapters on Practice and the Treatment Process.) West, W. (ed.): Changing Concepts and Practices in Occupational Therapy.

Theoretical References	Core Concepts	Focus of Practice	Clinical Treatment References
Note: Many of the treatment references include theoretical sections. Cumming, J., and Cumming, E.: Ego and Milieu (Part I). New York, Atherton Press, 1962. Gerth, H., and Mills, C. W.: Character and Social Structure. New York, Harcourt Brace, 1953. Coser, L.A., and Rosenberg, B.: Sociological Theory. New York, Macmillan, 1957.	Focus: the individual's participative relationship with his environment (both animate and inanimate) primary memberships	General – Milieu Therapy Specific approaches 1. Therapeutic community 2. Work therapy 3. Transactional analysis 4. Behavior modification 5. Recapitulation of ontogenesis 6. Use of groups	Stanton, A. H., and Schwartz, M. S.: The Mental Hospital. New York, Basic Books, 1954. Llorens, L., O.T. in an ego-oriented milieu. AJOT, Vol. XX, No. 4, 1966. Jones, M.: Therapeutic Community. New York, Basic Books, 1953. Cumming, J., and Cumming, E., Ego and Milieu (Part II & III). New York, Atherton Press, 1962. Reilly, M.: O.T. can be one of the greatest ideas of 20th century medicine. AJOT, Vol. XVI, No. 1, 1962. Berne, E.: Games People Play and Transactional Analysis. New York, Grove Press, 1961, 1964. Ullman, O.P., and Krasner, L.: Case Studies in Behavior Modification. New York, Holt, Rinehart & Winston, 1965. Smith, A., and Tempone, V. J.: Psychiatric occupational therapy within a learning theory context. AJOT, Vol. XXII, No. 5, 1968. Mosey, A.: Recapitulation of ontogenesis. AJOT, Vol. XXII, No. 5, 1968. Materials from National Training Laboratories for Applied Behavioral Science—NEA, Washington, D.C. Edelson, M.: Ego Psychology, Group Dynamics, and the Therapeutic Community. New York, Grune & Stratton, 1964. Fairweather, C.: Social Psychology in Treating Mental Illness. New York, Wiley & Sons, 1964. Fidler, G.: The task-oriented group as a context for treatment, AJOT, Vol. XXIII, No. 1, 1969.

CHART 5-2D   COMMUNITY MENTAL HEALTH

Theoretical References	Core Concepts	Focus of Practice	Clinical Treatment References
Barnouw, V.: Culture and Personality. Homewood, Dorsey Press, 1963. Kluckhohn, C.: Culture and Behavior. New York, Free Press, 1962. Duhl, L.: The Urban Condition. New York, Basic Books, 1963. Eaton, J., and Weil, R.: Culture and Mental Illness. Glencoe, Ill., Free Press, 1955. Duhl, L. J., and Leopold, R. L. (eds.): Mental Health and Urban Social Policy. San Francisco, Jossey-Bas, Inc., 1968.	Focus: Concepts about urban ecology and sociology (city planning, community organization, etc.) Role Theory: 1. Functional ascription (expectations) 2. Membership: accommodation mechanism 3. Functional achievement (realization)	Primary Prevention consultation and mental health education to: schools housing police community agencies, etc. Secondary Prevention crisis intervention day center programs continuity of care in geographical location available to population being served home programs Tertiary Prevention halfway houses sheltered workshops outpatient and followup groups	Caplan, G.: Principles of Preventive Psychiatry. New York, Basic Books, 1964. A.O.T.A.: Proceedings of Seminars on Community Psychiatry, 1966. Becker, E.: The Revolution in Psychiatry: The New Understanding of Man. Free Press of Glencoe, 1964. Dumont, M. P.: The Absurd Healer: Perspectives of a Community Psychiatrist. New York, Science House, 1968. Gillette, N. P.: Changing methods in the treatment of psychosocial dysfunction. AJOT, XXI, 4:23, 230, 1967. Watanabe, S.: Four Concepts Basic to the Occupational Therapy Process. AJOT, XXII, 5:439, 1968.

interpersonal relations and socialization processes; concepts of extrinsic and intrinsic motivation and environmental influences on behavior; and conscious and unconscious thought processes, defense mechanisms and symbolic or representative communications. The reader is referred to an effort at synthesizing these factors, edited by June Mazer.[28] This review emphasizes the need for an integrated theory and points to the difficulties in communication between therapists representing various empirically derived beliefs.

Ego Psychology

It may be that the missing link lies somewhere in the field of ego psychology. It is the function of the ego to organize and respond appropriately to both internal and external stimuli. Body, mind and society each pummel the ego, demanding instant response, mediation, gratification, change and synthesis. Insofar as the ego has the necessary strengths to respond flexibly and reasonably directly, the individual perceives himself and is perceived by others as being fairly well integrated, and he is viewed as being "healthy."

Despite the fact that "ego" is a psychoanalytic term, and in that way may create a communications barrier for some people, it would appear to be the fundamental concept which will allow the integration of the several existing partial theories of occupational therapy. Through its functions, the ego demonstrates the degree of competence and mastery which the individual has achieved over his environment. It perceives both internal instincts and externally derived sensory-motor stimuli and organizes and executes appropriate responses to each. It is limited by any existing biologic or neurophysiologic deficits within the individual, just as it is limited by the nature of the individual's developmental experiences; both of which may predispose the individual to certain maladaptive patterns of behavior. The ego synthesizes its own reality, mediating between primitive physiologic and psychologic urges, and those requirements which society imposes as a necessary prerequisite for continued participation. The ego appears to determine, therefore, the individual's response to the world of activities and interpersonal affairs which makes up the realm of occupational therapy.*

Whether or not ego psychology proves to be the integrating force, the development of a unified theory of practice should be of the highest priority within the profession.

---

*Two primary references which clarify the relationship between behavior and ego function, and which therefore are directly applicable to the occupational therapy process, are:
  1. Edelson, M.: Ego Psychology, Group Dynamics, and the Therapeutic Community. Grune & Stratton, New York, 1964.
  2. Cumming, J., and Cumming, E.: Ego and Milieu: Theory and Practice of Environmental Therapy. Atherton Press, New York, 1966.

WHO NEEDS OCCUPATIONAL THERAPY?

This is not only a question which students ask daily; it is a long-standing question within the profession, one which is often verbalized in an effort to determine when and how to offer services, what to offer, and to whom. The question may also be heard at a second level of meaning, one which is less often admitted to consciousness, but which has had at least equal impact on the development of the profession: if what we offer is automatically so much a part of the lives of all people—activities related to economic roles, leisure activities, family interactions, community projects, childhood play, and learning—who needs occupational therapy? When the question is recognized at this level, it causes occupational therapists to become somewhat anxious, for the answer requires an adequate rationale for the existence of the profession.

In the past, the profession attempted to find support and direction and a raison d'être through identification with the medical profession.[10] This orientation presumed that persons requiring occupational therapy had specific medical or psychiatric disabilities; they were felt to be sick and in need of medical supervision. Occupational therapy was thus assumed to require medical supervision, also, since the therapist's own medical education was obviously not adequate to diagnose and treat medical conditions. The concept of medical referral arose, and the therapist was directed as to which patients were to be seen in occupational therapy, as well as having doctor's orders regarding the nature of the therapeutic program. Therapists were eager to be identified as knowledgeable about medical and psychiatric issues, and adopted white uniforms and other practices which would bind them more closely to the medical model.

The major advantages derived from this period, in terms of the development of the profession of occupational therapy, are as follows:

It was a period in which to explore the relationships between health and illness, as exemplified through choice and mastery of activity, seen as an extension of the patient's self-concept, and his potential for recovery.

It was a period during which the therapist's security was bolstered by having medical authority upon which to rely while the profession of occupational therapy sought its own theoretical constructs.

And it was a period which spawned a growing awareness on the part of occupational therapy that medical practice did not really desire or require the supervisory-dependent relationship which existed, and that physicians and nurses were more eager to collaborate as peers in assessing patients' needs, determining objectives, and referring patients to each other as the need arose for different services for a given patient or group.

But then a second dilemma arose: if occupational therapists were not to be medically directed, wherein does the authority lie? "Who needs occupational therapy?" became a question of social relevance. And it is from the society-at-large that a profession must derive the mandate for its practice.

The occupational therapist has been described as being concerned with functions, with the strengths and abilities of those with whom the therapist works. Assisting persons to experience a normal developmental process or to master developmental tasks more satisfactorily is a major concern of the therapist. The activities of daily living and the pursuit of appropriate social and economic roles are issues which occupational therapists attempt to mediate for the handicapped, the sick or the disadvantaged. And finally, the profession is concerned with the quality of life in the community itself, because one's health is partially determined by standards of living, levels of education, opportunities for self-fulfillment and the availability of an adequate range of jobs.

Thus, occupational therapy is concerned with a much broader range of issues than appeared to be true during the medically oriented period of development. Whether or not this is a primary truth is not clear. It may be that the real concerns of the profession have always been as broad as they are now, and that they were only *apparently* narrowed, so as to find entry through medical channels. This would appear to be true because of the relative ease with which occupational therapists today slip into community health programs, seeing readily the relationships between family patterns, work conditions, learning and leisure, and overall health. So perhaps this has always been the strength of the profession and its real purpose. In either case, the practice of today reflects and is dependent upon a concern for man and his activities as they simultaneously express and determine his states of health and satisfaction.

Within the society at large, then, who needs—who can benefit from—occupational therapy? It would be easy to generalize that persons of all ages who experience difficulty in accomplishing their everyday tasks and who are unsatisfied with their lots in life, yet are unable to make satisfactory changes—that these vast numbers could benefit from occupational therapy. But efforts must be directed toward more limited objectives, while at the same time a system is developed through which the results of the occupational therapy methodologies can be assessed. It will then be possible to describe specific services and to predict their results, based on substantial evidence. On such a foundation, the service concepts of the profession could be expanded into social realms and be used to help prevent the development of personal-social dysfunction.

CHART 5-3   SEVEN ADAPTIVE SKILLS*

A. Perceptual-Motor Skill
    The ability to receive, integrate and organize sensory stimuli in a manner
      which allows for the planning of purposeful movement.
    The sub-skills required are the abilities
    1. To integrate primitive postural reflexes, to react appropriately to ves-
       tibular stimuli, to maintain a balance between the tactile subsystems,
       to perceive form and to be aware of auditory stimuli.
    2. To control extraocular musculature, to integrate the two sides of the
       body and to focus on auditory stimuli.
    3. To perceive visual and auditory figure-ground, to be aware of body
       parts and their relationships, and to plan gross motor movements.
    4. To perceive space, to plan fine motor movements and to discriminate
       auditory stimuli.
    5. To discriminate between right and left and to remember auditory
       stimuli.
    6. To use abstract concepts, to scan, integrate and synthesize auditory
       stimuli; and to give auditory feedback.
B. Cognitive Skill
    The ability to perceive, represent and organize objects, events and their
      relationships in a manner which is considered appropriate by one's
      cultural group.
    The sub-skills required are the abilities
    1. To use inherent behavioral patterns for environmental interaction.
    2. To interrelate visual, manual, auditory and oral responses.
    3. To attend to the environmental consequence of actions with interest,
       to represent objects in an exoceptual manner, to experience objects, to
       act on the bases of egocentric causality and to seriate events in which
       the self is involved.
    4. To establish a goal and intentionally carry out means, to recognize the
       independent existence of objects, to interpret signs, to imitate new
       behavior, to apprehend the influence of space and to perceive other
       objects as partially causal.
    5. To use trial and error problem solving, to use tools, to perceive vari-
       ability in spacial positions, to seriate events in which the self is not
       involved, and to perceive the causality of other objects.
    6. To represent objects in an image manner, to make believe, to infer a
       cause given its effect, to act on the bases of combined spatial relations,
       to attribute omnipotence to others and to perceive objects as perma-
       nent in time and space.
    7. To represent objects in an endoceptual manner, to differentiate be-
       tween thought and action and to recognize the need for causal sources.
    8. To represent objects in a denotative manner, to perceive the viewpoint
       of others and to decenter.
    9. To represent objects in a connotative manner, to use formal logic and
       to work in the realm of the hypothetical.

---

* Adapted from Mosey, A.C.: Three Frames of Reference for Mental Health.
Thorofare, N.J., Charles B. Slack, 1970

CHART 5–3 (Continued)

C. Drive-Object Skill

The ability to control drives and select objects in such a manner as to ensure adequate need satisfaction.

The sub-skills required are the abilities

1. To form a discontinuous, libidinal object relationship.
2. To form a continuous, part, libidinal object relationship.
3. To invest aggressive drive in an external object.
4. To transfer libidinal drive to objects other than the primary object.
5. To invest libidinal energy in appropriate abstract objects and to control aggressive drive.
6. To engage in total and diffuse libidinal object relationships.

D. Dyadic Interaction Skill

The ability to participate in a variety of dyadic relationships.

The sub-skills required are the abilities

1. To enter into association relationships.
2. To interact in an authority relationship.
3. To interact in a chum relationship.
4. To enter into a peer, authority relationship.
5. To enter into an intimate relationship.
6. To engage in a nurturing relationship.

E. Group Interaction Skill

The ability to be a productive member of a variety of primary groups.

The sub-skills required are the abilities

1. To participate in a parallel group.
2. To participate in a project group.
3. To participate in an egocentric-cooperative group.
4. To participate in a cooperative group.
5. To participate in a mature group.

F. Self-Identity Skill

The ability to perceive the self as an autonomous, holistic, and acceptable object which has permanence and continuity over time.

The sub-skills required are the abilities

1. To perceive the self as a worthy object.
2. To perceive the assets and limitations of the self.
3. To perceive the self as self-directed.
4. To perceive the self as a productive, contributing member of a social system.
5. To perceive the self.
6. To perceive the aging process of the self in a rational manner.

G. Sexual Identity Skill

The ability to perceive one's sexual nature as good and to participate in a heterosexual relationship which is oriented to the mutual satisfaction of sexual needs.

The sub-skills required are the abilities

1. To accept and act upon the bases of one's pregenital sexual nature.
2. To accept sexual maturation as a positive growth experience.
3. To give and receive sexual gratification.
4. To enter into a sustained heterosexual relationship.
5. To accept physiological and psychological changes which occur at the time of the climacteric.

But the question remains unanswered: who needs occupational therapy?

Empirically derived findings indicate that those persons who learn more easily through "doing" than through thinking and conceptualizing, those who express themselves more comfortably through actions than through words and those who have some neurophysiologic components to their problems that result in cognitive-perceptual-motor processes requiring training (i.e., learning through repetitive doing) seem to benefit most from occupational therapy.

Another scheme of reference states that persons with maturational or developmental deficits which lead to difficulty in mastering the social and economic tasks that are appropriate to their chronological age appear to benefit from occupational therapy. Activities graded through the physiological, psychosocial and work-related processes mastered in proper sequence help to insure lasting competence or assist in achieving health.

A similar theory is presented in detail (Chart 5–3) because it demonstrates the dynamic interrelatedness of the several parts of the developmental scheme. Mosey has proposed the concept of adaptive skills as the fundamental theory of occupational therapy: "Adapted skills are those learned abilities which enable man to satisfy human needs and meet environmental demands."[14] Failure to master any part results in difficulty as the next task is confronted, with total success being compromised until the several separate parts are mastered and integrated into the whole. This concept is supported by the work of Havighurst[20] and Erikson,[18] and it plays a significant part in determining which persons can benefit from the occupational therapy process.

The seven adaptive skills, with their sub-skill components, are listed in Chart 5–3. It is postulated that each sub-skill must be learned in proper sequence before mastery of the next sub-skill can be satisfactorily achieved, although learning of several sub-skills within one adaptive skill may be occurring simultaneously. Similarly, mastery of more than one adaptive skill may be in process at any given time. Skills are listed according to their relative developmental sequence.

In summary, then, given the state of knowledge within and the technics available to the profession, the following kinds of conditions appear to benefit from occupational therapy:

1. States of dysfunction which reflect difficulty in integrating developmental tasks.
2. Behavior disorders which reflect difficulty in communication, resulting in expression of primitive needs through action which attempts to provide direct gratification, rather than through verbalization and indirect or postponed rewards.

3. Cognitive-perceptual-motor deficits which force the individual to respond inappropriately, to a world of stimuli which cannot be perceived or understood by others.
4. States of regression or fixation at primitive, pre-verbal levels of communication.
5. Socially unsophisticated persons who express their needs more easily through activity than through abstract conversation.
6. Learning disorders, where the results of an act must be immediately and concretely available if learning is to take place.
7. And physical illnesses which impinge upon the individual's personal integrity, wherein the accomplishment of his activities of daily living provides reassurance and a needed sense of competence.

THE EVALUATION PROCESS

Evaluation as a Professional Responsibility

Just as any person responsible for creating or directing change must know from whence he begins, so must the occupational therapist evaluate the capabilities of the individuals with whom he works. The evaluation process determines the baseline, provides a springboard from which the objectives are formed, and thus serves as the foundation for the program of treatment or readjustment. It permits the identification of those problems which can and those which cannot be mediated through the occupational therapy process. It gives some indication of the potential for change, and thus helps set more realistic objectives. It enlists the cooperation of the client in beginning to assess not only his capabilities but his dreams, and it introduces him to a process through which he can help to initiate a course of action designed to master some of the difficulties with which he has previously struggled alone.

Evaluation also serves the purpose of keeping the therapist's work current, for it is a spiral, building process. Each treatment session should be assessed and each target area reviewed, in order to determine the effectiveness of the activities process and to revise the objectives as they are mastered or found to be unreachable. Treatment should not persist in a straight line. It is the system of evaluation which is built into the treatment process that ultimately determines the effectiveness of the treatment.

The evaluation process represents a commitment to a professional responsibility. It is the means by which the therapist determines what, if anything, he is to offer toward the individual's planned program. Findings of the evaluation are, in a sense, public property. They are most surely the concern of the client, who has helped to insure the success of the evaluation and upon whom much of the success of treatment depends. And they are of interest and value to other personnel who may be collaborating in the program of the individual in question. Exchange of evaluation results is, then, a professional responsibility, and these results must be recorded and made available appropriately, and in useful form.

The professional concept of the therapist may be one of the most crucial factors influencing the results of the evaluation. To judge or critically appraise another human being is not only fraught with dangers such as losing one's objectivity, it is a practice which is considered to be "impolite" and which is sometimes interpreted as an invasion of privacy. The therapist, in attempting to put himself in the patient's place, projects his own anxiety about "being uncovered" or having his most personal secrets revealed and assumes that the patient shares these feelings. The assumption may be true, as far as it goes. But the patient comes with another, equally strong set: he needs help. And only through discovering the areas which require change and identifying the strengths which can be used to produce change can the patient be relieved of the problem from which he is eager to be freed. Given a chance to collaborate in the evaluation process, patients generally lose their reluctance to be studied, for their motivation toward improving their adaptive skills is the stronger of the two forces. Freida Fromm-Reichman pointed out that man prefers health to illness. It is the therapist's job to help the individual move toward health without creating more anxiety than he can tolerate in the process.[29] Because the occupational therapy evaluation enlists the patient's active participation and reveals his capabilities in performance while letting him feel partially in control of the situation, it may be less threatening to him than some other types of evaluation procedures.

But the therapist's self-concept influences his role as evaluator in another way, too. To evaluate is to create a baseline, which then assumes some objectives to be achieved through the treatment modalities of the profession. In other words, one must be able to demonstrate that the occupational therapy methodologies do, in fact, accomplish predetermined claims or objectives. The degree and quality of change may then be further measured or evaluated. It thus becomes apparent that one's evaluation procedures measure not only patient performance and ability, but the therapist's own success and even, to some degree, the inherent worth of the occupational therapy process itself, with which the therapist feels so closely identified! While this concern is not usually a conscious one, it does have an influence on the behavior of the individual therapist.

There is a third aspect to the concept of professionalism, which must be mentioned briefly. During the period when occupational therapists working in psychiatry felt they should be medically directed, the need for evaluation technics was obviously less. The doctor determined which patients might benefit from occupational therapy and directed when and how they should participate in therapeutic activities. The objectives for the patient were established by the doctor, though sometimes this was done in conjunction with the therapist. These objectives were always *related to* and *stated in the terms* of the psychiatrist's own goals for the patient. The occupational therapy process was, therefore, clearly an adjunct to the psychiatrist's treatment program, and neither occupational therapist nor doctor assumed that there might be other objectives which would, in fact, be the prerogatives of the occupational therapist-patient pair. Reilly speaks of the challenge which now confronts the therapist: "It is the task of medicine to prevent and reduce illness; while the task of occupational therapy is to prevent and reduce the incapacities resulting from illness."[23] From this perspective, if the occupational therapist is to enjoy the rights and privileges of a true professional, he must establish his evaluation procedures and use them effectively as the basis for producing change or guiding the patient to more successful patterns of adaptation.

What Is an Evaluation?

An evaluation is an assessment of a given state of function. It is dependent upon a thorough knowledge of the norms — the usual level of function — relative to the condition being assessed. The evaluation determines the degree and amount (quality and quantity) of discrepancy between what is considered to be the norm and the functions being demonstrated during the evaluation process.

The judgments made by the therapist are based on facts, insofar as there are standardized tools for purposes of evaluating the functions in question. The evaluator relies heavily, too, on clinical judgment, which is the product of training and practice. His self-awareness mediates the evaluation process as it permits him to "see" or "hear" critical issues which may be as painful for him as they are for the client. The success and accuracy of the evaluation depends upon the therapist's knowledge of developmental theory, dysfunction and maladaptation, social pressures and conditions. Accuracy, too, is dependent upon the therapist's skill in administering the evaluation, observing and recording the data and summarizing the results. The final process requires an interpretation of all the data collected and a synthesis of these facts into a statement portraying the individual's current level of function. From this statement a plan for the ensuing occupational therapy process may be made.

What Does the Occupational Therapist Evaluate?

The occupational therapist evaluates the individual's ability to select and use his activities of daily living in such a way that he gains personal satisfaction and is comfortable and productive in an appropriate economic role. The capacity for expanding this competence is also assessed, as are the apparent limitations which may or may not respond to a therapeutic regime. Different theoretical assumptions require different methods of evaluation. The remainder of this section describes the evaluation technics which have derived from some of the theories discussed earlier.

In their text, *Occupational Therapy: A Communication Process in Psychiatry*, the Fidlers propose that the action processes, which are reflected through physical and creative activities, serve to communicate directly and symbolically certain otherwise unrecognized components of personality structure. They postulate that these actions plus the objects produced and the associations elicited through the activities process combine to produce a dynamic assessment of the individual. The following five areas of function* are assessed in order to derive the basic evaluation for occupational therapy purposes:

1. **Concept of Self:** To assess how the patient perceives himself and how he functions within this concept. The nature of his body image, identification, self-esteem, etc.

2. **Concept of Others:** How he perceives others and how he may be expected to relate to others. What expectations he has concerning relationships, how he views authority and peers, what interpersonal distortions exist, and how he behaves in relation to these.

3. **Ego Organization:** The nature and extent of his capacity for reality testing, the validity of his perceptions, the nature and degree of his capacity to organize, control, predict, follow through, etc. The extent of his recognition of the real-unreal, of the me-not me, and the quality of his defenses.

4. **Unconscious Conflicts:** A delineation of areas of unconscious conflict, of frustrated basic needs and drives, of conflicting impulses and needs and areas of functioning that generate anxiety, elicit defenses, etc.

5. **Communication:** The nature and manner of communicating feelings and thoughts. The nature and extent of verbal and nonverbal communication, his use of symbols, effectiveness of communication, areas of difficulty, etc.[16]

The technics derived from this theory rely heavily on an activities analysis process which allows the therapist to compare the patient's response to the activity—actions, manipulation of media, end-prod-

*Fidler, G. S., and Fidler, J. W.: Occupational Therapy—A Communication Process in Psychiatry. pp. 103-104, New York, Macmillan, 1963.

ucts, and verbal associations—to those of other individuals who are felt to represent a range of norms in response to these activities. Projective technics provide the basis for much of this evaluation process, but data is collected empirically on all aspects of communication and interaction, including relationship to the therapist, relationship to the group, and relationship to the activities as they are selected and handled.

Reilly's frame of reference is directed toward performance in socially determined roles, and she postulates that the achievement phenomenon which is basic to the occupational therapy process has a developmental core. She designates the developmental continuum of work and play as "occupational behavior," and proposes that the primary concern of the occupational therapist is the evaluation and strengthening of the individual's occupational role system.[23]

Moorhead, in developing this facet of the Reilly proposal, discusses the individual's self-concept as it is shaped through his life's experiences in attempting to master the occupational tasks and integrate those roles appropriate to his developmental level. Success leads to self-confidence and further expectations of success, while failure to accomplish gives rise to negative expectations and serves to make it progressively less likely that he will acquire the necessary adult occupational role.[30] Moorhead* offers the following variables to assist in identifying the degree to which appropriate occupational roles and functions have been mastered:

A. Autonomy and Independence
    a. Realistic perception of one's own assets and liabilities
    b. Ability to make stable decisions and implement them effectively
    c. Competence in management of time, space and personal needs
B. Implementation
    a. Motivation
    b. Orientation to:
        1. Own interests, choices and preferences
        2. Own requirements for rewards and satisfactions
        3. Range of possibilities for implementation, some appreciation for alternatives
    c. Job or position seeking ability, possession of training, education, etc.
C. Maintenance
    a. Adequate task/work behavior
        1. Continuity

* Moorhead, L.: The occupational history. Am. J. Occup. Therapy, 23:329-334, July/Aug., 1969.

  2. Stability
  3. Quality of performance
 b. Capacity to accept failure, perform under stress, and
    maintain flexibility
 c. Adequate interpersonal competence
 d. Balancing skills in work-play, activity-rest, etc.
 e. The capacity to handle conflicting role expectations

Moorhead notes that adequate test procedures have not yet been developed, but data collection in this frame of reference would appear to rely heavily on interview technic.

Mosey, whose adaptive skills are presented in Chart 5-3, creates an evaluation process which determines whether or not the individual has learned the various skill components. These findings are compared with information regarding the personal and social roles the individual is to assume, in order to determine if the acquired skills components are adequate. An *occupational therapy evaluation sheet* assists the therapist in checking off the level of sub-skills not yet acquired in each of the seven major skill components. [14]

This evaluation sheet is in interesting contrast to Moorhead's variables and the Fidlers' areas of function. Mosey presents patterns of dysfunctional or pathological behavior as the check points on her evaluation, while Moorhead and Fidler provide nearly neutral statements against which to measure the individual's performance. The implication is that the two latter procedures are more concerned with health and function, while Mosey's frame of reference is maladaptation and disability.

EVALUATION TECHNICS

The Interview

The methods used by the occupational therapist for evaluation purposes are dependent upon the kind of information it is necessary to obtain. No evaluation procedure is likely to be completed without including an interview. This may be the only means employed to collect the data, though that would be somewhat unusual for a profession specializing in human behavior and activities processes. There are many excellent references available on interview technics,[31,32] and only some fundamental principles relative to the use of the interview in occupational therapy will be offered here. It is a technic best learned through supervision, and role-playing may also provide some experience in integrating theories with on-the-spot learning.

It is essential to establish the purpose of the interview clearly in the minds of both the interviewer and the interviewee. While each has different roles and responsibilities, they are collaborating toward the same end. The interviewer bears the responsibility for establishing rapport, in order to insure that the interviewee can present himself and his problems as fully and clearly as possible. This also aids in the development of a sense of trust, which will assist them in establishing and working toward their objectives. The interview initiates the creation of a plan, which should become the automatic extension of the interview itself. The plan may actually establish long range goals, or it may be simply a design for a thorough evaluation process, based on the needs expressed through the interview.

There are several components to a good interview. Seldom are they in operation singly; usually they are coordinated into an operational whole; but they may be stated independently, even though the interviewer will need to develop skill in using them as a single fluid process. *Observation* is the first component. One observes what the patient does, hears what he says, and notes the behavioral or nonverbal communications which may or may not be so subtle. The careful observer will be able to restrict his own biases and attitudes and refrain from imposing his own expectations in such a way that the interviewee responds according to how he perceives what the interviewer wants to see or hear.

Listening is an equally important skill. The therapist must learn to listen actively and reflect genuine involvement with the concerns being expressed. This does not necessarily mean interjecting ideas or feelings, but making it clear that the other person's contributions to the interview are being fully shared. It is important to learn to listen before talking. The inexperienced interviewer may feel uncomfortable during silences, but the silence may contain messages of its own. Listen to the silences, and then proceed with the interview. *Active listening* also implies that the therapist is engaged in a directed interview process. As one listens actively, he anticipates the direction of the other's remarks and intervenes as necessary to insure that both are still working toward their established purpose.

The ability *to ask questions* which will evoke the necessary information is a third interviewing skill. Questions are the means by which the interviewee is guided through the maze of information he possesses, so that he shares those issues and concerns which are critical to this particular interview. Questions are not a legitimate means of satisfying the interviewer's curiosity about personal or embarrassing issues in the client's past. It may be necessary to phrase questions which do elicit such information, but it should be clear to both parties that this is within the requirements and purposes of the interview. Leading questions which stimulate the individual to talk freely about an idea or an incident are far more productive than questions which can be answered with one or two words. The questions must be posed so that the client is comfortable and feels that he has adequate time to present as much in response as he desires. And there are no magic questions! One cannot assume that a single imaginative inquiry will bring forth great insights for the individual. In fact, he should not be encouraged to reveal confidences until he is assured of your interest and support and ability to help him.

The interviewer may offer *comments* for purposes of encouraging the interviewee to elaborate on a point or to show that he understands what the other person is trying to say. The interview should not be considered an equal-opportunity kind of dialogue, however. The interviewer is responsible for obtaining a body of information which he will then use for a specific professional purpose; his ideas and opinions are irrelevant during the interview itself. The interviewee is responsible for clarifying his feelings and sharing as much data as he can, so that the purposes of the interview may be accomplished. He therefore should be the major contributor to the content of the interview guided by the therapist who is more knowledgeable about how to elicit the necessary information.

It is important that the interviewer *speak the language of the client.* Obviously, one must retain most of his usual style of speech or he will sound condescending. On the other hand, it would not be useful to impress upon the client the sophistication with which one customarily handles the subject at hand! The therapist who needs to rely on a battery of specialized jargon in order to make clear the distinction between himself and those who come to him for help demonstrates a sense of insecurity which is readily recognized. The professional interviewer speaks straightforwardly and clearly, modifying his usual style of conversation only when it becomes evident that the other person has not understood. A therapist takes into consideration also: Is the nature of the communications barrier which may be present an intellectual or educational impairment? A perceptual deficit? A lack of sophistication? A state of depression or drug-induced slowness? Or is it a preoccupation and a state of anxiety which misrepresents the individual's actual potential?

There is also the question of when and *how to answer personal questions.* Personal questions may be posed by the interviewee for several reasons, and the interviewer should listen carefully to ascertain the objective of the question. He may simply believe that he should show some interest in the interviewer, in order to be polite. He may be curious to know something more specific about the individual he is expected to trust. He may ask personal questions as a hostile defense when the interviewer has intruded too quickly. Or he may be interested in showing that he is ready to work closely (i.e., personally) with the interviewer.

Finally, the personal question may also be an indirect effort to introduce a topic about which the individual is somewhat reluctant to talk. If the interviewer can discuss such an embarrassing issue, then perhaps it will be all right to present one's own concerns about it. Only careful listening will assist the therapist in "hearing" this message. Before redirecting the interview toward its purpose, the interviewer should reply with a brief, honest statement in answer to the question.

CHART 5-4   BOSTON STATE HOSPITAL HOME TREATMENT SERVICE OCCUPATIONAL THERAPY EVALUATION

Name_____ #_____ Age_____ Date_____ Staff_____

Reason for Evaluation:

Impression of the Visit: (description of the patient and surroundings)

Educational Experience: (level attained, majors, interests, extracurricular activities, adjustment, relationships developed)

Work Experiences: (chronological list of jobs and dates, type of work, interest in jobs, why changes in positions)

Military History: (branch, dates, rank, duties, station, discharge, adjustment)

Avocational Interests: (social activities, hobbies, leisure time, friends, include past and present, why a change)

Activities of Daily Living: (what is a typical day, what responsibilities, duties, self-care, how has this recently changed?)

Other Information: (pertinent material related by the individual not applicable to other areas)

Implications: (based on information obtained, assess the following)
    Motivation: for activity, socialization, work

    Relationships: family, peers, social and business acquaintances, therapist

    Ego Functioning: strengths and weaknesses as seen through performance

    Areas of Conflicts: indicated by inability or breakdown of performance

    Communication: manner, effectiveness

Assessment of Potential: (what assets, what can we expect, what are the patient's expectations?)

Summary of Impressions and Functioning:

Recommendations:

Treatment Goals:

Treatment Program:

The student is urged to study the book[32] from which these principles are derived and to explore in detail that author's examples of the interview process.

An interview may be structured around an interview schedule which provides a series of topical guidelines to insure that the necessary information is obtained. Therapists working in programs which have sub-specialty services may devise a series of interview schedules and select the one related to the program for which the client is assumed to be ready. For example, Chart 5–4 presents the interview schedule developed by Watanabe for use in a home treatment service. It assists

CHART 5–5   ACTIVITY CONFIGURATION

Weekly Schedule of:_____   Therapist:_____
                          name

Typical week at home:_____   in hospital:_____   in day care:_____

Part I

Directions: List in detail *all* activities which are a part of your day.

Morning	Mon.	Tues.	Wed.	Thurs.	Fri.	Sat.	Sun.
7:00– 9:00							
9:00–11:00							
11:00– 1:00							
Afternoon							
1:00– 3:00							
3:00– 5:00							
5:00– 7:00							
Evening							
7:00– 9:00							
9:00–11:00							

CHART 5-5 (Continued)

Part II

Directions: List each activity (once) that you included in Part I. Use as many sheets as necessary. Rate all activities according to the rating scale attached.

	Function	Autonomy		Adequacy
List Activities	A	B_1	B_2	C

Rating Scale

A. Function
  1. Work
  2. Chore
  3. Education
  4. Skill practice
  5. Exercise
  6. Recreation
  7. Social activity
  8. Rest
  9. Therapy
 10. Your own
     designations

B_1. Autonomy
  1. Have to do it
  2. Want to do it
  3. Both

B_2. Autonomy
  1. IG—I want to do this and I think
     this is good
  2. IN—I want to do this and I think
     this is not good
  3. OG—Others make me do this and
     I'm glad they do
  4. ON—Others make me do this and
     I wish they didn't

C. Adequacy
  1. I do this very well
  2. I do this well enough
  3. I don't do this well enough

the therapist in collecting information about the client, the family, and the home, and provides a system of recording the facts and impressions, as well as indicating the implications for future service. Thus both the process of evaluation and the interpretation of the results are recorded on a single useful form.

Another interview style requires that the individual write certain information in response to an organized structure provided by the interviewer. Together they explore and the client elaborates upon those areas which the interviewer feels he must know more about. The "Activity Configuration" presented in Chart 5-5 is an interview method created specifically for occupational therapy.[33] Because the activity configuration records the patient's perception of what his day is like, it provides a glimpse into the world to which the patient is responding. In addition to the specific activities he engages in—work, play, self-care, service functions—it permits him to relate the amount of responsibility he assumes for his own life style, and the nature of his self-concept. For a theoretical frame of reference which appears to support this technic, see Watanabe's "Four Concepts Basic to the Occupational Therapy Process."[26]

The technics of interviewing, then, may be either the primary method of evaluation or a supplementary technic. Several additional brief examples will suffice.

The Play History. For a number of years, occupational therapists working in pediatrics have used the Gesell Developmental Schedules to determine the level of developmental function of patients referred for recreation or treatment.[34] The possibility always exists that the hospitalized child will suffer ill-effects from the traumatism of illness, hospital or surgical procedures, or separation from home and family. Similarly, the child living in a disturbed family or the child who suffers serious cultural deprivation may have his development interrupted in ways which result in poor mental health. For this reason, several evaluation procedures are reviewed which might be appropriate for use in occupational therapy or community programs serving children.

Two doing-oriented interviews which are especially suitable for an occupational therapy evaluation are the Gesell,[35] mentioned above, and the Denver Developmental Screening Test.[36] Each of these provides a series of rating scales appropriate from birth through approximately six years. They list specific activities which provide an opportunity to assess the child's gross and fine motor skills, language and social development, adaptive skills, and (DDST only) some fundamental cognitive-perceptual-motor areas of development. Since the activities upon which the scales are based are typical of the interests and everyday experiences of the child, he is seen in a setting which resembles the environment and the challenges which are natural to him. In addition, the informality of the DDST allows the mother to be present and to comment upon how differently the child may be performing for the examiner. Interview skills, appropriate to elicit additional information from the mother, are therefore required.

Takata has proposed a play questionnaire which may serve as an interview schedule. It could be used with either of the two rating scales just described or with an activities-of-daily-living inventory and other determinants of school progress or neuromuscular development.

The open-ended questionnaire was developed for use either in the home or in a clinical setting. It proposes six areas to be explored in order to evaluate the play behavior of the child: (1) availability of appropriate toys; (2) play space; (3) play ideals and play fellows; (4) nature of the child's play with toys and other non-toy objects, such as animals; (5) nature of the child's play with human beings; and (6) quantity of play.[37] The first part of the questionnaire is designed to elicit information regarding the nature and quality of the child's play, such as how, where and with whom he plays. The second part is concerned with quantitative play, the frequency of play, and the time allotted (or permitted) for play. The child's daily activity schedule is the focus for this part.

Such an evaluation process would permit the development of a play profile, against which to measure change through a course of pre-scribed activities. These might be carried out as treatment by the occupational therapist through a program of therapeutic management in the school, or in the home, where the primary emphasis was directed toward evoking change in the parents and the family constellation.

The Occupational History. At the other end of the developmental scale, Moorhead has proposed "The Occupational History" as the baseline for treatment planning for the adult.[30] Earlier, in the section on "What Does the Occupational Therapist Evaluate?", the critical variables to occupational function as derived from Moorhead's proposal were presented. The means of accumulating this data is an interview technic described as the data selection method. This form of history-taking relies on a semi-structured procedure wherein specific questions are asked and the interviewer persists in rephrasing and probing until the necessary information can be brought forth. Interview skill is, therefore, a requisite to successful use of this technic. Many persons who have been identified as patients are, in fact, occupational misfits — persons who are not prepared to assume occupational roles and functions which are required by and acceptable to their communities. This evaluation procedure is proposed, then, as being particularly valuable with dropouts, the chronically unemployed, long-term hospitalized patients, and senior citizens who deteriorate because of lack of purposeful involvement.

Activities as Evaluation Procedures

A profession must devise the procedures which are necessary to establish and support its basic tenets. The occupational therapy process stimulates interaction between selected persons, certain activities procedures, and non-human objects. Occupational therapy presupposes that corrective change can be brought about through these directed experiences, and it would appear that essentially the same procedures could be used to determine the individual's current level of functioning and to design the required therapeutic program.

The challenge has long been raised that the evaluation process must determine what is to be the entry point on the continuum of therapeutic activities. It is of more than historical interest that a very early formulation is included here. This outline describing a comprehensive evalu-

CHART 5–6   FUNCTIONS OF OCCUPATIONAL THERAPY

A. Preliminary therapeutics
   Object: To establish confidence of patient in hospital and in department
   Method: (1) From prescription card obtain former occupation
           (2) From prescription card determine limits imposed by psychosis
           (3) Relate interim therapy to known work patterns
           (4) Maintain a monotony of tempo
           (5) Maintain narrowness of range within perceptive capacity and limits of execution
           (6) Use clear cut figure against neutral background
           (7) Use few and sharply differentiated colors
B. Diagnostic or occupational survey
   Object: (1) To determine basic functional capacities
            (2) To determine level of total functional capacities
   Method: (1) History of occupation as:
               a. Child
               b. Youth showing (a) all occupations
               c. Adult   (b) degree of accomplishment
                                 (c) interest displayed
                                 (d) satisfaction and dissatisfaction
                                     in results
                                 (e) subjective evaluation of economic
                                     capacity
                                 (f) determine norms of individual
                                 (g) determine norms of individual training
                                     and environment
           (2) Testing of function (in regard to the individual determine
               for him)
               a. Normal patterns used in personal behavior and residual
                  level
               b. Normal patterns used in economic occupation and residual
                  level
               c. Normal patterns and residual level available for use in
                  hobbies
               d. Patterns available in latent talents and their availability for
                  compensatory training
           (3) Other interests and ambitions
               Where possible, have patient outline these and, if possible,
               test for basic and residual level patterns
           (4) Testing recreational and amusement levels (to be tested indi-
               vidually in small groups non-competitively and in large
               groups competitively)
               a. Limits of motorial and emotional capacity in relation to
                  physical exercises expressed as satisfaction or dissatis-
                  faction to different rhythms
               b. Response to music of varying rhythm
                  1. Hearing
                  2. Singing
                  3. Responding motorially: (a) Dancing
                                             (b) Marching
                                             (c) Games

CHART 5-6 (Continued)

C. Advanced therapeutics
    Object: From information in A and B, basic and residual levels of percep-
           tion, analysis, synthesis and adaptation have been determined. It
           is now necessary to use these available patterns in retraining in
           occupation and in evaluating patient-occupational-environmental
           relationship
    Method: Progressive alteration within known capacities
         (1) Variation in tempo of work, recreation, etc.
         (2) Variation in familiarity of motor patterns
         (3) Variation of figure-ground relationship. This also to include
             training of patient in recognition of his own altering rela-
             tionship. Figure-ground to become more difficult of contrast
             so that training in perception and analysis are obtained
         (4) Progressive variations in colors, gradually proceeding to many
             colors merging into ground-figure combination

From Lang, H. B.: Additional functional values in occupational therapy. Occupational Therapy and Rehabilitation, 17:317, 1938.

---

ation process was presented by Dr. H. Beckett Lang[9] in a paper entitled, "Additional Functional Values in Occupational Therapy," read at the Thirteenth Annual Institute of Chief Occupational Therapists, New York State Department of Mental Hygiene, May 2–5, 1938. Dr. Lang was concerned about the lack of structured, directed, diagnostic processes within occupational therapy and felt that the contributions of the profession would be greatly magnified if they were based on a systematic evaluation procedure. He outlined that procedure as shown in Chart 5–6. Therapists who study Dr. Lang's proposal carefully will recognize a number of familiar concepts which appeared throughout the section on the theoretical basis for occupational therapy. Much of what he proposed seems to be closely related to both the current emphasis on social psychiatry and the field of behavior therapy.

Free Choice. Perhaps the least sophisticated of the activities-based evaluation technics is the method of free choice.[38] Patients who are reasonably well integrated and capable of making choices, for example, may be allowed to select from a variety of controlled activities experiences in an informal setting. This method appears to be the least similar to a test procedure and has the advantage of giving some indication as to what — if anything — the individual would choose to do in his leisure time and how he perceives himself in the world of productive activity.

Free choice does not, however, imply lack of control. The activities available shall have been carefully selected by the therapist to represent a variety of action experiences; interpersonal demands ranging from isolation through group participation; activities which range from requiring nearly constant individual direction by the therapist to almost none at all; work roles representing specific groups of function and responsibility, and so forth. The range is endless, but each activity offered must have been carefully and thoroughly analyzed, and a means devised for evaluating the patient so that his choice and the qualities displayed through his work may be compared to some standardized norm.

This method would be particularly valuable in a community mental health program or as part of a pre-discharge evaluation before the patient leaves a hospital or day care center. It might be used as an initial evaluation procedure if the person in question is capable of making independent choices and is reasonably well integrated.

Projective Technics

In the late 1950's, references began appearing which challenged the profession of occupational therapy to establish a method of projective testing which would utilize the raw materials of creative activity.[22,39] Therapists with adequate knowledge of psychodynamic and projective theory, who worked in centers where such concepts were valued, began to explore the media from this perspective. The Azimas proposed the triad of pencil drawings, finger paints and ceramic clay. This became the fundamental grouping of media, though others elaborated on this combination in various ways.[16,40,41] While relative agreement prevailed as to *what* could be evaluated in this manner, it became obvious that the development of a set of standards through which the projections could be rated was far more difficult. Several so-called rating scales now exist, but none of them are, in fact, more than lists of things which may be *observed* and then *interpreted* (not rated on a scale) through the examiner's clinical judgment.

The material obtained through such procedures has been found to be extremely valuable for diagnostic purposes, and for use in planning and developing treatment programs in occupational therapy. Similarly, it is useful in detecting change in psychodynamic patterns. It is desirable that work proceed in this area, so that it may be determined how — and if — the occupational therapist can provide standardized ratings of the objects and actions observed through the projective test battery.

Principles

While there are elaborate bibliographies on the theory of projective testing,[42,43,44,45,46] only a few principles are presented here in order to focus attention on those aspects of the occupational therapy process which relate to this subject. *An individual's response to any stimulation is determined and predictable; it is not accidental.* It is determined both by present conditions and by past experiences. It is predictable in terms of his life style, or typical patterns of behavior. Since any response is limited by those past experiences in failure and success which have produced the individual's present-day self-concept, no response is accidental. It is the result of an image which can only respond in already established patterns. Unless the individual becomes overwhelmed by pressures so great as to be disorganizing, he cannot respond in a manner which is ego-alien; that is, his response must be congruent with his image of himself.

When unstructured or semi-structured materials are presented (drawing, painting, ceramics, carving), the response will be a spontaneous re-creation of the individual's life style and/or self-image. The response will be personalized in terms of the unique life experiences of the individual. It is difficult to hide things or to falsify the response, since there is no "right" or "wrong" answer to be given. The answer can be only a reflection of the sum total of the individual's experience.

An individual's basic personality structure finds expression in the private world of his creations. His responses to the unstructured media are thus consistent in quality and content, relative to the nature of the stimuli offered. The response to the challenge presented by the media is also typical of the individual's behavior in any setting, given similar stimuli. And his responses represent a clear statement of his feelings about himself in the immediate situation.

Examples

A few examples follow to illustrate how one projects himself, his abilities, thoughts, feelings and self-concept through the occupational therapy media.

The ability to deal with spatial relationships may be demonstrated through games and dance, drama, design, photography and chess. The use of the objects and their relative positions as they are spaced give clues as to the individual's concept of his size and importance, his mobility and stability. The placement of the objects also indicates how, or if, he uses structure in order to provide security and familiarity. Some cognitive-perceptual-motor functions may also be observed: Does he see the object as it is? Does he recognize it? Can he define its function? Can he use it appropriately?

The ability to organize fragments into a whole is another element of function which may be assessed through the projective media. Mosaic tiles, jewelry making, cooking and assembly line work provide examples of this function. One may view the ability to cope with multiple stimuli and note the degree, if any, to which this begins to be an overwhelming experience. Similar kinds of cognitive-perceptual-motor functions may be viewed, though it would be necessary to distinguish between the psychological and neurophysiological etiology of such dysfunction. Projected also may be the degree of one's ability to conceive of himself as a whole, not having to divide himself (behave in a fragmented way) in order to relate to or to control the several parts.

The ability to reduce a whole destructively, in order to create a new whole, is a third function which may be studied through projection. The use of a wood or metal lathe, the process of stone or wood sculpture, bookbinding, or cutting out a sewing pattern are examples of such activities. The individual can demonstrate the degree to which he is able to see aggression as a constructive force. The ability to conceptualize an invisible end product may also be noted. One's fear of his own aggressiveness as being potentially uncontrollable may interfere with the accomplishment of such tasks.

The fourth example is the direct opposite of the one preceding: *the ability to produce something out of nothing*. Clay, fingerpaints, and spontaneous dramatics offer such an experience. Such projections give an indication of the ability to set one's own limits regarding the work, the ability to conceptualize and be assured that there is a controllable end product within an amorphous shape, and the ability to engage with the unknown, which also demonstrates the defenses called into action in order to master such a situation.

The end result of a comprehensive evaluation procedure is the production of the individual's self-image, represented through the objects and actions involved. The following assumptions are made, based upon projective theory, assumed on empirical evidence to be significant for the occupational therapy process:

1. The individual's handling of and response to the inanimate objects is roughly analogous to the way he relates to and "handles" other people. The characteristics represented through some media — strength, pliability, resistiveness, organization — have their equivalents in human personality structure. The response to the characteristic is assumed to be similar, whether it is encountered in a human or an inanimate object.

2. The symbolic representation of self, as presented through the accomplished tasks, may be considered as a self-portrait — a view of the individual as he really sees himself. It may be refined, crude, sloppy, delicate, or unfinished; it may be in conflict with two or more opposing parts. It is the individual's projection of himself as he assumes others also see him.

3. The processes involved in completing the task, as well as the objects themselves, may also be viewed as a presentation of self in relation to others. Indicated here may be such things as his ability to be responsible for his own behavior, the degree of independence he is comfortable in displaying, and his internalized self-control versus his need to rely on externally derived controls. Freedom to experiment with feelings toward others and the ability to become involved in actions and relationships may also be assessed.

Some Guidelines

Several guidelines and precautions should be noted. Each of us has a personal, inner world which overlaps somewhat with that which most people identify as "reality." Projective technics demonstrate the uniqueness of the individual, separating his personal inner fantasies from the public reality. The exposure of thoughts and feelings usually felt to be too personal to be shared, and hence either repressed or selectively kept secret, is not to be considered lightly. The professional responsibility for maintaining confidentiality must accompany any interview or evaluation procedure.

One safeguard occurs in the use of projective tests, and the beginning therapist is cautioned against its exploitation. What one unconsciously allows to be projected may be interpreted only theoretically by the evaluator. No communication between two human beings is worthwhile unless it can be consensually validated. Therefore, only insofar as the individual is able to share his association to the tasks and objects with the evaluator, can the evaluator be certain that his interpretation of the data is accurate. It must be remembered that the fantasies of the client are the ones which are important, not those of the therapist! The technics of observing and recording accurately, specifically and objectively what is done in the activities process must be carefully separated from the technic of interpretation, which will be discussed under "Developing a Plan."

One further caution. The interpretation of data during the evaluation process is strictly contraindicated and inappropriate. When, during the course of therapy, the individual is able to deal with these materials, that readiness will be indicated. Even then, interpretations of functional processes (i.e., behavioral representations of thoughts and feelings) are usually the medium of confrontation, not the psychological raw material itself.

DEVELOPING A PLAN

Results of the Evaluation

The evaluation process may have included formal and informal observations, tests and other procedures. The findings must be carefully assembled, taking care to separate the objective data from the subjective data, and to note the absence of information in areas which still need to be explored. It may be possible to use information obtained from the nurse, family, social worker, employer or school teacher to complete the data, or it may be necessary to do further evaluations through occupational therapy media.

When the findings have been clearly recorded and studied they may be interpreted. The accuracy of the interpretation depends upon the accuracy of the data as recorded, as well as its completeness, the experience and knowledge of the evaluator, the appropriateness of the tools he used for the evaluation in light of his experience and ability, and upon his skill in collaborating with others in verifying his data. Interpretations are, of course, the impressions and assumptions of the evaluator, and, therefore, must be subjected to a process of validation as the program plan unfolds. The validation should be twofold; the interpretations should be based as much as possible on standardized norms and the patient himself should be asked to assist in the consensual validation of his experiences.

Each of the evaluation procedures described above results in a composite picture of the individual, usually stated in terms of functional capacities. To some extent, the technics used in the evaluation process were determined by the overt needs which were apparent as the individual presented himself to the therapist. In that way certain of the findings may have been predetermined, and the profile drawn from the total evaluation may be predisposed toward a plan of a certain nature. So long as this was done deliberately and not as an oversight, it is perfectly acceptable.

Each therapist develops his own method of establishing a plan for change. The following principles are suggested:

1. That an evaluation procedure serve as the basis for the plan.
2. That the findings of the evaluation be clearly and objectively recorded.
3. That these findings be verified as fully as possible.
4. That the total results of the evaluation be interpreted.
5. That a plan be made jointly between client and therapist, a plan which is consonant with the objectives of any other person or persons sharing the responsibility for the client's program.
6. That the plan be regularly reviewed and modified in light of accomplishments or new evidence derived through the occupational therapy process.

Objectives

The objectives toward which patient and therapist are working must be clearly established in the minds of both. They must also be shared with other persons who are either responsible for a portion of the patient's program or who, in some fashion, can influence the course of action. In this latter group are parents, spouses, peer groups, teachers, siblings and employers, for they represent the environmental influences which have contributed to the patient's difficulties. Unless they are adequately informed about the objectives toward which the patient is working, and assisted in understanding and accepting the necessary changes in his life style, they will continue to perpetuate many of the difficulties which brought the patient into therapy. Time is well spent, therefore, in collaborating with these persons to the end that they are in support of the overall objectives.

It may, however, be impossible for these people to accept the objectives established for the patient. Theories of social psychiatry suggest that the patient is often the victim of a way of life — the "weakest" link in the chain. He serves an important function for the group by being sick. So long as he remains sick, the other members of the group need not change their behaviors and can avoid looking at their relationships to each other. Change in the patient's behavior (i.e., improvement through therapy) upsets the apple cart. Anxiety is aroused in the other persons who make up the constellation, and they attempt to restructure the status quo ante. In a "sick" family constellation or group, some one person must be identified as sicker than the others, if the remaining members are to retain their independent abilities to function. Change threatens their security, and change will, therefore, be resisted. It is important to assess the significant groups with which the patient is affiliated, so that the objectives for change may be more realistically established.

A second consideration is the length of time required to attain certain objectives. Long-range objectives may provide a frame of reference, as they indicate the apparent potential for adaptation and improved function. But they may be so unattainable in the patient's eyes that they are worse than useless; they simply force him to recognize how far he is expected to go. And the way may appear to him to be too long and hazardous. Such global objectives, also, may reflect the therapist's grandiosity, his need to work miracles, or to succeed in "curing" this patient where others have failed. Should the patient identify such an attitude in the therapist (and they almost always do!), the ensuing power struggle leads only to defeat and disappointment for both parties.

Therefore, some concrete, realistic and quickly obtainable goals must be established as the plan is initiated. The therapist should explore with the patient what he *most* wants to change about his life and what things are most troublesome for him. Then, he should determine what skills the patient believes are his strongest, which behaviors he is proudest of, and which of these he believes could be applied toward effecting the desired change. This kind of planning enlists the patient as a positive force in bringing about gratifying change in his condition. The choice of the actual procedures and activities is still the responsibility of the therapist, but the objectives have been established through mutual agreement, and, therefore, the patient's self-respect has already received an important boost.

Regular review of the results of the evaluation and the changes accomplished through the immediate objectives should help to keep the working plan current. The potential for change, as established through the evaluation process and as stated in the long range objectives, can be more effectively accomplished through short-term, more specific goals, developed and shared by patient and therapist.

A Plan for What: Treatment or Learning?

Traditionally, the persons with whom occupational therapists work have been identified as patients. A patient usually is defined as someone in need of treatment, since the term "patient" implies illness. Other professional groups have called the persons with whom they work "clients." This term usually refers to someone who seeks a service, but not a medical service. Persons being seen by occupational therapists today fall into both categories. They include patients in institutions, psychiatric or medically-oriented day care or community programs, school children with learning problems, social misfits, troubled parents, displaced and unwanted oldsters. While these people may also have medical problems, their primary reason for being seen by the occupational therapist lies in the realm of interpersonal or social function. The term "mental health" may be used to describe the needs of either the psychiatrically ill patient or the social misfit. This chapter was named accordingly, as it attempts to explore the ways in which occupational therapists can meet the mental health needs of a variety of persons.

Whether patient or client, the occupational therapist must set some objectives for a course of action which they will share. Indeed, it has been suggested by several authors that perhaps the psychiatric patient needs re-education rather than treatment. The results of the evaluation process indicate *needs*, areas of function which are inadequate or inappropriate. Is occupational therapy to provide an attack on the etiological processes which led to the present state of function? And if so, is that treatment? Or does occupational therapy engage the individual in a program of problem-solving, of developing (learning) skills and attitudes which will enable him to function more effectively, and, thereby modify the image of himself as being an inadequate, helpless patient?

The answer to the first question cannot be given unequivocally. There is not yet enough data on the effects of the occupational therapy process. While that question must be answered through clinical studies and research as quickly as possible, the current lack of an answer does not prevent the second question from being answered with an emphatic "yes." Occupational therapy effects change through learning, by allowing the individual to see the consequences of his actions and by permitting him to establish patterns of behavior which are both satisfying and congruent with his wish to be a productive member of society. He *learns*, in other words, to behave in ways which are basically gratifying to his needs, and he integrates attitudes and patterns of behavior which are socially acceptable to the community in which he must reside.

In one of his last papers, Franz Alexander explored the dynamics of psychotherapy in light of learning theory.[47] He stated that since a patient's decision to seek psychotherapy was based on difficulty in dealing with critical issues confronting him daily, it seemed inappropriate that the therapist concentrate unduly on early etiological factors. Exploration of the past was valuable insofar as it provided information which could be useful in changing the ideas and behaviors which were troublesome to the patient. "To overcome repressions and thus be able to recall the past is one thing: to learn from it and be able to act on the new knowledge, another."[48] To Alexander, therapy was a process of relearning which included cognitive elements; it also included the learning which took place from the actual interpersonal experiences of therapy. He described emotional insight as the result of learning through therapy, indicating that *emotional* referred to the interpersonal experiences, and that *insight* indicated the cognitive element of the learning.

Other authors have also related therapy to learning. Redlich and Freedman point out that psychotherapeutic technics should be directed toward assisting the patient to change undesirable habits and to replace them with learned attitudes and behaviors which are more effective in accomplishing his everyday tasks. Viewed in this way, psychotherapy must be considered to be a learning process, but the authors differentiate psychotherapeutic learning from most educational experiences in the following way:

> "The nature of the behavior disorders that require such intervention is so severe that society usually grants the recipient a sick role; the psychological healer has the special status of a therapist; the subject matter for the patient's learning is the self, a person's private and basic patterns of response. In view of the latter consideration the model of parental function in fostering growth and development seems the educational mode most closely related to therapy.[49]*

Shimota has suggested that occupational therapists consider themselves as teachers, who enable others to acquire skill or knowledge about living.[50]

In challenging the somewhat symbiotic relationship between oc-

* Redlich, F.C., and Freedman, D.X.: The Theory and Practice of Psychiatry. New York, Basic Books, 1966.

cupational therapy and medicine, Bockoven suggests that the generic function of the occupational therapist belongs to the educational and economic life of the community.[51] It arises out of the interest in and respect for the integrity of the individual as he creates a social and economic role for himself. It would follow, therefore, that the occupational therapist should be involved in a teaching and learning transaction which permits the individual to explore those problems which prevent him from having a satisfying and productive socioeconomic role. Shannon has said: "The activities provided by occupational therapy must approximate life's activities in type and function, to be significantly useful in the restoration process."[52]

In view of the above, and in light of the fact that the practice of occupational therapy is currently expanding to include more non-medically oriented problems, it becomes difficult to describe the primary functions of the therapist solely in terms of a treatment process. It is a convenient and familiar term, however, and at times, obviously, the appropriate one. But for purposes of a better understanding of what transpires between therapist and patient or client, let us look to the area of ego psychology and study briefly the relationship between learning and ego functions. It is in this realm that occupational therapy may be most effective when the mental health needs of the individual have been identified as the primary concern of the therapist.

Learning and Ego Functions

There are innumerable references which identify ego functions. One* which is primarily concerned with brief psychotherapy and quick return of the patient to his role in the community lists the following ego functions which must be assessed in order to determine the primary targets of psychotherapy:

> *Adaptation to reality* — best viewed as adaptation to the cultural matrix, the appropriateness of one's role-playing.
>
> *Reality testing* — an integral part of role-playing, involving perceptions and judgment, the primary function being the differentiation of external (objective) data from internal (subjective) determinants.
>
> *Sense of reality* — the differentiation of self from the rest of the world of objects, places and time. When the function is strong there is an absence of conscious awareness of self.
>
> *Drive control* — the regulation of instinctual drives. Genetic endowments may vary here, as environmental factors also may influence the intensity of the drive. The strength of the superego affects drive intensity also, as the drives run counter to superego demands.
>
> *Object relations* — including both the quality and intensity of one's relationship with people. Manifest aspects of such relationships

---

* Small, L.: The Briefer Psychotherapies. New York, Brunner/Mazel, 1971.

should be supplemented by projective productions of the patient, his dreams and fantasies.

Thought process — dependent upon the maturation of an infant's perceptual ability, progressing from initial differences to increasing clarity and differentiation in all sensory modalities.

Defensive functions — the personality's barriers against both internal and external stimuli of threatening intensity or meaning. Repression was the first defense identified; many others have since been elaborated.

Autonomous functions — those activities (perception, intention, language, productivity, motor development) assumed to be independent of conflict. Closer examination finds that they are indeed likely to be involved, perhaps in a secondary way. They are, of course, susceptible to developmental deprivation and to organic damage.

The synthetic function — which tends to overlap most with the other functions since it involves the ego's ability to form *Gestalten*, to maintain the necessary functions of life, of adaptation.[53]

An example may demonstrate how learning can effect ego functioning. In the area of *drive control,* the individual needs practice in recognizing the effects of his inadequately controlled impulses. Learning sequences can be provided so that the individual moves slowly through this process:

a. Consciously identifying the problem, the urge, or the desire in such a way that he becomes more fully aware of what it is he really wants.

b. Weighing the consequences of each of the various alternatives for attaining the desired object or engaging in the desired behaviors.

c. Selecting one of the alternatives and implementing it in such a way that the actual consequences can be experienced.

d. Reviewing the outcome of this particular course of behavior in terms of the positive and negative forces which interacted to produce the end result.

e. Reappraising the desired goal in light of the social and environmental pressures and standards, as well as his own skills for handling a course of action.

f. Selecting a more manageable or realistic (less self-defeating) alternative and initiating the learning sequence again.

Repeated practice in this kind of problem-solving is effective through occupational therapy because of the immediate concrete evidence of the consequences of behavior. Both the therapist and the activities process serve to reinforce the learning through the consistent demonstration of how a particular behavior serves to be disappointing, degrading, or otherwise socially disapproved. Improved choices of behavior, appropriately related to attaining a clearly identified goal, may be rewarded through praise. But more important is the individual's concrete success, attained through his own resources: this is a positive reinforcer for behavioral change.

Becker states that "normal" must be considered to mean "not stupid"; normal is not relative to illness in the sense of mental health or mental function.[54] The normal individual is a creative person who is able to exercise maximum control over his choice of behaviors and responses. Relying heavily on John Dewey's educational theory, Becker points out that human need is really the need for the possibility of choice. The individual who is blocked, who cannot move ahead because he does not recognize the alternatives which lie before him, is one who suffers restriction of his sense of self-esteem, and of the growth and expansion of his other ego functions. In Becker's view, learning consists of exploring the widest possible range of human and nonhuman objects, in order to arrive at a formula for behavior which provides maximum security and satisfaction while the individual simultaneously develops the maximum range of choices for human interaction. The person who is in need of psychiatric help is thus in need of a learning experience, for he is "stupid" in the realm of human behavior. He has failed to develop the necessary skills for assessing the alternatives for action in a given situation, and he is perpetually confronted with overwhelming problems for which he has no solution. Withdrawal, in one of the several symptomatic ways so familiar in psychiatry, becomes his only alternative. Relearning, or therapy directed toward exploration of alternatives, becomes the method of choice for allowing him to re-engage satisfactorily with his society.

White[55] has developed the thesis that behavior may be motivated by energies which are independent of instinctual drives and are inherent in the ego structure. These energies must be utilized solely in the satisfaction of all drives, but at other times they are operant solely in regard to their own effects. His name for these energies is "effectance." Motivation, in the psychoanalytic frame of reference, has always been considered to be the result of the reduction of drives. White suggests instead that the dynamics of effectance are in response to the exploratory opportunities which the individual recognizes in his immediate situation. The manipulation of one's environment is inherently satisfying, and the tendency to explore and to try out means of making an impact on the environment, as well as on other human beings, is natural and spontaneous—a response not dependent upon the need for drive reduction.

The result of having caused an effect on the environment is that the individual experiences a "feeling of efficacy." White proposes that it is a primitive, biological endowment, as fundamental as the satisfactions that are gained through feeding or sexual activity, though not nearly as intense. Productive or playful activity may be inherently satisfying in itself, serving no other purpose than to cause a feeling of efficacy. Activity for its own sake is not insignificant; it is an important aspect of the adaptive process, and an essential core in the development of personality. Exploratory and playful activity done for its own sake reveals its significance for adaptation and survival, when we appreciate that it is through action and the consequences of action that we learn to become effective in dealing with our surroundings.

White also introduces two other terms, *competence* and *a sense of competence*. Competence describes the ability of the individual to interact effectively with his environment. It is the cumulative result of his past experiences with the human and nonhuman environment, irrespective of the ways in which those interactions had been motivated. The sense of competence describes one's subjective impression of his interaction with his environment. It does not always reflect accurately what others judge to be his level of competency. It is possible that in an instance where the individual felt it to be of primary importance that he succeed, the slightest indication that he was not 100 per cent successful leaves him with a feeling of incompetence, whereas in the eyes of those who observed his performance, it was carried out exceptionally well. The term *feeling of efficacy* describes the experience of each individual transaction with the environment, while the *sense of competence* is reserved for the accumulated, organized sequences which are the result of one's life-style.

White feels that one's expectations of the environment are closely determined by what kind of changes he is able to effect, and the sense of competence he has when he faces a new challenge in the outer world. One must be able to predict the consequences of his behavior, and the effects it will have upon others, if he is to venture forth into the outer world with any degree of self-assurance. Each individual has need for both self-esteem and self-love. White feels that the psychoanalytic theory has failed to differentiate adequately between these two. Self-esteem has more to do with respect than with love, and respect for one's self is acquired through successful mastery of effective skills. One's sense of competence; that is, his feeling about and accurate appraisal of what he can and cannot do to effect change, determines his level of self-esteem. White says, the "whole understanding of schizophrenia ... turns on recognizing the pathologically low sense of interpersonal confidence."[56]

The conclusions we might draw from the foregoing review of psychiatric theory provide direction for a discussion of the treatment or "change functions" of the occupational therapist. First, we have questioned whether or not therapy is treatment, or learning and relearning. Second, we have identified the major functions of the ego which apparently can be influenced through learning experiences. Third, we have explored Becker's concept of the relationship between failure to learn to recognize alternatives and to develop adequate responses to those alternatives, and his implication that these failures lead to what he calls "stupidity"; further, his accusation that it is society's failure to provide appropriate learning about objects that results in the personal failure which previously has been called mental illness. And fourth, we have looked at White's theory on effectance and competence as two major sources of energy which mediate a number of the functions of the ego. The relationship between one's sense of self-esteem and his ability to effect the desired change in his surroundings would seem to be a natural core for the occupational therapy process.

The Occupational Therapy Plan

The theoretical concepts reviewed above may be used to develop a description of occupational therapy functions. A problem of semantics does exist, and should be clearly recognized as such. For example, there is a great deal of similarity between the foregoing discussion of learning and the following outline for a treatment program, developed by Fidler and Fidler:*

1. What is the nature of the patient's pathology? What are the difficulties in thinking, perceiving and functioning? What unconscious needs and conflicts seem to be causing problems?
2. Which problems are to be of primary concern at this time?
3. Is the treatment process to be oriented toward uncovering, support, or repression?
4. What are the primary problems in the area of interpersonal relationships? How may the patient be expected to behave in relation to others? What constitutes the nature and quality of a relationship that can be expected to be of benefit at this time?
5. Which activities can be expected to meet treatment needs and elicit desired responses?[16]

White postulates that the energies of effectance and competence must be utilized in the maintenance of all other ego functions. The individual's difficulties in thinking, perceiving and functioning might well be dealt with, then, in light of learning experiences which required the mastery of progressively more complex skills, directed toward effecting change in the human and nonhuman environment. The integration of the appropriate interpersonal (peer and therapist) relationships with carefully selected activities processes (nonhuman objects and the concomitant actions) is the basis for the Fidlers' concept of treatment. In this frame of reference, treatment and learning would appear to be nearly synonymous.

*Fidler and Fidler: Occupational Therapy—A Communication Process in Psychiatry, pp. 160-161.

Another perspective on planning for change is provided by Shannon.* Working in a program modeled on the play-work continuum, based on Reilly's theory of occupational role behavior, he described an occupational therapy plan developed through this pattern:

> First, it is necessary to maintain and then gradually strengthen the existing skills of the individual;
> Second, work must be initiated toward the development of new skills which will assist the individual in resuming his life plan;
> Third, the entire nature of the individual's work-play scheme should be examined in order to provide a therapeutic program which leads to establishing a more positive balance between work and play in his life style.[52]

Shannon's plan for an occupational therapy program might be related to Moorhead's variables, described earlier in the section on "What Does the Occupational Therapist Evaluate?" Both are concerned with the individual's need to develop adequate behaviors in social interaction, and successful economically-required skills. Such mastery would lead to a sense of competence, and feelings of efficacy, more appropriate to the individual's age and current life-style.

A third scheme for developing a treatment plan or a program for learning is based on the developmental model. It would employ the results of the evaluation process by posing questions such as these:

> What are the strengths and qualities of the ego skills that this individual depends upon for his negotiations with other persons, and with his inanimate environment?
> How appropriate are these skills for his chronological age? What other (higher level) skills should he have acquired by now? And at what age were his present-level skills more appropriate?
> How does he relate to other persons, and what does he expect from them? Gain from them? Offer to them through the relationship? At what developmental stage would these interactions be deemed appropriate?
> What kinds of tasks provide a challenge for him? In what areas does he demonstrate autonomy? Competence? Effectance? What developmental level does this kind of behavior symbolize?

The plan which the therapist and client developed would include activities and relationships appropriate to the developmental needs demonstrated. These activities would be explored progressively in order to develop those ego skills which allowed the individual to (a) recognize alternatives for action; (b) select (for him) the best alternative; (c) carry it out appropriately; and (d) experience satisfaction and a feeling of achievement from each task.

*Shannon, P.D.: The work-play model: a basis for occupational therapy programming in Psychiatry. Am. J. Occup. Therapy, 24:215, 1970.

THE OCCUPATIONAL THERAPY PROGRAM

The Setting

The setting in which the individual's treatment or learning program takes place must approximate the real world in which he needs to learn to live more satisfactorily. Occupational therapy is a laboratory for living, a place where interpersonal skills and the mastery of task behaviors are the fundamental studies. Encounters with staff and peers as well as with the cultural objects of the environment should elicit responses and provide feedback which relate to the therapeutic process. In such a model community the individual should be challenged to assess each new situation and to learn from it. Immediate response from the human environment should help him to determine the effectiveness of his choice of behaviors.

People learn differently and at different rates of speed, but of most significance for the occupational therapy process is the developmental level through which the patient is currently working. The setting must provide an opportunity to select from and engage in age-appropriate tasks and relationships while permitting the re-exploration or mastery of a much earlier function, in a representative fashion. Difficulty in controlling one's rage when attempting to manipulate stubborn, resistive, unpliable objects (human or otherwise) is a behavioral indication of one of the typical struggles of the 3–5-year-old. When such behaviors are found in an adult male, and when they have contributed to his difficulty in holding a job, the learning experiences provided must allow for recognition of his adult male role, while permitting the mastery of more appropriate adult behaviors through practice in attaining earlier, prerequisite skills. The use of tools and equipment may be required, but the tasks themselves should be graded so that resistance and difficulty in controlling the task are gradually increased, until the adult level of control is achieved. Gratification, or reinforcement of the desired behavior, is provided by the mastery of each task throughout the learning scale.

The setting must permit a wide range of tasks and use of the appropriate tools. A significant determinant of the success of the occupational therapy program lies in the variety of structural variables which can be provided. Diasio* states:

> ...one of the distinguishing features of occupational therapy is its conscious emphasis and insistence that, in addition to man's need for meaningful engagement with his environment, there are *therapeutic properties inherent in the environment which may be structured for*

*Diasio, K.: Psychiatric occupational therapy; search for a conceptual framework in light of psychoanalytical ego psychology and learning theory. Am. J. Occup. Therapy, 22:400, 1968.

treatment purposes. These properties include not only the structuring of the patient-therapist relationship, but . . . the physical and complex social role environments as well.[24]

The ideal occupational therapy laboratory is the community itself. With increasing frequency, the real world is being used to provide learning experiences through which poorly functioning individuals may acquire better habits of living. When it is not possible to use the community itself, it is imperative that the values of that community be incorporated into the occupational therapy program. Working conditions, cultural values, economic realities, family patterns of interaction, peer groups, and leisure time pursuits must typify those of the patient's real world. The transition is otherwise too risky, the chances for failure too great. The individual either adopts patient-like roles and behaviors as a defense (i.e., chronicity takes over) or he becomes a "repeater," one who persistently takes hospital-oriented behaviors and tries to function with them in the community, returning regularly to remaster those very skills which serve him so poorly. The setting for the occupational therapy program is indeed a critical variable.

The Staff

Several levels of function are currently represented in the occupational therapy profession: the registered therapist (OTR); the certified occupational therapy assistant (COTA); and the occupational therapy aide. The roles and functions described throughout this chapter include those in common practice, as well as those which appear to be imminent with the changing demands of the health care system. These roles and functions may be viewed briefly from the administrative perspective.

A basic principle of management states that any function should be performed by personnel who are qualified at the most basic level possible. In other words, each function or technic should be carried out, under appropriate supervision, by persons who are *not* qualified to perform more complex functions nor to assume professional responsibility *greater* than that required by the particular task in question. In view of the immense shortage of qualified health personnel, it is essential that each occupational therapy program be assessed in terms of the functions it performs, the roles required to perform those functions, the personnel available and qualified to perform each function, and the personnel available who are qualified to supervise each function. While guidelines have been established by the American Occupational Therapy Association to assist in determining levels of function and responsibility, each service unit or department will have varying strengths and unique requirements which determine how certain tasks should be executed and supervised.

The nature of the services to be offered is determined by the overall objectives of the comprehensive program, of which occupational therapy is a single part. Total program emphasis may be on activities of daily living, on exploration of prevocational roles, on unconscious forces which can be elicited and studied through projective technics, or on development of leisure time pursuits for chronically maladapted citizens. Within each of these and many other areas, occupational therapy services can be offered at varying levels of sophistication. It does not necessarily follow, however, that the most sophisticated (i.e., verbal, highly educated, intellectually-oriented) therapist is the best person for a specific job. Social psychiatry research offers plentiful evidence that the empathic relationships which can emerge between worker and client who share common backgrounds and expectations may be far more productive of therapeutic goals than those wherein the therapist relies too heavily on knowledge, and not enough on shared real-life experience.

For other reasons, too, the delegation of functions must be made up and down the academic ladder. It appears to be increasingly unrealistic to assume that there will ever be adequate numbers of health professionals. Shortages of occupational therapy personnel, as with all disciplines, are acute, and efforts at recruitment yield dishearteningly small increases which are immediately offset by the population expansion. The training of a mental health worker (an aide, in former years) requires one-fifth the time as does the education of an OTR and perhaps one-twentieth the financial cost. The COTA currently completes his preparation in two years, compared with nearly five years for the OTR. A major challenge facing the occupational therapist in mental health today is to define the basic tasks which can be performed by persons having these other kinds of preparation, so that their recruitment and training may be facilitated.

It is conceivable that the OTR of the near future will not deal directly with patients, at least not in his primary role. Rather, the roles of consultation, supervision, in-service training, research and administration will be the prerogatives of the professionally-trained therapist. All other functions relative to mental health programming are likely to be planned and executed by the COTA and/or his associates, the mental health worker or occupational therapy aide. (Mental health worker refers to the generalist, usually recruited from the indigenous population surrounding the mental health center; occupational therapy aide refers to personnel trained more specifically in occupational therapy tasks, but the two roles usually are reasonably interchangeable, and carry similar status, responsibility and rewards.)

Professional judgments are the responsibility of the most highly trained member of any discipline. Establishing priorities, sequences and long range objectives for the total program requires the judgment of the OTR. Similarly, general supervision over the evaluation of clients and the program objectives developed for each should be retained by professional level personnel. But while the quality of care should be determined at the professional level, the experiences required to accomplish the individual's program objectives may be better planned, as well as implemented, by other members of the staff.

It is not possible to list those functions which should, or can be, delegated. Basically, they are those which are characterized by straightforward problem-solving tasks which may be objectively viewed in terms of the required activities of daily living; procedures which can be assessed through rating devices based on standardized scales, and which do not require judgments based on complex theoretical issues; and relationships developed through commonality of experience, similar community or personal values, and the ability to communicate in some essential style.

The Patient Population

Most mental health centers find that a majority of their patients have certain elements in common. Similarities in economic status, educational levels, cultural backgrounds, and age ranges are usually identifiable. A few centers, particularly those emphasizing educational programs for members of mental health professions, make an effort to serve a broader cross-section of the population. It is helpful even then to identify the commonalities of experience and the shared problems or symptoms of the group, for this should influence the major parts of the total program.

Shannon describes a therapeutic program developed for a 100-bed psychiatric unit in an Army hospital. Investigation of the work-play histories of his patients revealed that the majority had these four things in common: (1) difficulty in the area of occupational choice; (2) failure to complete high school; (3) history of unsatisfactory work experiences; and (4) difficulty in managing free time.[52] The program Shannon developed in response to these four problem areas was based on individually planned daily activities. The appropriate developmental sequences were incorporated, with tasks and relationships determined by the current need for mastery and social interaction. The day's program balanced work and play in accordance with the patient's need to experience these roles and tasks. Real work and a genuine recreation program provided the two extremes on the continuum, while activities such as playing musical instruments and assembling electronics kits replaced the more traditional occupational therapy activities.

The life-style of the individuals of this patient population, not diagnoses or descriptions of symptoms, determined the nature of their occupational therapy programs. Therapy was directed toward the development of appropriate occupational roles and behaviors, which could be transferred easily into community (army or civilian) life.

Metzker and Hyman, working on an emergency psychiatric service in an urban area, assessed their typical patients as: (1) coming from lower class socioeconomic situations; (2) being from minority racial, cultural and ethnic groups (with the language difficulties this implies); (3) rarely having completed high school; and (4) having had substantial deprivation in experiences with the human and nonhuman objects that usually contribute to learning.[57]

In response to these needs, they developed the following objectives as their general plan for an occupational therapy program, individualized according to each person's special needs:

1. Re-establishment of the patient's contact with reality
2. Increase of the patient's control over his own behavior, particularly the behavior that results in discomfort on the part of those in his social environment
3. Increase of the appropriateness of the patient's interaction with his environment, including the people in that environment
4. Increasing abrogation of the role of mental patient
5. Re-establishment of the patient's self-esteem
6. Support and reinforcement of the patient's adaptive defenses against his own fantasies, his own anxieties and his own impulses.

The media used to accomplish these objectives also had carefully selected properties. Projects were short-term in nature, providing quick and sure success; the activities were not complex, did not require much creativity, and utilized primarily gross motor skills; materials which were colorful and stimulating were used, and visual and auditory stimuli were appropriately controlled.[57] Since the average patient remained in this program less than two weeks, these kinds of structural decisions insured maximum individual gain without sacrificing large periods of time to more unique evaluation procedures. Assessment of *typical* needs allowed for good overall program planning, within which special individual needs could be met with a minimum of adjustment of the total program. The patient population, then, serves as one of the necessary dimensions when a total activities program is being planned.

Work or Play? . . . With Whom?

In the vernacular of the day, free choice activities in occupational therapy are a "cop-out." Therapists who fail to negotiate a contract with the patient which clearly states that the therapist has the knowledge, experience and responsibility for selecting the content of the therapeutic program, have clearly abdicated their professional roles. The selection of the activity is determined by the needs uncovered through the evaluation process, by the patient's interests and his preferred skills, and by the therapist's knowledge of the activities processes which might facilitate the accomplishment of the objectives they have established together.

If the occupational therapy process effects change through learning, what is it that the individual can learn through doing and interacting and studying the results? Fidler states that participation in the occupational therapy process can lead to the development of specific ego skills, and therapeutic activities may be particularly useful in:

> developing frustration tolerance, learning to rely on inner controls in the absence of external ones, assessing social reality, drawing inferences, learning to sublimate, using past satisfactory experiences as resources; developing realistic responses to failure, success and error; mastering feeling and developing and improving the ability to make decisions and problem solve.[58]

Stated more simply, one can learn

> To live and work with other people, individuals and groups, socially and economically;
> To satisfy his own needs, physical and social needs as well as the need for self-esteem;
> To communicate effectively with others, through perception of verbal and bodily messages, verbal and behavioral responses.

The program, then, must provide opportunities for

1. Working with individuals who can offer the significant kinds of relationship required for successful accomplishment of a developmental task.
2. Working with groups, which provide certain kinds of reality testing, and offer experiences in shared accomplishments.
3. Exploring the multiple facets of the activities processes which are a part of occupational therapy, to the end that he learns what challenges him, what he can master, what is satisfying, and which things are best left to others.
4. Developing efficacy and a sense of competency; the self-esteem required to face new tasks and economic roles is thus acquired.
5. Playing, as a means of relating to others as well as for its own sake, in the sense that play balances work, and play may be a necessary regression in the service of the ego.

These opportunities are outlined separately below.

Therapeutic relationships. Earlier in the chapter the subject of therapeutic role models was discussed from the developmental point of view. Other references throughout the chapter have referred to the relationship between therapy and learning, therapist and patient, and therapy through developmental encounters with age-appropriate objects and activities.

The most pertinent and complete discussion of individual therapeutic relationships in occupational therapy is found in the fourth chapter of Fidler and Fidler,[16] entitled, "The Dyadic Relationship." The basic problems encountered in the helping relationship are fully outlined from both the patient's and the therapist's point of view. Comparison of these concepts with the earlier discussion in this chapter on developmental models for the therapist's role should lead to a fairly complete understanding of what is involved when one individual attempts to help another overcome social and emotional problems.

The following example describes an individual therapeutic relationship. Jane, a young woman of twenty-seven, applied at the mental health center for guidance regarding the choice of a career. She stated that she had engaged in nine different occupations or training programs for occupations in the past ten years. Currently she was enrolled in a community junior college in a pre-social work curriculum. Her decision to enter this program was based on her experiences during the previous year while working as a secretary to the guidance counselor in the high school. She had found the contacts with the students interesting, and was intrigued by the thought of being able to discuss with them the problems which they shared with the guidance counselor. However, the college program was difficult to endure, as had been the other three educational programs she had attempted in preparation for a new career. She became obsessive about the assignments and most of her energy was devoted to organizing time and materials, planning how and when to get the work done, leaving little energy to deal with the assignments themselves. In addition, the basic courses in liberal arts and human development seemed too distantly related to social work or guidance and counseling, and her fellow students were also "distant."

Her secretarial skills were based on high school courses which she had found to be comforting in their structured way, and the teacher had been one who rewarded her students through a great deal of sensitive, personal attention. Consequently, Jane used her skills in this area as a security device, alternately taking jobs which used these skills to boost her sense of competence and then attempting to engage in other, more challenging jobs which were more appropriate to her intellectual abilities. The other jobs included work as an assistant to a junior executive in an advertising firm, receptionist at a men's university club, and cashier at a small hotel. Previous efforts at education and training included advanced secretarial training (which included some bookkeeping), dietetics, radiologic technology, and nursery school education.

This information was collected through the intake interview and Jane was referred to the occupational therapist for further evaluation and recommendations to be made at the intake staff meeting the following week. The evaluation revealed a woman who had minimum self-esteem and whose sense of competence was considerably lower than her actual skills would imply. Her ability to invest in human relationships was grossly underdeveloped, and she saw herself as lonely and unapproachable. The search for a career appeared to be a search, instead, for human companionship, yet her preoccupation with details and structure served to counteract any impulse to seek friendships.

These findings were reported to the intake staff and it was agreed that the occupational therapist should serve as primary therapist for Jane. Team review of the case was scheduled for the following month.

In discussing a treatment program with Jane, the therapist attempted to discover which problems Jane was most interested in correcting first. Jane was able to agree that another disruption in her education would serve only to avoid dealing with the problem of career choice, and agreed to stay on in school.

She identified her need for support (i.e., companionship) as being her greatest concern. The choice of a pre-social work career appeared to have been an indirect effort to find guidance for herself, and through tactfully phrased questions, the therapist helped Jane validate this assumption. They agreed, therefore, to work together so that Jane could use the relationship to gain understanding about her difficulty in career selection and her unmet needs for companionship and human affection.

The therapist's relationship with Jane centered around the core problem of vocational choice and identity, a developmental task of late adolescence. Jane's reliance on secretarial skills for security seemed related to the experience with a warm and understanding role model, the high school teacher. The therapist sought to establish a learning situation which would allow Jane to explore her feelings about work, independence, adult femininity, and gratification through friendships or partnerships. Because Jane was comfortable with highly structured activities which did not require independent creative judgments, the therapist suggested that they begin with sewing. This activity offered the necessary structure; it appealed to the "adolescent's" need to become more familiar with herself and to explore the adult feminine role from the point of view of sexual identity. The therapist's initial role was that of mother-teacher; as Jane began to see that the therapist was concerned about her as a person, she began to discuss the loneliness she had felt in her own home. Productivity and orderliness had been praised, but not rewarded through affection or physical demon-

CHART 5–7   A COMPARATIVE ANALYSIS OF PSYCHOANALYTIC GROUP THERAPY, THE TRANS-ACTIONAL GROUP, AND GROUP DYNAMIC PROCESSES

Developed for the AOTA Regional Institutes, 1966, by Kenneth V. Skrivanek, O.T.R.

"DEFINITION AND CHARACTERISTICS"

1. **Psychoanalytic Group Therapy:** The application of psychoanalytic theory and principles through which several persons are treated simultaneously, but not necessarily in the same way. Technics may vary, but they are primarily concerned with interpersonal issues, their intrapsychic determinants, with the purpose of attaining characterological change in each member. There is minimal involvement with the environment; no manifest task to be accomplished; and the process of socialization is generally contraindicated.

Examples:
Group therapy
Group Psycho-therapy
Interactional group therapy
Analytically-oriented group therapy

2. **The Trans-Actional Group:** The incorporation of both psychoanalytic and group process theory and principles to provide a "living experience" which is subject to exploration and analysis by the participants. The "living experience" demands an involvement with the environment in which the group transacts, and an active participation in the "doing" of a task. The exploration of the interpersonal issues, which arise in the "doing," is directed toward increased self-awareness; self-actualization, and behavioral change for each member. The active involvement with the environment and the participation in the task provide a microcosm of a "living experience" through which each member can be confronted, and can explore his behavior.

Examples:
Activity-oriented group therapy
Task-oriented treatment groups
(Sensitivity training groups)

3. **Group Dynamics:** Denotes the study of the structure and functioning of groups (group processes), notably the psychological aspects of "small groups," with special reference to the changing pattern of intra-group adjustment, tension, conflict, cohesion and relationships. It emphasizes eliciting from members some behavior that will bring about the desired change in group structure which will facilitate the attainment of the group goal, without primary concern for consequent, more or less permanent, change in the members as individuals. Group dynamics is primarily concerned with the development of effective group leadership and member participation so that the group can more effectively attain its given goal.

Examples:
Activity groups
Patient councils
Student governments
Planning committees
Executive boards

CHART 5-7 (Continued)

Psychoanalytic Group Therapy

Purpose: To work through individual intra-psychic conflicts.

Methodology: The exploration of intra-psychic processes via the multiple transference phenomenon.

Role of Therapist: To validate reality, clarify distortions, guide toward individuation.

Focus of Group: On the intra-psychic determinants of individual reactions within the group.

Member-Leadership: Leadership role contraindicated. Cohesiveness a negative factor. Individuation of primary importance.

Goal of Member Roles: Individuation of each member through the analytic group process.

The Trans-Actional Group

Purpose: To work through problems of interpersonal relations. To increase self-understanding and the perception of self in relationship to others.

Methodology: The exploration of the "cause and effect" relationships inherent in participating in the task experience.

Role of Therapist: To help group members relate the task experience to the purpose of the group.

Focus of Group: On the interpersonal effect each member's actions have on the others while participating in the task experience.

Member-Leadership: Exploration of the evolution of leadership role within the group and its significance and effect on group members. Consideration of other alternatives.

Goal of Member Roles: The evolution of flexibility in roles, and a diminution of their stereotypy, as interpersonal problems are worked through, alternative courses of action are considered, and more interdependent functioning develops.

Group Dynamic Processes

Purpose: The accomplishment of tasks in the most meaningful and expedient manner.

Methodology: The use of process analysis: member roles, power structures, flow charts, etc.

Role of Therapist: Group trainer, process analyst, observer (no feedback on psychic issues!).

Focus of Group: On cohesiveness, the development of a group ego, and effective democratic leadership and delimitation of member roles, all directed toward the accomplishment of the task.

Member-Leadership: Leader is selected for the task; authoritative, laissez-faire; or, ideally, democratic.

Goal of Member Roles: Delimited by the purpose and structure of the group. Ideally they are designated so that each member has a meaningful and productive experience.

strations of love. Jane had felt that she needed to succeed in order to be loved, but her mother had never indicated just what kind of success would bring the evasive love rewards.

The therapist gradually structured the relationship so that Jane made more and more decisions, each rewarded by praise of genuine accomplishments, praise which clearly said that it was Jane who was lovable, not her skills and productivity. Discussions developed around the topic of independence and what it was like to succeed and be on your own — "Wasn't that just more loneliness?" Jane asked.

As the relationship developed, the therapist moved into the role of the superego ideal, the "other" adult who replaces the parent as the child's standard for adult behavior. The therapist worked now as an older companion, one with whom Jane could identify as a successful career woman. They shared tasks, including some of Jane's school assignments, and Jane learned that success did not always lead to empty praise, but might be a means to a sense of closeness and intimacy. The next phase of her program saw Jane enter a task-oriented group, where she explored peer relationships and vocational choices under the guidance of the therapist whom she had learned to trust.

Task-oriented groups. The use of task-oriented groups in occupational therapy has been a major development within the field. This technic allows patients to work with peers who are functioning at the patients' developmental level, and to explore the tasks and relationships which are appropriate to learning at this stage of development. The therapist provides some reality testing for the group, and assists in maintaining an adequate structure within which the group can progress. The therapist does not function as a leader or authority figure, but provides group membership roles as they are required in order for the group to operate. In this way, the necessary role models for group behavior are demonstrated. Peer groups provide maximum learning at several stages in normal development. It is essential to capitalize on this in the therapeutic process.

Mosey[59] outlines the concept of developmental groups in a most useful way. Fidler[60] has elaborated on the technics of group process as they are utilized in occupational therapy. Skrivanek developed a comparative analysis of several types of learning groups, shown in Chart 5-7. Gillette and Mayer[61] offer the following examples of the kinds of learning which can be achieved through the task-oriented group.

> When interpersonal closeness becomes threatening, verbal and intellectual defenses may be used to keep other people at a distance. In a task-oriented activity group, each member is confronted with the expectation that he contribute to the completion of the task at hand. Efforts at evading demands or attempts to isolate oneself are more

easily demonstrable in this setting; group members help each other assume responsibility more appropriately by insisting that each one do his share of the task. What one does, in such a setting, speaks more loudly than what one says.

With intellectual defenses removed or blocked by others, the individual may resort to more primitive ways of maintaining his security and comfort. Thus psychopathology may be graphically demonstrated in a setting where therapist and fellow group members can offer immediate support in exploration and understanding of the conflict. The patient who maintains that he is able to function without treatment and should be allowed to do so can be helped to accept his need for treatment when the group points out how poorly he carries out directions, is unable to be punctual, and presents his needs so inappropriately.

Conversely, some patients are so overwhelmed by the prospect of being with other people that the opportunity to use a task in order to create an interpersonal distance is welcomed. Accepting help with an activity from the group may be the initial step in reversing the process of isolation and withdrawal. Many activities require joint efforts of two or more persons. Being forced to ask another person to hold the end of a board so that it can be sawed may be an acceptable way to ask for help without the risk of giving in to strong dependency needs. Experiencing support in such instances may eventually lead the patient to be able to ask for emotional support.

Certain aspects of task-oriented activity groups provide needed structure and limits for some patients. There is safety and comfort in the predictability of response to the media, tools and work plan being used. A patient who struggles to control his impulsive aggression may be able to use his energies more constructively when there are clearly visible limits within which to work: pounding nails into a bookcase is an example. Both media and fellow members, as well as the therapist, can help to give this feeling of security. Working together on the printing of a newspaper, where each person has specific assignments, offers the opportunity to express critical or provocative ideas within safe limits.

The task sets definite limits and boundaries on what the group can do, and on how it can be done. These restrictions are realistic and are determined by the nature of the activity rather than by an arbitrary authority figure. They assure group members that emotions and impulses will be kept under control. Such experiences, where strong emotions may be expressed and accepted for the first time, lend support to the member in trying out similar behavior in other settings as well. It also helps persons recognize limits which are available for help, as well as those which are unduly restrictive and must be dealt with in another way.

The importance of feeling a part of a group—for the first time, perhaps—should not be overlooked. For people with limited interpersonal skills a sense of belonging to a group is facilitated by having a task on which to focus. When a "we" feeling has been too threatening because of the struggle to maintain one's ego boundaries, it is pleasing to be able to identify oneself indirectly as a member of the group by referring for example, to "my music group." Relating to each other through the catalytic task eases the problem of too much closeness. The group members can measure their growth in learning to relate to each other by noting the increasingly complex nature of the tasks which they are able to complete as a group. Indirect communication of ideas and feelings can be expressed through what one does and says in relation to the task at hand. These messages can then be understood in the terms of interpersonal relations, the restrictive defenses against direct expression of conflicts or anxiety having been by-passed.

Another aspect of the task-oriented activity group is also related to solving problems in communication. There are multiple opportunities in such a setting for nonverbal or symbolic (representational) communication. The most obvious of these occur when the group is involved in an artistic production of some sort. Puppetry and other kinds of dramatics offer unlimited paths toward expression of thoughts and feelings disguised as belonging to someone else. If the feeling is accepted, or if the authority figure does not react punitively, perhaps it is safe to acknowledge such feelings in oneself. Art media of all kinds also provide outlets for communicating materials which one is reluctant to express verbally. Group members often discover similarities in the manner in which they paint or draw emotional scenes. It provides an amazing sense of relief to learn that feelings and conflicts and anxiety may be had in common with others. The realization that one is not alone in his plight is tremendously reassuring.

Activities and the Self

It is inherent in the occupational therapy process that the individual can both experience the human and nonhuman environment through his active participation in them and can begin to assess the quality and quantity of his object relations to the end that he makes some necessary modifications in his attitudes and behavior. The activities process itself assists him in communicating both his present characteristic responses to objects, and his wishes and preferences for other means of relating.

It is important that the individual's interests be tapped at a meaningful level, in order to determine the extent to which his behavior is inner or outer directed, congruent or alien to his self-image, and consequently how readily it may be modified through therapy.

Matsutsuyu[62] presents six propositions relevant to studying interests. Their application to occupational therapy is readily apparent:

Proposition 1. Interests Are Family Influenced.
Interests are determined by early developmental contingencies that are primarily localized in the family unit where early intra-familial experience influences direction.

Proposition 2. Interests Evoke Affective Response.
Interest can evoke affective response with persons, things and ideas, and can be expressed as likes, dislikes, indifferences or as preferences.

Proposition 3. Interests Are Choice States.
The capacity to make interests choices serves the process of commitment to life roles for work, through occupational choice, and for play, through recreation and leisure.

Proposition 4. Interests Can Be Manifest in Effective Action.
Interest as a subjective experience can lead the individual to engage in pertinent activities that can be satisfying and have adaptive value.

Proposition 5. Interest Can Sustain Action.
Degree or strength of interests varies according to the level and type of interaction with the event and can serve to sustain action during the learning stages or to maintain functional achievement.

Proposition 6. Interests Reflect Self-Perception.
Expressed interests are subjective statements which reflect self-perception.*

Recognition of motivation to change and of the processes which the individual can tolerate as he works toward change, must be an integral part of the therapeutic plan. Matsutsuyu devised an Interest Check List, composed of eighty common leisure time activities; it allows the individual's interests to be categorized for use in program planning. The categories are: Manual Skills, Physical Sports, Social Recreation, Activities of Daily Living, and Cultural/Educational. Identifying major areas of interests gives a perspective on the individual's feelings of competence, as well as an indication of the kinds of activities he may feel compelled to pursue. Understanding of such forces is useful in attempting to redevelop former skills and roles or learning to adapt to new requirements for occupational and social behaviors. Attitudes toward activities, feelings about one's abilities and limitations, and the sense of being inner or outer directed must all be considered when the activities are chosen.

The purpose of the NPI [Neuropsychiatric Institute, U.C.L.A.] Interest Check List is to classify and describe the interest state of psychiatric patients by: (1) classifying the intensity of interest according to item responses, (2) classifying types of interest according to the category

* Matsutsuyu, J. S.: The interest check list. Am. J. Occup. Therapy, 23:323, 1969.

system, (3) describing the individual's ability to express personal preference, and (4) describing the individual's capacity to discriminate type and intensity.[63]*

Combined use of such an interest check list and the Activities Configuration presented in the section on interview procedures might lead to a sound planning basis on which to construct a weekly program for persons attending occupational therapy. It would be equally appropriate for community and day care programs or the chronic care wards of the state hospital. Matching life tasks (via therapeutic activity) to needs for learning, achievement, and personal development is the key to good occupational therapy.

Play

The need to play, in a truly re-creative way, has possibly never been greater than during the present decade. Man struggles to maintain his integrity against the encroachments of automation, mobility, impersonalized mass communications and non-personal human relations. There is evidence that work, as it is now perceived, is ego-alien; it is superimposed by social custom and demand, and freedom to choose one's occupation and means of earning his daily bread is, in reality, freedom in name only. Custom and conditioning have long since predetermined the roles and functions which the individual sees as his narrow, inevitable choice.

In contrast, play is purely ego-syntonic, congruent with the individual's sense of well-being, a purposeful and healing pursuit which balances the stresses of the work situation's demands. Haun summarizes this with the following proposition†:

> 1. Man is so constituted that the normal functioning of his central nervous system is critically dependent upon the maintenance of sensory input.
> 2. In origin, the bulk of this sensory input can be operationally divided among housekeeping, work and recreation.
> 3. Sensory input derived from housekeeping tends to be affectively neutral; from work, ego-dystonic; from recreation, always ego-syntonic.
> 4. Man's normal function is related to the balance between ego-syntonic and ego-dystonic sensory input.[64]

Work, of course, need not be the antithesis of pleasure; it is what we, collectively, have made of it. By the same token, we have influenced recreation so that for many, it cannot be a pleasurable, no-strings-attached experience. It is common to find that persons need excuses to

---

* Matsutsuyu, p. 326.
†Haun, P.: Recreation: A Medical Viewpoint. New York Bureau of Publications, Teachers College, Columbia University, 1968.

play, reasons such as maintaining health, socializing for business purposes, or playing to "let off steam." Mental health needs are poorly served by any of these attitudes regarding work and play: that work is dull, self-destructive, a necessary evil; that play is frivolous, wasteful of time, and perhaps a bit sinful in its pleasures. The typical mental patient has a history of unsatisfactory experiences in both realms. Neither work nor play provides pleasure or satisfaction.

Both White[55] and Erikson[18] discuss the learning that takes place through play. White emphasizes that the fundamental sense of competence is derived through the mastery of play activities. Through play, one learns what effects he can make on the environment and how he is, in turn, affected by the environment. Florey* paraphrases White in presenting these variables which must be available if learning is to take place through play:

> ...(1) The environment should provide both human and non-human objects ... (2) The non-human object environment should provide novelty ... (3) The environment should allow for and provide the opportunity for exploration, repetition and imitation ... (4) The play environment should be free of such stresses as hunger, anxiety or fear, since these interfere with exploratory play ... (5) The play environment should not be associated with isolation, fear or pain ...[65]

As the child moves along the developmental scale, he begins to effect change in his environment in ways which reward him with a sense of having done well—having accomplished a planned task. Florey reviews Erikson's account of the latency period—his stage of industry versus inferiority—and suggests these variables as necessary to the learning process†:

> ...(1) The environment should provide systematic instruction ... (2) The environment should provide the child with the opportunity to make things and deal with things that have significance in the adult world ... (3) There should be role models who know things and know how to do things ... (4) There should be opportunity for association with peers ...[66]

Both sets of variables imply preparation for work as well as for play. Mastery of tasks, the feeling of effectance and the ensuing sense of competence are important prerequisites for a healthy personality. When mental health needs are threatened, the occupational therapist must look to the balance between work and play. The areas of need may be symptomatic of deficiencies in role behaviors or skills required to do either successfully.

---

* From Florey, L. L.: Intrinsic motivation: the dynamics of occupational therapy theory. Am. J. Occup. Therapy, 24:321, 1969.
† Florey, p. 323.

The need for balance between re-creative leisure experiences and sustaining, productive economic pursuits cannot be over-emphasized. Nor will this balance often be found in persons referred for mental health services. The activities and relationships provided through the therapeutic program must maintain this balanced perspective. As the individual increases his sense of self-esteem, he will be able to pursue a gradually widening range of activities. It is important that he be helped to recognize how and why certain activities bring pleasure, and that others are alien to his self-concept and, therefore, unpleasant. Only through recognition of what he hopes to gain and is able to gain through his own skills can he identify the potential gratification to be had through any activities process, be it work or play.

Planned learning experiences leading to improved play functions may be offered in a variety of ways in the occupational therapy program. Characteristically, leisure time pursuits are entirely voluntary and spontaneous, and take place with one's neighbors or friends; there are strong tones of neighborhood values in one's recreational choices. Therefore, it is recommended that the leisure time improvement program be a function of the ward, the Patients Activities Committee, or a patient-citizens advisory group which operates in the community. Through such an organizational structure, persons learn to identify what it is they really want to do; how to select the partners with whom to pursue such an activity; to make decisions about the time involvement, the win-lose intensity that is required; to deal with the issues of being responsible, dependable and responsive to the needs of others. These and many other opportunities for learning to structure one's own life in a balanced way, should be provided through a recreation program which is conceived, planned and executed by the persons whom it serves. In no other way can the realities of self-gratification be so easily provided.

Work

Play is the antecedent to work. This is true of the normal developmental process and it follows logically that it should be the sequence of learning through therapy.[67] Choices of play or leisure time activities represent the most ego-syntonic patterns of behavior. The occupational therapy program which initiates learning and exploration of attitudes and skills at the play level can move forward more easily to study those activities and attitudes gradually acquired through the developmental process, labeled in the adult role as work, or occupational behaviors.

Shannon, in reviewing Neff's book, Work and Human Behavior, states that "work is defined as a function of two interrelated variables: the work environment and the work personality. . . . The work personality is a product of social learning over a prolonged period and a semi-autonomous area of the general personality."[68]

Fidler* speaks of the needs which are a part of mature functioning, needs which customarily are both identified and gratified through the work process.[69]

1. The need for identity; to perceive oneself as an individual uniquely human, distinct from others, with worth and value. From this need emerges the need for self-actualization and the need to be self-determining and self-directed.

2. The need for relatedness: to experience a mutual sharing collaborative relationship with one's fellow men as well as a relatedness to one's environment.

3. The need to perceive oneself as a productive, contributing member of one's society.

4. The need for consensual validation: to validate one's concepts and perceptions of self and others, of one's external world and the inter-relationship of these.

The developmental tasks which precede the formation of the adult work personality must be mastered in sequence if the occupational behaviors are to be successful and appropriate. Experiences related to occupational choice dominate a major proportion of the adolescent period of development. Many adolescents and young adults referred for treatment on the basis of widely divergent problems or symptoms are primarily troubled about occupational roles, and the inability to identify and engage in work which satisfies the needs Fidler describes.

Shannon[52] points out the significance of an individually planned program which creates the appropriate balance between play and work experiences, determined by the current level of developmental tasks to be reviewed or re-accomplished. The task-oriented group would appear to be a particularly meaningful way in which to explore and resolve some of the basic issues surrounding work adjustment.

The concept of treatment by means of peer group experiences plus mastery of occupational behaviors is perhaps easier to grasp in relation to the adolescent or young adult. The example which follows is meant to show the application of these principles to a later developmental period.

A task-oriented group has been created to meet the needs of eight chronically underemployed men, ages ranging from 33 to 56. They have been marginally adjusted in their occupational and social roles throughout their adult lives. Two have histories of several brief admissions to state hospitals and three received early medical discharges from the

_____
* Fidler, G. S.: A second look at work as a primary force in rehabilitation and treatment. Am. J. Occup. Therapy, 20:72, 1966.

armed services on grounds of inability to adopt appropriate military attitudes and behaviors. Five of the eight were high school dropouts with low achievement records throughout their educational histories. Six of the men grew up in lower class socioeconomic families, though four of those families showed records of adequate occupational behaviors on the part of the father. The other two men were products of white collar families with middle class orientation to work and its value.

The group has chosen to construct some playground equipment for the underprivileged children in the neighborhood. Funds for the project have been solicited by the group from the community action committee, and materials as well as basic minimum wages are provided. The group members, throughout the life of the task, will explore their relationships to each other (Fidler, second need, above[69]); become aware of their individual responses to the task and its requirements (the third need); each will be supported in recognizing and gratifying his own needs and uniqueness (the first need above); and the group itself will provide the security and validation necessary for growth and change (the fourth need).

Through such an experience, typical of the play-work activities of the adolescent and his peer group, these men will re-assess their attitudes and skills in the area of occupational behaviors. In addition, opportunity is made for developing the sense of social and community responsibility which is a necessary part of the adult personality and a developmental task of adulthood, according to Havighurst[20] and Erikson.[18] Mastery of these tasks will lead to the development of a self-concept appropriate to the chronological age, and a resultant ability to assume the necessary personal and social commitments.

THREE LEVELS OF PREVENTION

The primary concern of the occupational therapist is, and always has been, health. The functional aspects of an individual's health, not the disease processes which destroy health, have been the focus of this profession. Occupational therapy has few life-saving technics, but many life-prolonging services; little skill in intervention in acute and devastating but quickly passing illness, yet much to offer the chronically handicapped person and the patient who is overwhelmed by the prospects (real or imagined) of permanent disability. The occupational therapy philosophy states that man can, through the use of his own hands in an activities process, influence the state of his own health. It is essential that this concept become an integral part of the nation's health care system.

From the perspective of maintaining health, services related to medical-social problems can be outlined on a continuum of prevention. Primary prevention includes those services which intervene in the social, economic and family conditions leading to illness. Inadequate housing, unequal job opportunities, poor and unequal educational programs, inadequate public health measures, poorly designed and managed recreational facilities, and social tensions resulting from discrimination are problems which have a serious, destructive impact on health. These social problems require professional intervention in order to prevent physical and psychosocial illness and disability.

Secondary prevention has a clearer relationship to medicine. Professional duties center around detection of potential or early illness and intervention in the process so that dysfunction and chronicity are avoided. Skillful medical processes prevent the disabling effects of the illness, identifying the illness as a crisis in itself, but preventing the complications and the residual effects which are the really dreaded aspects of a medical problem. Prevention at this level also insures that the life-style of the patient need not be significantly altered following the illness, unless, of course, such a change is desirable as a means of preventing further illness.

The third level of prevention is the area of rehabilitation. It has been in this realm that occupational therapy has traditionally contributed to health. Rehabilitation starts at the point where the patient is unable to recover all that he had previously, or is unable to attain the skills normally considered to be within the human potential. This level of care is directed toward preventing fixation and regression, loss of function and self-esteem. It may require that certain aspects of chronicity be accepted, but it denies that man is unable to better his lot, and must passively accept the aftereffects of illness or trauma.

Excellent suggestions for the kinds of occupational therapy services which can be developed in these three areas have been made by West[70,71] and Wiemer.[72]

"It might be argued that the responsibilities and judgment required by a program of preventive care, directed toward basic living conditions and social processes, constitute a higher level of professionalism than do programs based on the medical model. The professional is charged to view his society broadly and to develop services or philosophies which will help to improve the quality of that society. It does indeed seem unwise to be so involved in trying to undo the results of disease or social process that we forget to try to stop the problem at its source. Treatment requires skilled technics based on sound theory. Those same theories, in conjunction with an understanding of the social, economic and environmental issues facing mankind, might become the basis for a program of preventive services which could significantly raise the health standards of a community."[73]

Occupational therapy must move in the direction of identifying services which can be used in the continuum of preventive care. The directions were clearly stated by Dr. Adolph Meyer and have been echoed by thinking members of the profession ever since. The occupational therapy philosophy speaks directly to the ills of today's society. We must not lose the opportunity to provide leadership to those who seek to improve the quality of life and to destroy the influences which in turn destroy health. No other profession has such a history of concern for man's uniqueness as demonstrated through his productivity and the resulting state of health.

REFERENCES

1. Meyer, A.: The philosophy of occupational therapy. Arch. Occup. Therapy, 1:1, 1922.
2. Ibid., p. 5.
3. Ibid., p. 8.
4. Slagle, E. C.: Training aides for mental patients. Arch. Occup. Therapy, 1:11, 1922.
5. Ibid., p. 14.
6. Ibid., p. 15.
7. Haas, L. J.: Practical Occupational Therapy, ed. 2. Milwaukee, Bruce, 1946.
8. Marsh, L. C.: Shall we apply industrial psychiatry to psychiatry? Occup. Therapy and Rehab. 12:1, 1932.
9. Lang, H. B.: Additional functional values in occupational therapy. Occup. Therapy and Rehab., 17:317, 1938.
10. Wade, B. D.: Occupational Therapy for Patients with Mental Disease, In Willard, H. S., and Spackman, C. S.: Principles of Occupational Therapy, ed. 1. Philadelphia, Lippincott, 1947.
11. West, W. L.: Changing Concepts and Practices in Psychiatric Occupational Therapy. New York, American Occupational Therapy Association, 1959.
12. Frank, J.: Therapeutic use of self. Am. J. Occup. Therapy, 12:215, 1958.
13. Josselyn, I.: The Adolescent and His World. New York, Family Service Association of America, 1949.
14. Mosey, A. C.: Three Frames of Reference for Mental Health. Thorofare, New Jersey, C. B. Slack, 1970.
15. Occupational Therapy Manual on Administration, revised 1965. Kendall/ Hunt, Dubuque, Iowa.
16. Fidler, G. S., and Fidler, J. W.: Occupational Therapy: A Communication Process in Psychiatry. New York, Macmillan, 1963.
17. Chart developed for the American Occupational Therapy Association Regional Institutes of 1968, under Grant #123-T-68, Rehabilitation Services Administration.
18. Erikson, E. H.: Childhood and Society. New York, W. W. Norton, 1963.
19. Pearce, J., and Newton, S.: The Conditions of Human Growth. New York, Citadel Press, 1963.
20. Havighurst, R.: Developmental Tasks and Education. New York, McKay, 1952.

21. Gillette, N. P.: Changing methods in the treatment of psycho-social dysfunction. Am. J. Occup. Therapy, 21:230, 1967.
22. Azima, H., and Azima, F. J.: Outline of a dynamic theory of occupational therapy. Am. J. Occup. Therapy, 23:215, 1959.
23. Reilly, M.: The educational process. Am. J. Occup. Therapy, 23:299, 1969.
24. Diasio, K.: Psychiatric occupational therapy: search for a conceptual framework in light of psycho-analytic ego psychology and learning theory. Am. J. Occup. Therapy, 22:400, 1968.
25. Smith, A. R., and Tempone, V. J.: Psychiatric occupational therapy within a learning theory context. Am. J. Occup. Therapy, 22:415, 1968.
26. Watanabe, S.: Four concepts basic to the occupational therapy process. Am. J. Occup. Therapy, 22:439, 1968.
27. Mosey, A. C.: Recapitulation of ontogenesis: a theory for practice of occupational therapy. Am. J. Occup. Therapy, 22:426, 1968.
28. Mazer, June: Toward an integrated theory of occupational therapy. Am. J. Occup. Therapy, 22:451, 1968.
29. Fromm-Reichman, F.: Principles of Intensive Psychotherapy. University of Chicago Press, 1950.
30. Moorhead, L.: The occupational history. Am. J. Occup. Therapy, 23:329, 1969.
31. Richardson, S. A., Dohrenwend, B. S., and Klein, D.: Interviewing: Its Forms and Functions. New York, Basic Books, Inc., 1965.
32. Garrett, A.: Interviewing: Its Principles and Methods. New York, Family Service Association of America, 1964.
33. "Activity Configuration" was adapted by Sandra Watanabe from a form and an interview process developed by Richard Spahn of the Austin-Riggs Foundation, Stockbridge, Massachusetts, 1968.
34. Schad, C. J.: Occupational Therapy and Pediatrics, In Willard, H. S., and Spackman, C. S.: Occupational Therapy, ed. 3. Philadelphia, Lippincott, 1963.
35. Gesell, A. L., and Armatruda, C. S.: Developmental Diagnosis. New York, Hoeber, 1941.
36. Denver Developmental Screening Test, by Frankenburg, W. K., and Dodds, J. B. Denver, University of Colorado Medical Center, 1967.
37. Takata, N.: The Play History. Am. J. Occup. Therapy, 23:314, 1969.
38. Gillette, N. P.: Standardizing Observation Techniques through Available Occupational Therapy Media. Proceedings of the American Occupational Therapy Association Sub-Committee on Psychiatry, October, 1964.
39. Linn, L. S., Weinroth, L. A., and Shamak, R.: Occupational Therapy in Dynamic Psychiatry. Washington, D.C., American Psychiatric Association, 1962.
40. O'Kane, C. P.: The Development of a Projective Technique for Use in Psychiatric Occupational Therapy. Buffalo, State University of New York, 1968.
41. Shoemyen, C. W.: A study of procedure and media: occupational therapy orientation and evaluation. Am. J. Occup. Therapy, 24:276, 1970.
42. Anderson, H. H., and Anderson, G. L. (eds.): An Introduction to Projective Techniques. New York, Prentice-Hall, 1951.

43. Buck, J. N.: The House-Tree-Person Technique, revised manual. Beverly Hills, Western Psychological Services, 1966.
44. Frank, L. K.: Projective Methods. Springfield, Illinois, C. C Thomas, 1948.
45. Hammer, E. F. (ed.): The Clinical Application of Projective Drawings. Springfield, Illinois, C. C Thomas, 1958.
46. Machover, K. A.: Personality Projection in the Drawing of the Human Figure: A Method of Personality Investigation, ed. 1. Springfield, Illinois, C. C Thomas, 1949.
47. Alexander, F.: The dynamics of psychotherapy in the light of learning theory. Am. J. Psychiatry, 120:440, 1963.
48. Ibid., p. 445.
49. Redlich, F. C., and Freedman, D. X.: The Theory and Practice of Psychiatry. New York, Basic Books, Inc., 1966.
50. Shimota, H. E.: Psychiatric occupational therapy. Am. J. Occup. Therapy, 19:79, 1965.
51. Bockoven, J. S.: Challenge of the new clinical approaches. Am. J. Occup. Therapy, 22:23, 1968.
52. Shannon, P. D.: The work-play model: a basis for occupational therapy programming in psychiatry. Am. J. Occup. Therapy, 24:215, 1970. 1970.
53. Small, L.: The Briefer Psychotherapies. New York, Brunner/Mazel, 1971.
54. Becker, E.: The Revolution in Psychiatry. New York, The Free Press of Glencoe, 1964.
55. White, R. W.: Ego and Reality in Psychoanalytic Theory: A Proposal Regarding Independent Ego Energies. Psychological Issues, Vol. III, No. 3, Monograph 11. New York, International Universities Press, Inc., 1963.
56. Ibid., p. 131.
57. Hyman, M., and Metzker, J.: Occupational therapy in an emergency psychiatric setting. Am. J. Occup. Therapy, 24:280, 1970.
58. Fidler, G. S.: unpublished statement, The Philosophy and Structure of the Activities Therapy Department, Hillside (New York) Hospital. 1969.
59. Mosey, A. C.: The concept and use of developmental groups. Am. J. Occup. Therapy, 24:272, 1970.
60. Fidler, G. S.: The task-oriented group as a context for treatment. Am. J. Occup. Therapy, 23:43, 1969.
61. Gillette, N., and Mayer, P.: Draft for a planned monograph on group processes for occupational therapists. 1966.
62. Matsutsuyu, J. S.: The interest check list. Am. J. Occup. Therapy, 23:323, 1969.
63. Ibid., p. 326.
64. Haun, P.: Recreation: A Medical Viewpoint. New York, Bureau of Publications, Teachers College, Columbia University, 1968.
65. Florey, L. L.: Intrinsic motivation: the dynamics of occupational therapy theory. Am. J. Occup. Therapy, 23:319, 1969.
66. Ibid., p. 321.
67. Shannon, P. D.: Work adjustment and the adolescent soldier. Am. J. Occup. Therapy, 24:111, 1970.

68. Shannon, P. D., in a book review published in American Journal of Occupational Therapy, *23*:350, 1969, of Work and Human Behavior, by W. S. Neff, New York, Atherton Press, 1968.
69. Fidler, G. S.: A second look at work as a primary force in rehabilitation and treatment. Am. J. Occup. Therapy, *20*:72, 1966.
70. West, W. L.: The growing importance of prevention. Am. J. Occup. Therapy, *23*:226, 1969.
71. West, W. L.: Professional responsibility in times of change. Am. J. Occup. Therapy, *22*:9, 1968.
72. Wiemer, R. B.: Some Concepts of Prevention as an Aspect of Community Health: A Foundation for Development of the Occupational Therapist's Role. Paper presented at the Annual Conference of the American Occupational Therapy Association, New York, November, 1970.
73. Gillette, N. P.: Occupational Therapy Belongs in the Community. Paper presented to The World Federation of Occupational Therapists, Zurich, Switzerland, June, 1970.

6

Occupational Therapy as a Supportive Measure

CLARE S. SPACKMAN, M.S., O.T.R.

Occupational therapy may be used as a supportive measure. Its purpose is to act as a psychic cushion and to help the patient to adjust to his stay in a hospital, convalescent or nursing home. For many patients enforced idleness, unfamiliar routine and surroundings, separation from their families and worry over their own physical condition cause a state of anxiety. This may be increased by apprehensiveness as to the future. Such anxiety may retard recovery. For those patients whose illness is psychosomatic in origin, occupational therapy is one of the most important means of treatment. A program of activity guided by a skilled occupational therapist can help the patient in his adjustment. Even more important is the interpersonal relationship between the occupational therapist and the patient, which in itself is therapeutic. The importance of the psychological aspects of illness cannot be overemphasized.

Of all phases of occupational therapy a supportive program offers the greatest challenge to the therapist and requires the greatest medical knowledge and understanding of the patient's psychological reactions both to his illness and to treatment. Medicine today is a constantly changing field. Methods of treatment learned 2 years ago are frequently obsolete. The therapist must be continually alert to such changes, modifying the program of occupational therapy accordingly.

Occupational therapy may be used as a supportive measure for a number of different types of patients, such as geriatric cases and those persons hospitalized or homebound by chronic diseases, as well as those in a general hospital.

Occupational therapy as a supportive procedure helps the patient to use his period of convalescence constructively and helps to prepare him for return to normal activities or for transfer to an intensive program of rehabilitation. The objectives may be divided into two categories: psychological and physical.

OBJECTIVES

Psychological:

To help the patient to adjust to hospitalization and to his illness.
To aid in alleviating worry and distress.
To maintain and to stimulate normal interests and social contacts.
To give an outlet for irritation and resentment.
To divert the mind from concentrating on the physical functioning of the body.
To assess vocational potentials when indicated.

Physical:

To aid in inducing sleep through controlled fatigue.
To provide an outlet for restlessness.
To aid in preventing contractures by provision of special splints.
To improve circulation and muscle tone.
To maintain correct posture in bed or chair.
To maintain and/or to develop general physical strength.
To aid in preparing the patient for ambulation.
To teach activities of daily living when indicated.

MEDICAL REFERRAL

The physician, in referring patients for occupational therapy, should select only those who are in need of a medically directed, planned program of activity. The types of patients most often in need of this are long-term cases (those hospitalized for 3 or more weeks and not acutely ill); those with psychological problems or with illness of psychosomatic origin; those needing special services such as activities of daily living or adapted equipment; and, in some instances, terminal cases when such a program can do much to ease both the patient and his family.

PLANNING AN OCCUPATIONAL THERAPY PROGRAM

The occupational therapist in planning a program must consider first the patient's psychological needs. However, any program to meet these needs must consider also the medical aspects of the case. The physician's referral should state both psychological and physical objectives to be achieved and precautions to be observed, adapted equipment or special splints needed. However, it is the therapist's responsibility to read the patient's medical chart carefully, so that the fullest possible knowledge of the patient and his condition may be obtained. The patient's psychological reaction to hospitalization and to his illness is of prime importance. Much additional information may be gathered from the nursing staff and the social worker, but the occupational therapist must observe the patient's behavior and attitude carefully as treatment continues.

Major Medical Points To Be Considered in Planning the Program:

1. The diagnosis, if known. Some patients are hospitalized for observation and diagnosis.
2. The usual symptoms and those which the patient has or may develop.
3. The usual course of the disease or injury. If the therapist does not know this, it must be ascertained by reading or by discussion with the patient's doctor.
4. The complications which may occur, such as cardiac involvement or infection.
5. The medical treatment and medications being given or diagnostic studies being done, such as sedatives or antibiotics; intravenous feedings or lumbar punctures.
6. Other services with which occupational therapy must be coordinated, such as nursing, physical therapy, social case work, school.
7. Other medical conditions of the patient, such as allergies, defective vision or diabetes.
8. Precautions and limitations, such as the position in which the patient must remain, limitations on activity or the posture of the patient.
9. The prognosis. Is complete recovery expected? Will there be a prolonged convalescence? Will there be permanent limitations of activity?

In addition to the medical aspects certain other points must also be considered, such as the patient's sex, age, marital status, educational background and mental ability.

In selecting an activity to suggest to the patient the therapist should ask himself the following questions:

1. Is it suitable only to meet the patient's immediate needs or will it be of value to him during convalescence or in the total rehabilitation plan?

2. Is it within the scope of the patient's mental and/or manual ability?
3. Will it interest the patient?
4. Is it within his financial means to continue at home?
5. Is it suitable for the patient to do in bed, on the ward, or in the clinic? Will it disturb the other patients?
6. How much of the activity can the patient do himself? Can he do at least 4/5th of it?
7. Is it within the prescribed physical limitations?

TYPES OF ACTIVITIES

The activities which may be used to meet the patient's needs are many and varied. For patients confined to bed, with only limited activity permitted, adapted games, guided reading or study, or light hand skills may be used. A program which combines recreation, study and manual activity will provide a better-rounded routine than one alone.

The greatest challenge comes when the patient is extremely limited in activity and has a prolonged period of hospitalization. Such cases will require the greatest degree of ingenuity and imagination on the part of the therapist. If possible, such patients should be stimulated to undertake intellectual or educational pursuits.

For patients who will need to use crutches for ambulation, the occupational therapy program may supplement that of physical therapy in order to strengthen the muscles of the shoulder, the arm and the hand. Such activities as leather punching, which places pressure on the hyperthenar eminence and develops grasp, are excellent.

Instruction in activities of daily living should be considered for all patients who may return home in a cast or are unable to use a leg or an arm, even if for only a few weeks. Simple adapted equipment, such as a small cardboard box used as a card holder, or a table with casters may greatly assist a convalescent patient. Too often such assistance is given only to the severely disabled, while the housewife with a fractured ankle in a cast is ignored because it is a temporary handicap.

For patients with cardiac conditions or other disabilities which will impose permanent restriction on activity, instruction in methods of work simplification is indicated. If the patient's interest can be aroused, this can be a fascinating subject to study and one which is primarily an intellectual pursuit. Any busy mother, with many household duties would profit by an introduction to work simplification, even though she may have no limitation on activity.

Any activity to be done in bed should in most instances be such that it does not interfere with the nursing routine; it should not stain the bed clothes, as may oil paint or shellac; it should not leave chips or pieces in the bed; and it should not disturb other patients in the room. A prolonged period in bed is an excellent time in which to learn touchtyping. It is a useful accomplishment which may enhance the patient's employability, yet the noise of the typewriter may be exceedingly annoying to the patient in the next bed. A small portable sewing machine may be operated easily in bed and usually does not irritate persons nearby.

PROGRAMS FOR DIFFERENT GROUPS OF PATIENTS

Programs planned for different groups of patients may vary considerably. The program for the patient who will make a rapid recovery need meet only his immediate needs. The patient who will have a prolonged convalescence at home should learn to do a number of practical projects with which he can continue his program after discharge from the hospital. He should be taught how to start and finish projects and should be given written directions and sources for the purchase of supplies and tools. In planning such a home program careful consideration must be given to the patient's ability and financial status and to the home itself. The plan for an entire day should be discussed with him. Household activities about the home should be included in the program whenever possible.

The chronically ill patient who will remain a semi-invalid when at home needs to have the same type of program. However, greater stress should be laid on doing household activities and on adhering to a regular daily schedule. Any projects which can be sold either in the neighborhood or at an outlet should be encouraged, since even a small sum of money may do much to improve the patient's morale. Emphasis also should be placed on the development of an inexpensive hobby.

A few patients while still in the hospital will need prevocational evaluation and/or a vocationally oriented program. Every effort should be made to recognize this need as early as possible and to meet it.

THE APPROACH TO THE HOSPITAL PATIENT

The approach to the hospital patient is often simplified if the therapist has been treating other patients in the ward or a semiprivate room, or if the referral is made on rounds. In each instance the therapist should first read the patient's medical chart carefully and should discuss the case with the nurse when feasible. The therapist should introduce himself to the patient, stating that the doctor has ordered occupational therapy. As the patient rarely knows what occupational therapy is, an explanation suited to his comprehension will need to be given. The therapist will have to talk with him to find out his interests and problems and to judge his ability. This is essentially an initial interview, and interview technics should be used accordingly.

The first impression which the patient receives is of the therapist's personal appearance, his voice and manner. The well-groomed, confident therapist who shows a warm personal interest in the patient and takes time to explain will have little difficulty with approach.

Guidelines for Working With Patients in Bed or on the Ward:

The therapist should keep in mind the following points:

1. Know the other treatments that the patient is receiving and fit occupational therapy into his schedule. Do not interrupt other treatments.
2. Know when visitors are allowed or expected and do not visit the patient at that time.
3. Be punctual in keeping appointments. Keep promises that have been made and do not make promises that cannot be kept.
4. Respect confidences but report important ones to the appropriate authority.
5. Be impersonally personal, tolerant and tactful.
6. Be able to talk interestingly if the patient prefers to listen, but be a good listener if he prefers to talk. Adjust conversation to the patient's interests. Avoid controversial subjects, such as race, religion or politics.
7. Speak clearly but in a low voice.
8. Show interest in the patient and in what he is doing or is planning to do.
9. Address the adult patient by his correct title and last name. Exceptions may be made according to custom. Show respect to elderly patients.
10. At all times behave professionally to the patient and to other hospital personnel.
11. Encourage the patient's confidence in his doctor and in other hospital personnel.
12. Avoid letting the patient talk continually about his illness. Do not discuss depressing or morbid subjects with him.
13. Avoid showing reactions of alarm, of horror or of sorrow.
14. Avoid hitting or jarring the bed. Do not sit on it, or interfere with special adjustments. Do not lay your own things on the bed or on the patient's bedside table.
15. Observe aseptic technics when indicated and sterilize occupational therapy equipment used.
16. Watch for signs of fatigue and do not stay too long, thus overtiring the patient.

17. Do not force an activity on the patient, but rather consider why he refuses it and what would be of interest to him.
18. Do not give the patient medication, water or anything to eat. Do not interfere in the nursing routine.
19. Do not take the patient from the ward without the doctor's permission and the nurses' knowledge.

Great responsibility rests on the therapist to check daily on the patient's condition so that the activities can be stopped or graded as may be indicated. Although the physician originally refers the patient, he rarely indicates changes. It is the therapist's responsibility to contact the physician when needed and to keep him informed by progress notes on the patient's medical chart, as well as by reports on rounds.

PLAN OF A TREATMENT PROGRAM

An occupational therapy program for a patient is made by listing the objectives of treatment and how the therapist plans to achieve them. For example: Mrs. X is a 65-year-old housewife hospitalized because of a coronary infarction. In addition to her cardiac condition she has limited vision due to cataracts. She will be in the hospital 6 weeks and then is planning to return home to her apartment. Her husband, who is 70, can help her with marketing and heavier housework.

Objectives:

1. To provide an activity to lessen her apprehensiveness. She is fearful that she will never recover sufficiently so as not to be a burden on her husband.
2. To help her to learn how to keep house, using the minimum of physical effort, and to help her to regain her confidence in her ability to do it.
3. When she is ambulatory, to have her practice cooking and other activities in the kitchen in the occupational therapy clinic.
4. To have her work out with her husband rearrangements of shelves and furniture in their apartment in order to conserve energy.

Program:

1. The patient is to be started on knitting 6″ squares for a baby blanket for her new granddaughter. This will require little use of her arms. She has done knitting previously and should be able to do it in spite of her limited vision. She has not tried to knit for several years.
2. Her husband is to be asked to bring in the floor plan of their apartment with the furniture and the doors drawn to scale. The

therapist is to discuss with the patient those household activities which will be too heavy and to help her work out ways of making the housework lighter. She is to be introduced to methods of work simplification to conserve energy.

3. After she is ambulatory she is to go to the occupational therapy clinic to try out the methods discussed in doing housework. This should give her confidence upon discharge.

4. Her husband is to come to visit her and the occupational therapist in the clinic to see the kitchen and discuss adaptations which can be made at home. The patient, her husband and the therapist are to discuss the problems and to plan what he can do to help, such as doing the marketing or running the vacuum cleaner.

5. Upon discharge the patient is to come to the occupational therapy department upon her first visit to the cardiac outpatient clinic 2 weeks later. Then the therapist will give further advice if necessary.

TYPES OF CONDITIONS TREATED

The various types of disorders that the occupational therapist is called upon to treat or which are complicating secondary conditions demand some particular knowledge, special precautions and some understanding of psychosomatic medicine. While no scientific classification of physical disorders is attempted here, for the convenience of the student, most of them are placed in one of the three following classes: medical, surgical and neurological. Orthopedic, ophthalmologic, and bronchoscopic conditions are presented separately.

OCCUPATIONAL THERAPY FOR MEDICAL CONDITIONS

Cardiac Conditions

Occupational therapy is frequently used prior to and following cardiac surgery and with patients who have rheumatic heart disease or coronary infarctions, arteriosclerosis and hypertension.

Most patients can return to a normal life with possible restrictions on competitive sports and limitations on lifting or stair-climbing. Many can return to their former jobs. Others will need retraining in jobs within their limitations. For all patients the development of an interest in a sedentary type of hobby can greatly increase the breadth of their interests and aid in their adjustment to restrictions.

Exercise within the limits specified by the patient's physician is essential in the management of a cardiac case. However, most patients fail to interpret the meaning of "light work." The therapist can be of assistance in planning with the patient a daily routine to be followed upon discharge.

For patients who will have a permanent limitation of activity, instruction in methods of work simplification and/or home-making is most helpful. The American Heart Association provides assistance and publishes excellent material which should be of help to these patients. This can usually be obtained through the local chapter of the Association.

In planning a program for a patient with a cardiac condition the therapist should be fully aware of the patient's present condition and prognosis. The program may be graded to activities requiring increased motion and strength, but only under the supervision of the patient's physician. Signs of fatigue for which the therapist should watch are increased pulse rate, dyspnea and palpitation.

Frequently the patient is first seen when on complete bed rest. It should be noted that if the head of the bed is kept so that the patient is in a sitting position, it is not necessarily an indication of improvement. The sitting position requires the least effort on the part of the heart. It is a safe rule that, if occupational therapy is ordered for such a patient, the program should be limited to fingertip, intellectual or passive activities with frequent rest periods. Motion of the elbows and the shoulders is contraindicated. Activities such as leather-tooling, copper-tooling and link-belts, although requiring a limited range of motion, use too much strength and pressure. Passive activities such as reading, listening to music, or selected radio and television programs may be of great value. Light activities such as sketching, writing or crossword puzzles may be used.

Patients who are on extremely limited activity as described in the previous paragraph are referred to occupational therapy because their anxiety and fear may prevent the needed rest. Closely supervised activity can and does relieve this situation.

As the patient improves, a program of gradually increased activity will enable him to regain strength and confidence. It will also help him to learn to judge his own limitations and need for rest. The patient who develops cardiac neurosis presents a serious problem. Activity started early can do much to prevent the development of such a condition.

Metabolic Disorders

Diabetes. Some diabetic patients who are hospitalized for standardization may be referred to occupational therapy. Nonstandardized diabetics are more prone to infection than other persons. Any cuts or abrasions occurring while in the occupational therapy clinic should be reported to the charge nurse for first aid.

Diabetic patients hospitalized for other medical conditions are apt to become unstandardized. Therefore, precautions should be taken against infection as stated above. It is more often the patient hospitalized for complications of his diabetic condition who is referred to occupational therapy.

A patient who has had diabetes for a number of years may develop circulatory problems resulting in ulcers and ultimately in gangrene, particularly of the feet and the legs. Prolonged hospitalization often is needed to heal these, and amputation may be necessary. As most diabetics are well aware of the possible outcome, the patient is apprehensive. Any program of activity which will help to distract his mind from his fears is of marked benefit.

If amputation is necessary and it is impossible for the patient to wear a prosthesis, or if it will be some time before he can be fitted for one, assistance and instruction in activities of daily living are indicated. If the patient is a housewife, instruction in homemaking, using crutches or a wheelchair, is most helpful.

Gastrointestinal Conditions

Gastrointestinal conditions may be divided into two groups: (1) those in which the cause is primarily physical in origin and (2) those in which the cause is primarily psychosomatic. In the latter group, although the cause is emotional, the resulting gastrointestinal disturbances produce organic changes, frequently serious in nature and requiring surgical procedures.

Intestinal Obstructions. A patient with intestinal obstructions usually comes into the hospital for observation, tending to be in a fair physical condition on admission but often following a downward course. This should be considered in planning the occupational therapy program so that it will remain within his physical capabilities. Fatigue should be avoided. Usually these cases are treated surgically.

Hepatitis. An infection involving the liver, may be due to various causes (e.g., homologous serum hepatitis or infectious hepatitis). The latter is usually on isolation, and aseptic technics should be observed. The common symptoms are jaundice, loss of appetite, nausea and vomiting. The hepatitis patient in the acute stage is on bed rest for approximately 3 to 4 weeks and should be given only light activities permitting frequent rest periods. Usually, there is a convalescent period of approximately 3 to 4 weeks, during which his program should be graded according to the changes in his physical condition. Activities involving the use of odorous materials, such as oil paints, turpentine and lacquer, should be avoided.

Psychosomatic Factors. Gastrointestinal conditions commonly considered as being psychosomatic in origin are peptic ulcers, ileitis, colitis and ulcerative colitis.

These cases tend to occur in late adolescence but may develop at any time. Frequently, the patient is immature and has no outlets for his anxiety and hostility other than physical reactions which affect the gastrointestinal tract. When seen in the hospital, in most instances he is suffering from marked debility and is depressed and tearful. Frequently, he is unwilling to undertake new activities for fear of failure. Essentially, he needs both absorbing and creative outside interests, yet he cannot focus his attention on anything but himself.

The treatment for these cases may include psychotherapy as well as medical and surgical methods. The program of occupational therapy should be planned to relieve emotional tension by offering an outlet for anxiety and hostility. Creative activities help the patient to develop another means of self-expression and to divert his mind from thinking only of his physical reactions.

Malignancies — Cancer and Sarcoma

As cancer may affect any part of the body and may occur at any age, it is impossible to give specific precautions. It should be noted that cancer patients are found on all services in the hospital. At no time should the therapist indicate to the patient that he has cancer. It is the physician's decision as to how much the patient should be told. In most instances surgery is indicated, but the patient may be hospitalized for radiologic treatment as well as surgery, or both. The patient is often referred to occupational therapy postoperatively. Terminal cases are also given occupational therapy, when it will be of assistance to them and their families.

In cases of sarcoma which affects the bones, amputation of the affected part is the usual treatment. These cases will need occupational therapy to maintain morale and for activities of daily living. If use of a prosthesis is feasible, they will be referred at a later date for training in the use of the upper extremity prosthesis.

The program for these cases must be geared to meet their psychological need and to aid them as much as possible to adjust to their condition and prognosis. As patients react differently to different forms of medical treatment, the therapist must observe each and arrange the occupational therapy program accordingly.

Rheumatoid Arthritis

Although occupational therapy is more often ordered for the arthritic patient to maintain or to restore function, an "active" case may be referred not for exercise but for a supportive program. Care must be taken to select activities for this patient so that only the noninvolved joints are used. The patient tires easily and often is depressed and fearful of activity because of the resulting pain. A program which encourages intellectual as well as manual and recreational activity is indicated, since many of these patients will have long periods of convalescence or may be permanently limited in activity. The therapist may be asked to make hand splints to prevent deformity.

Respiratory Conditions

Asthma, emphysema, cancer, tuberculosis, silicosis, sarcoidosis, lung abscess, chronic bronchitis and bronchiectasis make up this group. During the acute stages of disease, occupational therapy is contraindicated, but during convalescence it can be beneficial. Gradual resistance to fatigue can be developed, depression prevented, circulation improved, and adjustment to the disability made. The choice of materials to work with is perhaps the most important single factor here, as nothing must be used that is irritating to the respiratory passages. The use of certain materials, such as strong acids, paints, cotton and kapok, should be avoided. Occupational therapy for patients with these conditions may include redirection of avocational interests, prevocational evaluation, and energy saving techniques. Many of these patients are also elderly and have secondary conditions such as arthritis and cardiovascular or neuromuscular disorders.

Dermatologic Conditions

Many dermatologic disorders are merely the symptoms of a disease and as such are not infectious. Occupational therapy for patients suffering from skin diseases is of definite psychological value, because many of these diseases are disfiguring as well as painful. Often the hands are affected so badly that patients are unable to do much except read or tune in the radio or the television. This furnishes a fine opportunity to help the patient outline a constructive educational and recreational program through passive activity. If the hands are well enough to be used, the materials employed must be nonirritating. Patients with scleroderma may require graded occupational activities to help prevent contractures of the joints or to stretch them, particularly in the hands. Impetigo, scabies and ringworm are infectious and precautions should be taken against their spread.

Blood Conditions

Anemia, leukemia, hemophilia and Hodgkin's disease come under this classification.

With this entire group of patients there should be strict precautions to prevent cuts, abrasions or injury of any kind, especially in the case of the hemophiliac. Symptoms of most blood ailments are exhaustion, rapid pulse, shortness of breath, weakness, dizziness and a general slowing up in physical activities; leukemia, by enlarged glands; Hodgkin's disease, by enlarged lymph nodes. Mild and graded activities affording mental stimulus are provided for these patients through the use of arts and crafts, recreation, music and reading.

Surgical Conditions

Surgery may be divided into several categories: general, chest, neurologic, orthopedic, gynecologic, proctologic, ophthalmologic, otolaryngologic, bronchoscopic and plastic surgery. In many instances the general surgeon may work with a number of these, but in a large city hospital each is a specialty in itself.

Many patients hospitalized for surgery may be in the hospital only a few days. Others may need occupational therapy as a supportive measure prior to surgery as well as following it. Some patients will have prolonged periods of hospitalization following surgery because of immobilization in a cast, amputation of a part, plastic surgery or neurosurgery. The precautions for and the aims of occupational therapy will differ, depending on the reason for and the type of surgery done as well as on the patient's age and on his condition prior to surgery. Maintenance of morale is of vital importance.

In no instance should the occupational therapist, who has been treating the patient prior to surgery, resume treatment without the permission of the surgeon or without ascertaining whether there are special precautions to be observed. In cases when the patient is in traction or when he must maintain a special position, care must be taken not to interfere with the apparatus and to insist that the position be maintained while he is receiving occupational therapy.

Patients undergoing surgery for gastrointestinal conditions may profit greatly by a well coordinated program of occupational therapy. The psychosomatic factors involved should be considered carefully, and all treatment plans discussed with the physician and the social worker.

A patient's psychological reaction to serious burns may be extreme. The burned patient worries about his appearance and his economic and social adjustment. When skin grafting is necessary, the process may be prolonged, and during this period the patient needs encouragement and reassurance. When burns involve several joints, the first object of occupational therapy is to help overcome the secondary stiffness resulting from immobilization; the next is to help bring about a gradual stretching of the primary contracture. The stretching must not be abrupt, since the scar tissue and the new skin are sensitive and must not be torn or irritated; special splints are often indicated for hand cases. The materials used in therapeutic activities must be smooth and nonirritating.

Neurologic Conditions

Epilepsy, brain injuries, encephalitis, muscular dystrophy and multiple sclerosis belong in this category.

In some hospitals patients with neuroses or mild psychoses are treated on the neurologic service. In others they are on a separate psychiatric service. If the patient is on the neurologic service the occupational therapist should obtain specific instruction from his physician regarding precautions to be observed.

The patient when first seen by the occupational therapist may have been admitted for diagnostic studies. Occupational therapy for this type of patient may be of great value as he is frequently afraid, and many of the tests are unpleasant.

Patients with neurologic conditions may be classified into two groups: (1) those with a temporary condition from which they will recover, such as concussion or Guillain-Barré syndrome; and (2) those with a progressive disease such as muscular dystrophy or Parkinson's disease.

Patients with nonprogressive conditions benefit from a well-rounded program. Consideration must be given by the therapist to the patient's symptoms, such as pain, loss of muscle power and incoordination. Some of this group may be referred for specific treatment to improve physical function. The precautions to be observed will depend on the patient's condition and symptoms.

In progressive conditions such as multiple sclerosis or muscular dystrophy, if seen early in onset, the patient will need primarily a supportive program. His psychological reaction to his condition is of prime importance. It is essential to help him to continue normal activity in order to prevent disuse disability and to retain normal muscular action insofar as possible. Assistance in activities of daily living may be indicated, especially if his reaction to his disease is to give up. In actuality he often can continue to lead a normal life for many years. The treatment of these conditions in order to improve or to maintain physical function is covered in Chapter 7.

More severely involved patients with marked limitations need a program geared to meet their progressive condition and to help them to maintain a positive attitude toward life.

Patients with epilepsy, if the occurrence of the seizures is unpredictable, and if they take place during the daytime, should not be given activities requiring tools or equipment with which they might hurt themselves or others. Patients with frequent and severe seizures often appear dazed and retarded. These symptoms may disappear once the seizures are controlled. However, some patients, due to the drugs used, are slow in reaction and are drowsy. The patient's psychological reactions and fears must always be considered by the therapist in planning his approach. The importance of developing appropriate recreational interests and of providing proper vocational guidance cannot be over-emphasized.

The physical rehabilitation of patients with hemiplegia, paraplegia, and quadriplegia is discussed in Chapters 11 and 10. However, these patients may be referred for a supportive program prior to referral for physical rehabilitation. Patients should be encouraged to use the non-affected parts, be given assistive devices when indicated and be en-couraged to perform the normal activities of daily living. Every effort should be made to provide a program which will maintain the patient's normal interests and, if possible, develop new ones compatible with his probable permanent handicap. Care should be taken to assure that the patient maintains the correct position in bed or wheelchair, to prevent contractures or pressure sores. Hemiplegic cases may show signs of con-fusion and may have aphasia. In the early treatment of cases with aphasia prior to the beginning of speech therapy, conversation with the patient should be in the form of questions which can be answered with a nod of the head or by simple words within his ability. The therapist should ascertain, if possible, whether the patient understands what is said to him.

The patient's psychological reaction to his condition will vary, de-pending on his realization of the degree of probable handicap, his pre-vious emotional adjustment and his philosophy of life. Anything that can help to promote or maintain a good psychological adjustment is invaluable.

Tumors of the brain and the spinal cord usually are transferred to the neurosurgical service. These may first be referred for occupational ther-apy by the neurologic service while the diagnosis is still undetermined. The precautions indicated depend on the existing symptoms. A patient with a brain tumor may have severe headaches and vomiting, diplopia, or a decrease in visual acuity. Following surgery, the occupational ther-apist may be asked to visit the patient regularly, even though no planned program of activity is yet feasible. Most cases in the first week postoperatively will have some degree of aphasia, confusion, visual disturbance and muscle incoordination. These symptoms usually are transient. In many instances the prognosis for life is poor. This does not relieve the occupational therapist of the responsibility for instructing the patient or his family in activities of daily living and for providing simple adapted equipment which will do much to ease his last months of life and will greatly relieve the family situation. A patient with a tumor of the spinal cord will have resulting paralysis, either flaccid or spastic or both, and often this grows increasingly worse. The achievement of even limited activity is most encouraging to the patient. Following surgery, the recovery may be very rapid, or there may be a residual handicap needing physical rehabilitation.

Cases of concussion and/or fracture of the skull may have symptoms of postconcussion syndrome for some time. These usually include dizziness, especially on stooping, headache, difficulty in concentration, and irritability. The occupational therapy program must be graded carefully so as not to overfatigue the patient and increase his symptoms. At times the patient is depressed because of the slowness of recovery.

Herniated intervertebral discs are frequently referred for occupational therapy both in the period of establishing the diagnosis and during conservative treatment when the patient is on bed rest and may be in traction. These cases may be on either the neurologic or the orthopedic service. Activities which increase pain, or interfere with the prescribed position should be avoided. When the patient becomes ambulatory, emphasis on correct posture is essential. These patients are usually referred as outpatients for physical rehabilitation.

OCCUPATIONAL THERAPY FOR SPECIAL CONDITIONS

Orthopedic Conditions

Patients with traumatic injuries, disease, or deformities of the musculoskeletal system are treated on this service. Examples are: fractures, strains, dislocations, tuberculosis of the bone, sarcoma, scoliosis and other deformities.

Patients with orthopedic conditions are referred to occupational therapy for a supportive program because of the need of maintaining a positive outlook during long periods of inactivity.

Ophthalmologic Conditions

A number of patients are referred for occupational therapy with conditions of the eyes, such as glaucoma, cataracts, detached retinas or traumatic injuries. These do not necessarily lead to blindness but may do so. In such cases activities are indicated which will increase the sense of touch and will be of value should the patient become blind. Examples of these are touch-typing and manual activities which require the patient to distinguish between different sizes and textures. If the patient's eyes are bandaged, with the doctor's permission he should be encouraged to carry out normal activities of daily living such as eating, dressing, and walking around the room or the ward. Special instruction may be necessary. The Talking Book, a special long-playing phonograph, which reads aloud to the patient may be a comfort to persons accustomed to reading. Precautions with eye cases are to permit use of the eyes only when indicated.

The patient's psychological reaction to his condition may result in marked restlessness, irritability, resentment and depression. Fear of blindness is a predominating factor, though often not admitted. The therapist should be careful in his approach, being sure to identify himself each time. He should select and teach activities well within the patient's ability to accomplish.

The treatment of the newly blinded is discussed in Chapter 16. For instruction technics see Chapter 4.

Bronchoscopic Conditions

A number of hospitals have a bronchoscopic service on which patients are treated for such conditions as strictures of the esophagus and trachea, and cancer of the larynx. Many of these patients are long-term cases who need a supportive program. Patients with strictures of the esophagus are usually tube-fed, and no food or liquid may be taken orally. Patients with tracheotomies should be watched for need of aspiration. Dust and lint should be avoided.

BIBLIOGRAPHY

Allison, R. D.: The screening approach to cardiopulmonary disease. Am. J. Occup. Therapy 34:3, 1970.

Appleby, L., Morton, J. E. C., Lawson, R. A., Loudon, R. G., and Brown, J.: Toward a therapeutic community in a tuberculosis hospital. Am. J. Occup. Therapy 14:117, 1960.

Arthritis Special Issues. Am. J. Occup. Therapy 19:125, 243, 1965.

Berzins, G. F.: An occupational therapy program for the chronic obstructive pulmonary disease patient. Am. J. Occup. Therapy 34:3, 1970.

Choren, B. G.: The initial interview as a treatment procedure in occupational therapy. Am. J. Occup. Therapy 13:88,92, 1959.

Deissler, K. J.: The psychosomatic approach in prescribing occupational therapy. Am. J. Occup. Therapy 10:240, 1956.

Feallock, B.: Dermatomyositis: a case study. Am. J. Occup. Therapy 19:279, 1965.

Gellman, W.: Attitudes toward rehabilitation of the disabled. Am. J. Occup. Therapy 14:188, 1960.

Gilbert, D. C.: Energy expenditures for the disabled homemaker: review of studies. Am. J. Occup. Therapy 19:321, 1965.

Gregg, J. R., and Sherrill, S. S.: Eye problems of aging patients. Am. J. Occup. Therapy 11:313, 1957.

Hagen, Sister M. P.: Nursing home residents: a challenge to the occupational therapist. Am. J. Occup. Therapy 21:151, 1967.

Hendrickson, D., Anderson, J., and Gordon, E.: A physiological approach to the regulation of activity in the cardiac convalescent. Am. J. Occup. Therapy 14:292, 1960.

Institute: The patient's point of view. Am. J. Occup. Therapy 10:181, 1956.

Jensen, I.: The occupational therapist in a home care program. Am. J. Occup. Therapy 20:298, 1966.

Johnson, A. M.: The adolescent and his problems. Am. J. Occup. Therapy 11:255, 1957.

Kaplan, A. S.: Rehabilitation in chronic obstructive pulmonary disease. Am. J. Occup. Therapy 34:3, 1970.

Kovell, J.: A home care program. Am. J. Occup. Therapy 18:255, 1964.

Lakin, M., and Dray, M.: The psychological aspects of activity for the aged. Am. J. Occup. Therapy 12:172, 1958.

Myerson, L.: Some observations on the psychological role of the occupational therapist. Am. J. Occup. Therapy 11:131, 1957.

Newman, L. B., Wasserman, R. R., and Borden, C.: Productive living for those with heart disease: the role of physical medicine and rehabilitation. Arch. Phys. Med. & Rehab., 37:137, 1956.

Roberts, S. W.: Occupational therapy for the chronically ill. Am. J. Occup. Therapy 14:171, 1960.

Walker, A. D.: A treatment program for rheumatoid arthritis. Am. J. Occup. Therapy 14:209, 1960.

7

Occupational Therapy for the Restoration of Physical Function

CLARE S. SPACKMAN, M.S., O.T.R.

In the restoration of physical function the value of occupational therapy lies in the patient's mental and physical involvement in a constructive activity which provides the needed exercise and helps to develop normal use of the part. Therapeutic exercise lies in the province of physical therapy.

Occupational therapy is utilized extensively in treating patients with residual disabilities following disease or injury. Its aims are to restore physical function insofar as possible; to help the patient to adjust to and/or compensate for loss of function; to help to prepare the patient upon discharge to lead a normal life and, if of employable age, to return to gainful employment.

As indicated by the physician's referral the treatment program should be planned to achieve one or more of the following objectives:

1. Increase of coordination, muscle strength and endurance
2. Increase of range of motion of affected joints
3. Retraining in activities of daily living
4. Development of work tolerance
5. Prevocational evaluation

The patient's psychological reaction to his residual disability must be given as much consideration in planning the treatment program as is given to the selection of the activities which provide the needed exercise. The goal set for the patient to achieve serves as a guide to the therapist.

TYPES OF RESIDUAL DISABILITIES TREATED AND OBJECTIVES OF TREATMENT

Limitation of motion in a joint or joints

This may be due to injury to or to changes in the structure of the joint. For example, any of the following may produce limitation: contractures of the muscles and the tendons passing over the joint and/or contractures of the joint capsule and the ligaments; adhesions of the tendons, the ligaments and the joint capsule; excess callus formation or faulty alignment of bones following fractures; scar tissue over the area of the joint. The motion of the joint may also be restricted because of pain with resultant muscle spasm.

Causative factors which may result in a limitation of the motion of a joint are immobilization of the joint for any reason or the patient's failure to move the joint. Fractures, dislocations, infections, arthritis, bursitis, lacerations with or without severed tendons, and paralyses are common conditions which may result in such limitation. Edema of a part will restrict motion and, if it persists, may result in a limitation of motion in the joints involved.

The objective of occupational therapy is to restore motion in a joint through the use of constructive activity which stretches contractures, loosens adhesions, strengthens weakened muscles and reduces edema.

Muscle Weakness

This may occur following immobilization or prolonged bed rest. In such cases there is general weakness of all the muscles of the part. Other causes are flaccid paralysis, traumatic defects and pathological changes.

Flaccid paralysis may be caused by an injury to the lower motor neuron either to the cell in the anterior horn of the spinal cord or to the axone leading to the periphery. Injury to the cells in the anterior horn will result in flaccid paralysis of the muscles which are supplied by the axones forming the peripheral nerve. The paralysis is characterized by varying degrees of weakness of the affected muscles from a rating of zero, which indicates absolutely no muscle power, to a rating of *good*; by atrophy of the muscle; and by a nonpatterned distribution of the affected muscles. An injury to a peripheral nerve, on the contrary, will show a patterned distribution of muscles affected (i.e., all those muscles which are supplied by the nerve will be affected provided that the bellies of the muscles lie below the site of the injury). Also, since peripheral nerves are mixed nerves with both sensory and motor fibers, there will be a loss or diminution of sensation in the area supplied by the sensory fibers.

Examples of conditions causing flaccid paralysis due to involvement of the cells of the anterior horn are anterior poliomyelitis, Guillain-Barre syndrome, tumors and injuries to the cord. Examples of conditions affecting peripheral nerves are severance or bruising of the nerves.

The objectives of occupational therapy are to restore balance of power by developing coordinated muscle action and then greater muscle strength and endurance. Instruction in activities of daily living are important regardless of the prognosis.

Traumatic Defects in Muscles. Loss of motion and strength may be due to traumatic injuries to the muscle itself, such as rupture of the fascia or of the tendon, or severed tendons. These are usually treated by surgery. Occupational therapy is used following surgery to regain muscle strength and range of motion.

Progressive Conditions Affecting Motor Function. Pathologic changes may occur in the muscles themselves. The muscular dystrophies are typical of this group.

Patients with these types of conditions show a gradually progressive deterioration of motor function. Occupational therapy may be used to prevent disuse disability, to teach activities of daily living and to retard deterioration through a program of constructive activity.

Paraplegias and Quadriplegias. These may be due to conditions already listed or to traumatic injuries to the spinal cord, but because of the severity of the condition they have to be considered as separate entities. These are discussed in Chapter 10.

Loss of Coordination

Spastic paralysis is characterized by hypercontractility of the affected muscles, which will contract on any stimulus but especially upon stretching. For this reason it is said that a marked stretch reflex is the diagnostic sign of spasticity. This results in the development of strong hyperactive spastic muscles and weak antagonists. This condition is caused by any injury to the upper motor neuron, either in the cells of the motor area of the cerebral cortex, or the axones which form the pyramidal tract passing down through the brain and crossing to the opposite side at the decussation of the pyramids and down the cord to the point at which a synapse occurs with the anterior horn cell. The left motor area controls the right side of the body and the right motor area the left side of the body.

It should be noted that in some cases of spastic paralysis, especially in cerebral palsy cases, cerebral flaccid paralysis of certain muscles may occur. This is believed to be due to an injury in area 4 of the motor area and results in cerebral flaccid paralysis of the muscles. The muscle rating is always zero. Therefore, these are called "zero cerebral" or "OC." muscles. These muscles do not show marked signs of atrophy.

Spastic paralysis as seen in cerebral palsy occurring before, at or shortly after birth, may be caused by developmental defects, injuries at birth or conditions developing shortly after birth. The treatment of these is discussed in Chapter 12. Spastic paralysis occurring later in life may be due to cerebral vascular accident, trauma, encephalitis or brain abscess or tumor. The treatment of these is discussed in Chapter 11.

The objective of treatment is to restore balance of power by strengthening the weakened antagonists and by inhibiting or relaxing the spastic muscles, to prevent contractures or deformities, and to give instruction in activities of daily living.

Incoordination of muscle function resulting in involuntary motion or a tremor may occur because of disease or injury to the basal ganglion. If the cerebellum is affected there is a resultant ataxia. This may affect the balance, the sense of position of a part in space, and eye and hand coordination. As the cerebellum is the older part of the brain developmentally, an adult patient with a condition affecting the cerebellum may be unable to do activities which normally are controlled by the cerebellum but he may still be able to do those which were learned and are thus controlled cortically.

Some of the conditions which cause involuntary motion are athetosis, tremor and rigidity which are types of cerebral palsy, or Huntington's chorea, which usually affects adults, Sydenham's chorea which usually affects children, or Parkinson's disease. Ataxia is one of the types of cerebral palsy. Tumors of the cerebellum and toxic substances may also result in ataxia.

Loss of a Part

Amputations of part of an extremity may be necessary because of trauma or may be elective to save the life as in cases of sarcoma or circulatory diseases. Amputations of the upper and the lower extremities are discussed in Chapter 9.

APPROACH TO THE PATIENT

Two factors of vital importance in the use of occupational therapy for physical disabilities are (1) winning the confidence and the cooperation of the patient and (2) instructing the patient in the activity to be performed so that he will get the necessary exercise.

It is important that the person be considered as a whole, a human being with problems and interests, not merely as a case. In some instances information is available before the first interview, but more often than not this is purely medical in character. Much can be deduced from such information as age, education, occupation and marital status. However, these facts do not disclose fears, reactions, prejudices and beliefs, which are important points to be considered in the management of the patient.

A knowledge of human nature in general and of mental mechanisms is of great advantage, for patients may be fearful, dubious or critical. It is important to learn to recognize and to deal with each reaction. To do this requires experience, the ability to estimate a person's character on first meeting and an insight into the problems of others.

Frequently, a patient comes to the occupational therapy department with little or no understanding of the purpose of the treatment, and sometimes he comes with a definite antagonism, so that the value of occupational therapy must be explained and demonstrated to him. At times this is difficult, for he may have no idea, or an erroneous one, of what occupational therapy is, and he may fail to see how it will help a stiff knee or a useless hand. The average person, although he may be skeptical, carries out the physician's orders, and after the first or second treatment further effort seldom is required to convince him that directed activity can help him to regain physical function. Perhaps the best salesman for occupational therapy is the satisfied patient who tells the doubtful newcomer how the treatment has been helpful to him.

Most persons with physical disabilities, whether obvious ones or not, suffer from fears that may hinder greatly their ultimate recovery as well as their acceptance of occupational therapy. The most common fear is that of further pain. One of the advantages of occupational therapy is the fact that the patient is "the architect of his own reconstruction," and such pain as is caused by the performance of the activity to obtain the necessary exercise is self-inflicted and, therefore, is within his control. Tension is relaxed gradually, resulting in greater ease and freedom of movement. The focus of the patient's attention is changed from the painful motion to the accomplishment of an interesting project. Many patients who are completely sincere in their belief that they cannot move an injured joint without great pain find to their astonishment that, when they have become absorbed in an interesting task, motion becomes less painful and freer than before.

The fear of disfigurement is frequent. Many patients are embarrassed because of a disabled part and may try to hide it. Until the patient realizes that this reaction tends to draw attention to the condition, it is often difficult to gain full cooperation. The association with other patients having similar or worse conditions does much to help the patient to adjust. Many fail to recognize that time does much to reduce scars and that skillful use of a part disguises a disability.

Fear of permanent disability is a very definite problem in the rehabilitation of a patient. When a handicap is permanent the patient must adjust to it and learn to live with it. Psychologically, he must be handled very differently from the patient whose recovery will be complete or nearly so. One who never has been ill before is more apt to despair at the slowness of convalescence than one who has suffered other similar experiences. The therapist must know the prognosis before attempting to deal with this type of fear. If there will be a permanent handicap, he should encourage the patient to minimize it by teaching knacks of handling the part or compensatory motions that will decrease the degree of disability.

Fear of returning to work on the machine at which the injury occurred is found in some patients. If this fear exists, it is advisable at first to use an activity completely unrelated to the patient's job but one involving the use of the same skill and motions. Later, he may use power-driven machinery until he regains his confidence, and eventually he may return to the type of work that he did before being injured. However, it is noteworthy that the use of power-driven machinery seldom is indicated as exercise but usually is employed primarily for its psychological effect.

The confidence of the patient in the therapist's ability to treat his condition is of prime importance. Therefore, an attitude of experimentation is to be avoided. The patient should be handled with assurance so that he will believe in the efficacy of the treatment. Lack of confidence, uncertainty or indecision on the part of the therapist produces these same reactions in the patient. The therapist must have a thorough knowledge of the patient's condition, of the specific prognosis and of the proper application of the treatment. The patient reacts best when he feels that the therapist is vitally interested in his condition, his problems and his recovery. The words "vitally interested" give a clue to the secret of the successful approach. If the interest is genuine, the patient senses it and responds to it. Although it is the physician who recommends the treatment, it is the therapist who comes into intimate contact with the patient. It is upon the therapist that the success of the treatment largely depends.

In the treatment of patients with physical disabilities, it is of first importance that the patient get the exercise that he needs. The best way to see that he actually does so is to arouse his interest in the activity. Often tact and ingenuity are called for to persuade him that a certain thing must be done only in a certain way and for a specified number of times. The fact that the physician has ordered occupational therapy helps the patient to realize that it is part of his medical treatment. If its special purpose is explained clearly, it is seldom difficult to enlist his

CHART 7–1. POINTS TO BE CONSIDERED IN PLANNING AN OCCUPATIONAL THERAPY PROGRAM FOR A PATIENT REFERRED FOR THE RESTORATION OF PHYSICAL FUNCTION

MEDICAL FACTORS

Medical Referral	Physical Evaluation	Other Treatments	Health
Diagnosis	Joint measurements	Physical therapy	General health
Medical history	Presence of pain or swelling	Home exercise	Diabetic and heart conditions
Present condition	Tests of activities of daily living	Speech therapy	Allergies
Objectives of treatment	Tests of sensation	Social casework	Asthma
Precautions	Manual muscle tests	School	Previous injuries
Prognosis	Tests of reaction of degeneration	Vocational training	
INDICATE	INDICATE	INDICATE	INDICATE
Treatment to be given	Patient's abilities	Coordination with other programs	Conditions modifying or restricting treatment program
Frequency and duration of treatment	Patient's disabilities	Strenuousness of activity to be given	
Precautions to be observed	Progress shown by tests	Supplementation of other programs	
Possible extent of recovery			

PERSONAL FACTORS

Job requirements, such as standing, sitting, climbing, stooping, lifting, manual dexterity, special skills	Interests Education	Psychological attitude: fears; attitude toward others; toward disability; toward returning to work; enjoyment of ill health	Socioeconomic status, age, dependents, wages, vocational history, insurance, settlements pending
INDICATE	INDICATE	INDICATE	INDICATE
Work tolerance and special skills required to do job	Patient's interests Possible achievements Avocational needs Retraining needs	Effort, cooperation Approach	Drive to return to work, financial need, work experience

cooperation and later to arouse real interest. The average person wants to get well and enters with enthusiasm upon a course of treatment that combines interest with effectiveness.

PLANNING A TREATMENT PROGRAM

In planning a program of occupational therapy for a patient referred for the restoration of physical function a number of factors must be considered. These may be divided into two general groups: medical and personal. These are shown in Chart 7-1.

MEDICAL FACTORS

Medical Referral

The physician's referral serves as the guide for the treatment program. No patient may be treated by an occupational therapist without a medical referral. This should include the diagnosis. The medical history may be stated briefly, but usually this is obtained from the patient's medical chart and in part from the patient. The physician should indicate the patient's present condition. If there is a fracture he should state whether or not there is bony union. If the patient is wearing a support of any type, such as a brace or an Ace bandage, he should state whether it is to be removed during treatment. The objectives to be achieved in occupational therapy should be given, and parts to be exercised should be specified. Any precautions to be observed should be noted. The prognosis, the degree of recovery which the physician expects and, when possible, knowledge of the length of time recovery may take is of great assistance to the therapist in planning the program. It is not customary for the physician to indicate the activities to be used to achieve the desired results. He expects the therapist to use his professional knowledge and discretion. The therapist will usually have to supplement his knowledge of the patient's condition by reading the medical chart, by his own evaluation of the patient and by discussion with other services working with the patient, such as nursing, physical and speech therapy.

The following are examples of questions the therapist should ask himself and, if indicated, he should obtain the necessary information.

Fractures. What was the type of the fracture (such as compound, or comminuted)? How long was the part immobilized and how? In what position was it immobilized? Is there good alignment? Is there bony union? Does the fracture line extend into a joint? Is the part still in a half cast? If so, is it to be removed for treatment? Is the patient wearing a support or a brace? Is it to be removed for treatment? If the injury is to a leg and the patient is on crutches, is weight bearing permitted? Is there nerve involvement? Is there osteoporosis?

Infections. Is there active infection still present? Is there an open wound? Is there a loss of joint space, or is there ankylosis? Have tendons been destroyed? How much swelling remains? Is the skin tender to the touch?

Sutured Tendon. When was it sutured? Is the tendon likely to tear if stretched? Were sensory or motor nerves affected as well?

Burns. Has the burned area healed? Is there danger of tearing the newly healed skin? Are there severe contractures? Is there marked tenderness of the skin? What type of skin graft was used?

Arthritis. Which type of arthritis? Is the condition acute or chronic? Is there danger of a flare-up of the disease? Are certain joints not to be exercised? Is there much pain and swelling? Is there much deformity?

Dislocations. Is there danger of redislocation? Should certain motions be avoided.

Osteomyelitis. Is there likely to be a flare-up of the infection? Is the wound healed? If so, how long has it been healed?

Amputations of Fingers or Toes. Is the stump healed? Is there a danger of breaking the wound open? Is there marked tenderness of the stump?

Flaccid Paralysis. Where is the site of injury? Is it due to involvement of the anterior horn cells? Is it a peripheral nerve injury? What muscles are affected? What is the rating of the affected muscles? Is there a loss of sensation? How long has it been since the onset of the condition?

Neurologic Conditions. What are the symptoms shown? How do they interfere with the action of the patient's muscles? How much of the patient's condition may be due to disuse? Does the patient know his diagnosis and prognosis? What changes may be expected to occur? Does the patient have perceptual disturbances? Are there other related disabilities which will affect the treatment?

Head Injuries, Brain Tumors and Abscesses. Is the patient confused? Is he dizzy? Does he have headaches? Is there a resultant locomotor disturbance? Has the patient had or does he have aphasia? Are there personality changes? Is there a change in his intelligence?

Physical Evaluation

The occupational therapist must evaluate the patient's abilities, in order to plan the program. Even if recent measurements of range of motion and tests of muscle strength are available, the therapist should have him demonstrate what he can do and should note the findings in the occupational therapy record. The patient's ability to perform the activities of daily living should also be checked. If a test of activities of daily living has been done, the therapist should question him as to any changes in his abilities. With the person who does not have a severe disability this aspect of evaluation is often overlooked. Such a patient should be questioned as to whether he has problems in this area. For example, a person with a stiff knee may have difficulty in putting on his shoes; a patient with a hand injury may have difficulty in writing or in buttoning his cuff button. The questions asked should be related to those activities which his disability would make difficult, and the other questions should be omitted. In flaccid paralysis, electromyographic test results, if they are available, supply information that is helpful in determining the patient's probable rate of improvement. The therapist should check for loss of sensation, especially in the hands and feet. He should question the patient in regard to the presence of pain. How severe is it and where does it occur?

Other Treatments

It is important for the occupational therapist to know if the patient is receiving physical therapy and, if so, what treatment he is having. A patient with "low back pain" may be receiving only some form of heat in physical therapy to relieve the pain and the muscle spasm; another one may be on a program of resistive exercise and practice in correct weight lifting. The occupational therapy program for the first patient would differ widely from that for the second.

The exercise the patient has been told to do at home or on the ward by either his doctor or the physical therapist or by both will affect the occupational therapy program. For outpatients the distance the patient must travel, especially if by public transportation, must be considered. A patient with a disability of the lower extremity may get more than half the needed exercise in traveling to or from the clinic for treatment. However, if he drives a car or is driven this may not be the case. With all types of patients it is wise to discover what "treatment" they have invented for themselves in addition to that advised. The therapist must also decide whether the patient is really carrying out the program as directed.

If speech therapy is being given, the occupational therapist should discuss with the speech therapist the patient's speech problems and progress. In occupational therapy the speech training may be reinforced, provided that the occupational therapist is fully conversant with the aims of the program. In cases of aphasia it is important to find out from the speech therapist how well the patient comprehends spoken and written directions.

If the patient is known to the social service department, much helpful information regarding his problems, his psychological adjustment and his home environment may be obtained. There should be close coordination between the two services, especially when the social worker is working closely with the patient, seeing him once a week or more often, to help him recognize, to accept and to solve his problems. The social worker may be able to help the patient to make better use of occupational therapy. The occupational therapist may be able to report to the social worker his observations of the patient's reactions and special problems of adjustment.

If the patient is attending the hospital school, regular school or vocational school, it is important to plan the treatment schedule so that he loses as little time as possible and so that he is never absent from those sessions which are important to his education.

When a hospitalized patient is receiving occupational and physical therapy and has appointments with the social worker and is attending the hospital school or has scheduled periods of private tutoring, the making of a schedule to include all aspects of his program is quite a feat. If there are 20 or 30 patients to schedule, it may actually require special meetings of the staff to work out the schedules. Such meetings should include a representative from the nursing staff.

Health

One of the most important medical factors to be considered is the patient's general health. His medical chart should be studied carefully. In a rehabilitation center the patient receives a complete medical examination. However, on referrals from other services or specialists to the outpatient department other medical conditions may exist which affect the planning of the occupational therapy program and the precautions to be observed. Allergies, asthma, epilepsy, diabetes and heart conditions are often overlooked. Previous injuries also present a problem. Examples of this are: a patient sent for treatment of a severely disabled hand which is complicated by an old injury which may be mistaken for the present injury; a patient with a "frozen shoulder" who may have a limitation of extension of the elbow due to a fracture which occurred in boyhood; or a patient with a fracture of the patella who has a marked limitation of hip motion due to tuberculosis of the hip in childhood. In the last example it may be inadvisable to force hip motion and, therefore, the use of the bicycle saw to increase the range of motion in the knee may be contraindicated.

PERSONAL FACTORS AFFECTING THE TREATMENT PROGRAM

Job Requirements

Essentially all patients have occupations, although only some of them have remunerative jobs. Homemaking is the largest job category. It is as important to consider the needs of the housewife or the school child as it is those of the worker employed in industry. Equally, a patient may be doing work with which his disability will not interfere but cannot perform normal everyday activities such as carrying a suitcase or driving a car. The therapist should ascertain what motions and how much strength the patient needs to develop and how much work tolerance (that is, the ability to work a 7, 8 or 9-hour day) is necessary. Special requirements such as kneeling, crawling, lifting and ladder climbing should be ascertained. The treatment program should be graded so that upon discharge the patient can fulfill these requirements or is able to continue to develop strength and endurance under his own initiative.

Interests

The patient's interest and educational background also affect program planning. For those whose disability will force them to readjust or to change their jobs, the occupational therapy program should be geared to assess these even if the referral was for specific exercise. Patients' hobbies and avocational pursuits are important to consider, for the patient is often more interested in regaining the physical ability to do these than to do his job. If the patient fails to regain enough physical function to do his job and retraining is necessary, the occupational therapist, on the basis of his observations during treatment, should be able to make realistic recommendations in regard to the patient's vocational potentialities, or to the need for prevocational evaluation.

Psychological Attitude

The patient's psychological attitude toward his disability is of prime importance. This has already been discussed under "Approach to the Patient." The therapist should be alert to changes in the patient's attitude and should adjust the program accordingly. This is particularly true in cases with a functional overlay, when complaints of pain or loss of function are out of proportion to the physical findings.

Socioeconomic Status

The patient's socioeconomic status, his age and the number of persons whom he must support all affect program planning. The older patient tends to take longer to regain function than a younger one with a similar condition. A patient with a good work record tends to wish to return to work, while one who enjoys unemployment will welcome his disability as a bona fide excuse for "doing nothing." The person who is receiving illness benefits and/or workman's compensation and may be covered also by other types of benefits may find it pays him financially not to recover. For this reason the ratio between benefits paid and actual take-home wages should be considered. It should be noted that some forms of benefits are not taxed, while wages are. In assessing the financial pressure to return to work, it is always wise to find out whether the patient's wife or older children have taken jobs because of his illness. Suits pending or insurance settlements may affect subconsciously the patient's willingness to admit improvement.

FACTORS TO BE CONSIDERED IN THE SELECTION OF THE ACTIVITY

In order to select an appropriate activity to be used as treatment the occupational therapist must know the types of exercise which the patient should be given. These may be defined as follows:

Passive Motion. Performed by an outside agent and requiring no muscle contraction on the part of the patient.

Assistive Motion. Performed by the patient to the limit of his ability, the range then being completed by the operator or by apparatus.

Active Motion. Requiring no more strength than is used in making a movement through the complete range of action.

Resistive Motion. Performed against outside resistance. Activities in which tools are used come under this classification.

In occupational therapy, active and resistive exercises usually are employed, except for certain types of conditions as noted below.

Type of Exercise Indicated For Limitation of Motion of Joints

This type of exercise depends on the nature and the duration of the injury and the results desired.

Active Exercise. In the initial treatment of patients with recent injuries, such as fractures that are still in the cast or from which the cast has been removed very recently, or of patients with burns, newly healed infections or arthritis, only very light exercise should be given. Active exercise within the limits of motion, such as is obtained in braid weaving or swinging the pedal of the bicycle saw, may be used. Such work neither stretches nor strengthens muscle but it does prevent further limitation of motion of the joint and atrophy of the muscles through disuse.

Many patients when referred for treatment have recovered sufficiently to begin more strenuous active motion. This may be obtained by moving the injured joint through the greatest possible range of motion, thus stretching the contractures. For example, a patient with limited extension of the elbow may achieve increased extension in cord knotting by pulling out the cords to the side if each time he extends his elbow he consciously stretches it as far as he can. The muscles thus get active exercise that both stretches the contractures and strengthens the triceps as the contractures limiting the motion of the joint give some resistance to the triceps.

Resistive Exercise. For patients who have progressed beyond the acute stage, activities permitting gradation of resistance and range of motion should be given. The work should be carefully graded from light to heavy, using tools of increased weight, longer work periods and shorter rest periods as the patient improves. The range of motion should be increased by adjustments in the position of the work or in the type of tools. A patient with a limited range of motion in the elbow may be started using a hand saw on ¼-inch poplar and, as motion and strength improve, may be graded up to sawing 1-inch maple. Thus, by changing the thickness and the kind of wood the resistance is increased.

Resistive Exercise Combined with Stretching. For patients needing more drastic treatment this can be provided in the form of resistive exercise combined with stretching caused by the weight of the tool. In treating an injury of the wrist, metal hammering may be used to increase flexion. Depending on the position of the metal, the exercise may be simply resistive, or the resistive exercise may be combined with stretching. If the metal is placed exactly at the limit of flexion, the exercise is resistive. If the metal is placed a little beyond the limit of flexion, the force of the blow and the weight of the hammer will stretch the extensor muscles.

Passive Stretching. For patients with contractures, sutured tendons or burns, gentle stretching of the contracted muscles, tendons or scar tissue is necessary. With the muscles relaxed, the joint may be flexed passively or extended by pressure exerted by the parts above. Stretching of the flexor muscles of the wrist is obtained by passive hyperextension of the wrist in block printing, when the print is made by pressing on the block with the palm of the hand; or stretching of the flexor muscles of the fingers is obtained by passive extension of the fingers by holding down a piece of wood in sawing.

Type of Exercise for Flaccid Paralysis.

In the treatment of flaccid paralysis, it is necessary to know not only the type of exercise obtained but what gradation of muscle strength is required. A flaccid muscle is rated by manual muscle testing as having ratings from zero to *normal*. These are defined as follows:

If a muscle has no power whatever, it is rated as zero. If there is palpable contraction but no movement of the part, it is rated as *trace*. A muscle rated as *poor* can move the part through the range of motion with gravity eliminated but cannot move it against gravity. If the extensor muscles of the wrist are paralyzed and have a rating of *poor*, the patient can extend his wrist if his hand is on a slippery surface in neutral position, but he cannot extend it if his hand is hanging palm down over the table edge.

A muscle rated as *fair* can move the part through the range of motion against gravity but not against gravity and resistance. If the strength of the extensors of the wrist is rated as *fair*, the patient can extend his wrist from the position of flexion when the hand is hanging down over the edge of the table, but he is unable to do so if he is holding a tool in his hand.

A muscle rated as *good* can move the part through the range of motion against gravity and some resistance, the amount of resistance depending on the strength of the muscle. The patient may be able to lift only 1 ounce or as much as 5 to 10 pounds.

In occupational therapy there are few activities which can be used for zero or *trace* muscles. Those that may be used are passive, such as using a glove to strap a hand to a printing press handle or on a sand block. Finger painting, braid weaving and checkers made of light aluminum may be used for *poor* muscles. Any activity, provided that it is not resisted by the weight of the tool, may be used for *fair muscles;* for example, oil painting or sketching which may be used to obtain shoulder flexion. Any activity using tools, depending on the weight of the tool and the strength of the muscle, can be used for *good* muscles.

The following case illustrates increasing gradations in activity and muscle strength. When the patient was referred for occupational therapy for the extensor muscles of the wrist, their strength was rated as *poor*. He was given braid weaving to do. A polished piece of ⅛-inch plywood was placed over the weaving, which lay flat on the table. This arrangement enabled the patient to extend his wrist with gravity eliminated as he pulled the weft through the warp, the polished wood removing the friction of his hand against the weaving. When the manual muscle test showed a rating of *fair*, the position in which he worked was changed so that he extended his wrist against gravity. When his muscle test showed a rating of *good*, the activity was changed to block printing, in which he obtained extension of the wrist in inking the roller. As the muscle strength improved, the weight of the roller was increased from 2 ounces to ½ pound.

Localization of Exercise

At times it is important to exercise or to strengthen primarily only one muscle group and not its normal antagonists. Localization of the exercise in one group of muscles may be achieved by two methods in occupational therapy: eccentric contraction or return motion.

In physical therapy it is possible to exercise individual muscles by electrical stimulation or by specific exercises. In occupational therapy the performance of an activity necessitates the interplay of muscles and muscle groups.

Eccentric Contraction. The term *eccentric contraction* or *lengthen-*

ing contraction denotes the gradual relaxation of the contracted muscle as it resists the pull of gravity and the weight of the part of the body or of the tool in returning slowly to the position from which it was moved. In raising the arm forward above the head, the action obtained is contraction of the flexor muscles of the shoulder. When the arm is returned slowly to the side, there is *eccentric contraction* of the flexor muscles of the shoulder. Thus, although the shoulder has been flexed and the arm returned to the side, only the flexor muscles of the shoulder, not the extensor muscles, have been exercised. However, if the arm is brought down with a forceful blow, as in chopping wood, concentric contraction of the extensor muscles of the shoulder is obtained. In the use of activities as exercise, *eccentric contraction* or gradual relaxation of contracted muscles can be obtained best when the part is lowered slowly, resisting the pull of gravity. In using an electric hand sander pulling it toward the body exercises elbow flexors and shoulder extensors. As it is allowed to move forward eccentric contraction occurs as these muscles gradually relax.

Return Motion. Because exercise without heavy resistance will not strengthen a normal muscle but merely will keep it in condition, it is possible to exercise weakened muscles by giving them resistance and allowing the part to return to the initial position by contraction of the antagonistic muscles thus giving only minimal resistance (i.e., *return motion*). *Return motion* without resistance or with some resistance may be used for localizing exercise in affected muscle groups.

An example of an activity affording exercise for *poor* extensor muscles is finger painting for extension of the wrist. The moving of the wrist into flexion is a *return motion*. An appropriate activity for a *good* triceps is sawing with a hand saw, which gives strong resistance to the triceps. Pulling the saw back into position for the next stroke, using the hyperextensor muscles of the shoulder and the flexor muscles of the elbow is a *return motion* with only a little resistance to the normal antagonists. Thus the weakened triceps is strengthened, but the already strong flexor muscles of the elbow get only enough exercise to keep them in good condition.

These two methods, *eccentric contraction* and *return motion*, for localizing muscle exercise may be used in treating a single case. For example, a patient referred to occupational therapy for exercise for the wrist and the hand had the following muscle ratings on admission: flexor carpi ulnaris, *fair*; flexor carpi radialis, *fair*; palmaris longus, *fair*; flexor digitorum profundus, *fair*; flexor digitorum superficialis, *fair*; lumbricales, *poor*; interossei, *poor*; flexor pollicis longus, *poor*; flexor pollicis brevis, *poor*; abductor pollicis brevis, *poor*; special little finger muscles, *poor*. Braid weaving was used as the first therapeutic activity. The frame was laid flat on the table. The flexor muscles of the distal joints of the fingers, the lumbricales, the interossei, the flexor muscles of the thumb and the special flexor muscles of the little finger were exercised in grasping the weft and in packing down the weaving. The extensor digitorum communis and the extensor muscles of the thumb were not strengthened because the exercise given was not sufficiently resisted to strengthen them. The flexor muscles of the wrist were exercised by pulling through the weft with the forearm supinated and the palm upward on the weaving. The wrist was flexed and then returned slowly to the original position. Thus the patient used *eccentric contraction* of the flexor muscles rather than extension of the wrist.

Importance of Position for Proper Exercise

In the treatment of a patient, it is necessary to place him or his work in such a position that other motions cannot be substituted for the desired movement. Compensatory motions may be eliminated by stabilization of the joint proximal to the one to be exercised. In the treatment of both limitations of joint motion and muscle weakness, certain positions are more favorable than others for moving a joint. These are as follows:

1. **Position for Exercise of the Fingers.** For flexion of the fingers, the wrist should be slightly hyperextended. This relaxes the tendons of the extensor digitorum communis and permits greater finger flexion. For extension of the fingers, the wrist should be slightly flexed, thereby relaxing the long flexor muscles and permitting greater extension of the fingers.

2. **Position for Exercise of the Wrist.** In flexion and extension of the wrist, the elbow should be either rested on the table or held at the side to prevent compensatory elbow motion. Grasping a tool tightly will tend to stabilize the wrist and will limit its motion markedly because of tendon action. In hammering, the handle should be grasped with the index finger extended along the handle so that true flexion and extension of the wrist are obtained rather than abduction and adduction.

3. **Position for Exercise of the Forearm.** In pronation and supination, the elbow should be bent to 90° to prevent the substitution of internal and external rotation of the shoulder.

4. **Position for Exercise of the Elbow.** To obtain flexion and extension of the elbow, the arm should be held at the side to prevent compensatory motion of the shoulder, or both arms should be used in a bilateral activity. The motion of the back should be eliminated when possible.

5. **Position for Exercise of the Shoulder.** To obtain flexion and lateral abduction of the shoulder, compensatory back motions can be

avoided by using a straight-backed chair or by carefully instructing the patient to hold his back straight. Rotation of the shoulder is accomplished most easily when the arm is at an angle of 40° lateral abduction. Abduction is done more easily if the shoulder joint is externally rotated, at least partially. In some instances there is as much as 40° more range of motion in abduction if it is done with the shoulder externally rotated.

6. **Special Finger Motions.** The use of grasp to develop flexion of the fingers may be indicated in conditions in which this action can cause stretching of muscle contractures. The effort of a patient to grasp a tool handle tightly results in maintained contraction, but it may increase flexion of the fingers. The pressure of the tool in the palm of the hand produces passive flexion which, combined with the effort of grasp, stretches the extensor muscles of the fingers and strengthens the flexor muscles. When the limitation of motion is due to contractures of the long muscles of the fingers, active flexion and extension of the wrist stretches these and promotes finger motion. In all treatment of hand injuries it should be remembered that a strong grasp is one of the essential motions of the hand. In cases with flexor contractures, passive stretching may be indicated. In both instances special equipment such as built-up tool handles or special sand blocks may be of value.

Adaptation of Activities To Obtain Special Motions

Special adaptations of the methods of doing the activity or in the position of the work are frequently necessary even to the point of development of special equipment. Certain rules may be suggested as a guide when making adaptations of an activity:

1. The patient at all times must be in good posture.
2. If the patient is accustomed to doing the activity in a normal fashion, be sure that he understands why it should be done in a different way.
3. Except when necessary, avoid peculiar adaptations of equipment and the building up of tools because of the poor psychological effect on the patient.
4. Avoid complicated adaptations that require adjustment and readjustment, which are a waste of time.

Gradation of Activity

In directing the patient through the course of his treatment, care must be taken to grade the activity properly. The patient should progress as quickly as possible from light to heavy work and to longer work periods and shorter rest periods. Gradation of the range of motion of a joint and of the amount of coordination is also necessary. A patient whose treatment is begun with active exercise should progress as soon as possible to resistive exercise, which, in turn, should be graded from light to heavy work until he has achieved normal strength. Too much emphasis cannot be placed on the importance of graded activity.

Symptoms of Overfatigue

The physician referring the patient indicates the length and the frequency of treatments. A constant watch should be kept for symptoms of overfatigue, which usually are:

1. *Local:* redness, pain, swelling, heat and tremor in the affected part and decrease in range of motion.
2. *General:* restlessness, sighing, perspiration on forehead and upper lip, lack of attention and irritability.

The patient should be questioned as to whether or not any unusual symptoms occurred following a change in treatment. If there are complaints, his other activities should be checked, as well as his treatment in occupational therapy.

Principles in Grading Activities

In grading a treatment the following principles should serve as a guide:

1. *To strengthen muscles:*

A. A muscle must be tired by exercise if it is to become stronger, but overfatigue should be avoided.

B. Exercise against heavy resistance is required to exercise all fibers of a muscle.

C. The part must go through the complete range of motion against heavy resistance in order to exercise all muscle fibers.

D. The aim of the treatment should be to help to develop as much strength and endurance in the affected part as there was before injury. It is not enough for the patient to be able to lift 50 pounds if his job requires that he lift 100, or to lift it 5 times an hour if he must lift it 20 times.

2. *To increase the range of joint movement:*

A. To obtain an increase in the range of motion of a joint, the range of motion used in the activity must be increased. The joint should pass through the fullest possible range of motion every time the part is moved.

B. When the acute stage of injury is passed, the activity should require stretching of the affected joint or joints in the direction of the limitation (i.e., if there is a limitation of extension of the elbow, the stretch or the pull should come on the motion of extension as in using a hand saw).

3. *To increase muscle coordination.* The amount of muscle coor-

dination required by the activity should be increased as the condition under treatment improves.

4. *To develop special skills.* Special skills or unusual motions normally used by the patient on his regular job should be incorporated in the patient's activities as soon as he is able to do them.

In the treatment of injuries of the hand, the problem of special skills arises most frequently. The degree of grasp required and the use of fine tools such as tweezers, as well as combinations of hand and wrist activities used by the patient in his work, should be noted and given special attention.

5. *To develop work tolerance.* If the patient is employed, the general requirements of his job should be considered in grading his treatment. Patients having jobs requiring standing, stair climbing, ladder climbing or heavy lifting need to do these to develop work tolerance.

Combining Activities. In order to fulfill all the requirements of the patient in occupational therapy it is usually necessary to use more than one activity for him; for example, a patient with an injury of the hand may require exercise to increase flexion of the fingers, to strengthen the grasp and to promote muscle coordination and general strengthening of the arm. In addition, he may need to develop standing tolerance. The patient may be given printing for developing flexion of the fingers and use of the entire upper extremity, whereas woodworking may be used for general strengthening of the arm and ability to grasp. The patient is in the standing position for the entire period of his treatment.

Utilization of Recreation Periods. Recreation or rest periods of varying lengths may be necessary during the first stages of treatment. With the exception of those cases in which actual rest of the part should be emphasized, it is important to keep the patient occupied all the time that he is in the clinic. At first an entirely different activity may be used at this time. Later the rest period may be used to complete those parts of the project that do not give specific exercise.

Home Exercise. In many instances it is advisable to prescribe exercises to be done at home or on the ward. The patient who receives treatment daily usually progresses more rapidly than the one who receives it only every other day. This is particularly true in the treatment of patients with arthritis. In giving the patient activities to do at home the following should be considered:

1. Know whether the patient is one who is overzealous or indifferent in performing an activity or if he follows directions explicitly.
2. Be sure that the patient understands what he is to do. Have him both show and tell you; do not merely tell him.
3. At each treatment, check how much has been done at home and how he is doing it.

4. Grade the exercise and the effort in homework as in other treatment activities.
5. Insofar as possible make the exercise done at home a part of normal activities, such as dusting, washing dishes, painting or gardening.
6. If the patient needs this type of work but cannot be trusted to do it at home, give him an assignment for homework that he can bring to the clinic each time.
7. In giving home exercises, explain carefully why the activity should be done in a certain way to help ensure correct exercise.

Some patients after a period of instruction can continue their own treatment very adequately. As the patient improves he often may be able to return to work and he may get excellent exercise on his regular job. Then he comes to the occupational therapy clinic only for a periodic check-up and further direction. When there is a possibility that this can be done, the patient should be taught from the beginning to guide his own treatment, so that by the time he can return to work he will be able to recognize substitution and compensatory motion.

ACTIVITIES USED TO PROVIDE TREATMENT

The activities used to provide treatment must be constructive, as well as giving the desired exercise. Therapists who have a patient ride a bicycle saw without sawing out a project because it provides a greater range of motion than the stationary bicycle in physical therapy, or who have a patient sand a piece of scrap wood and then throw it back on the wood pile are not giving occupational therapy. More specific exercise may always be obtained by physical therapy. The value of occupational therapy lies in obtaining the exercise by constructive activity which enables the patient to transfer the motion, the strength and the coordination gained to normal activity. As the patient develops interest in his occupation he uses the part more naturally and with less fatigue. The psychological value of occupational therapy lies in utilizing the injured parts to do productive or creative work so that the patient satisfies basic needs. As treatment is graded to meet the requirements of his job he gains not only the work tolerance but also the self-confidence to return to work.

Interest Appeal of Activities. It is important that the activity selected be adapted to the patient's interests, age and sex. Woodwork and metalwork are almost universally interesting to men, women and children. Block printing is of interest to persons with some artistic tendencies and to those in the printing and the textile trades. Weaving is far more generally liked by men than is realized. In cities in which there are large textile factories, many of the male patients have worked on looms and are interested in weaving. The activities selected will depend primarily on whether the occupational therapy department takes care of men, women and children or of only one of these groups. A clinic equipped for the care of industrial patients would necessarily be very different from one in a general hospital. Activities such as gardening, digging, painting walls, masonry and carpentry and industrial skills such as assembly work and machine-shop work are most valuable, but their use is not possible in the usual hospital.

Adaptability of an Activity

Many of the activities used in occupational therapy are not of special value in the treatment of physical disabilities because they fail to meet the criteria set up to determine the adaptability of an activity for such treatment. To be adaptable for a specific exercise an occupation must allow motion to be localized primarily in the affected joint or joints or must strengthen certain muscle groups. It must also have a majority of the following characteristics:

1. **Provide Action Rather Than Position**
2. **Require Repetition of the Motion**
3. **Permit Gradation in the**
   A. Range of motion of the joint
   B. Resistance
   C. Coordination of muscle action

1. **Action Rather Than Position.** To increase range of motion and muscle strength, an activity should provide for the alternate contraction and relaxation of muscles. For instance if the purpose is to reestablish shoulder flexion, the patient should not work with his arm held constantly in the position of the greatest possible shoulder flexion but should alternately bring his arm to his side, the position of shoulder extension. The maintained contraction of muscles that occurs in grasping tools, such as a hammer or a sandblock, or that occurs in standing should not be used to increase range of motion but may be used to develop endurance.

2. **Repetition of Motion.** The activity should permit repetition of the required motion for an indefinite but controllable number of times. For instance, the bicycle saw permits exercise of the knee and the hip for as short or as long an interval as is indicated.

3. **Gradation.** The activity should permit grading in:

A. Range of Motion. The activity should afford opportunity for a greater range of motion than that permitted by the limitation of the joint. This allows for an increase of motion of the joint as the range of motion improves, until approximately normal motion is regained. If a patient has a stiff elbow with flexion of 120° and extension of 60° — range of 60° — use of a hand saw would provide the necessary exercise for increasing the range of motion.

B. Resistance. In order to strengthen muscles it is necessary to increase the amount of resistance given by the materials or the tools that the patient uses in an activity. Metal hammering on pewter, using a hammer weighing ¼ pound, requires much less effort than is required when a 1-pound hammer is used on aluminum.

C. Coordination. When coordination of muscles has been affected, the muscle exercise required by the activity should be graded from gross to fine movements.

Activities Having All or Some of the Requirements for Treatment of Patients with Physical Disabilities. If these criteria are applied to a given activity to determine its usefulness, then it is evident that only a small number of activities meet all requirements. Others meet the majority and, therefore, are valuable. Those that possess only one characteristic may be useful for brief periods, to give variety.

Woodwork is one of the most valuable occupations used for treatment, as it may be modified to meet all the requirements. It provides action rather than maintained contraction, with the exception of finger flexion in holding tools. For hand injuries, woodwork is useful primarily for developing grasp. Sawing and sanding give excellent opportunity for repetition of motion and they can be graded in range of motion, resistance and coordination.

Braid weaving fulfills all but one of the requirements mentioned. It is almost impossible to furnish any real resistance in the normal performance of braid weaving.

Weaving of various types, block printing, metal work, cord knotting, gardening, printing and many games are excellent.

Activities, such as knitting, sewing, chair caning, bookbinding, fly tying and chip carving are of doubtful value for specific exercise because they fulfill so few of the requirements. In leatherwork, with the possible exception of elbow extension and shoulder abduction in pulling out the lacing and of finger flexion in punching, there is neither action nor range of motion, but maintained contraction. It also lacks gradation of resistance. In bookbinding there is a variety of activities that afford exercise but these usually are repeated too infrequently to be of much value. Similar objections may be made to chip carving, knitting and chair caning.

Activities Affording Specific and General Exercise. An activity may afford excellent opportunity for both specific and general exercise. Woodwork is in this category. A patient with a fractured ankle may be given specific exercise on the treadle saw on which the parts of his project are prepared and then may be given good general exercise in sanding and assembling the parts. Weaving on a large floor loom likewise gives both specific and general exercise. The exercise obtained in braid weaving is primarily specific in contrast with the activities cited.

Activities Suggested to Provide Treatment

Part	Objective	Activities & Gradation
ANKLE *Diagnoses* Fractures of metatarsal & tarsal bones; malleoli; tibia & fibula lower 1/3 Contusions Sprains Flaccid paralysis Lacerations Crush injuries Burns Arthritis	Increase of range of motion-dorsi & plantar flexion Development of strength	Treadle saw – r.o.m.* (strengthens only plantar flexors) Treadle sander – same as saw but greater resistance Alexander bicycle saw – † r.o.m. if knee is also affected (only for fair + muscles to increase strength) Floor press – pumping with affected leg, quadriceps strengthening & co-contraction of ankle muscles Floor checkers – quadriceps strengthening – forcing of ankle dorsiflexion
	Standing tolerance Any activity can be used for standing tolerance as long as patient stands to do it Work tolerance requirements of job	Woodwork – assembly and use of power tools Floor press – pumping with nonaffected leg Shuffleboard Floor checkers Weight lifting as on job All weight lifting done in correct posture not bending over but flexing knees & hips, back straight Stair climbing, carrying weights Ladder climbing Kneeling and crawling
KNEE and HIP *Diagnoses* Fractures – in & around joints & shaft of femur or tibia Bursitis Internal derangement Minesectomies	Increase of range of motion: flexion & extension, hip abduction & adduction Development of muscle strength	Alexander bicycle saw – r.o.m. (only strengthens fair + muscles) Floor press – pumping with affected leg (strengthens quadriceps particularly) Weaving – floor loom for abduction & adduction, adaptation for other motions

* r.o.m. = range of motion.
† Other saws are now available with added resistance.

Activities Suggested to Provide Treatment

Part	Objective	Activities & Gradation
Arthritis Flaccid paralysis Burns Contusions		Floor checkers — particularly strengthens quadriceps — forces hip & knee flexion Potter's wheel — abduction of right hip Weaving — flexion of trunk on thigh
	Standing tolerance Work tolerance	As in **ANKLE** Standing activities in addition give co-contraction of muscles of lower extremities

BACK
Diagnoses
Fractures of
  vertebra
Slipped discs
  (pre- and post-
  operative)
Contusions
Strains
"Low back pain"
Flaccid paralysis
Arthritis
Sciatica
	Increased tone &
	  strength of back &
	  abdominal muscles
	Cervical extension
	Maintenance of correct posture while
	  working
		Alexander bicycle saw — tone and strength of trunk muscles
		Hand printing press — bilateral handles, strengthening of upper back muscles
		
		Cord knotting (cervical extension)
		Sanding — co-contraction of back muscles
		Floor press — alternating legs, strengthening knee, hip and trunk muscles
		Floor checkers — maintenance of correct posture for lifting
		Weaving — floor loom — trunk muscles

	Standing tolerance Work tolerance	As in **ANKLE** and **KNEE** and **HIP** Emphasis placed on correct lifting procedure & correct posture when standing or sitting

SHOULDER
Diagnoses
Arthritis
Bursitis
Fractures of
  Scapula
  Clavicle
  Humerus
Dislocations
Frozen shoulders
Tear of rotator
  cuff
Contusions
	Increase of range of
	  motion, muscle
	  strength
		Checkers
		Braid weaving — combining flexion, abduction, external rotation or for horizontal abduction & adduction
		Cord knotting — combining flexion, abduction, external rotation or for horizontal abduction & adduction
		Hand press — flexion or extension or abduction

Activities Suggested to Provide Treatment

Part	Objective	Activities & Gradation
SHOULDERS (continued)		
Rupture of muscles		Weaving – adapted loom
Axillary nerve injuries		Vertical or horizontal sanding – flexion, hyperextension or abduction
Brachial palsy & other flaccid paralyses		Metal hammering (internal & external rotation)
		Bag toss – circumduction
		Shuffleboard – forceful flexion to 40°
	Work tolerance – including standing tolerance if required on job	Any activity at normal working level such as woodwork
		Weight-lifting as done on job – any special motions used on job, such as external rotation, or reach-above head
ELBOW	Increase of range of motion and muscle strength	Metal tapping – for marked limitation of motion
Diagnoses		Weaving – adapted loom
Arthritis		Horizontal sanding
Bursitis		Hand sawing – for extension
Fractures		Extension drill
Dislocations		Hand press, forced extension
Burns		Shuffleboard, extension
Contusions		Weighted vertical or horizontal sanding or use of electric sander
Rupture of muscles		
Flaccid paralysis		
Lacerations	Work tolerance including standing tolerance	As in **SHOULDER**
FOREARM	Increase of range of motion, pronation & supination & muscle strength	Hand checkers
Diagnoses		Cord knotting
Fractures		Sanding
Flaccid paralysis		Block printing – hammering
Burns		Screwing
Arthritis		Metal hammering
		Weaving – adapted loom
		Hand press
	Work tolerance	As in **SHOULDER**
WRIST	Increase of range of motion and muscle strength	Braid weaving – poor & fair muscles
Diagnoses		Metal tapping – flexion & extension
Fractures		
Radial nerve injuries & other flaccid paralyses		Metal hammering
Arthritis		Stenciling – flexion & extension

Activities Suggested to Provide Treatment

Part	Objective	Activities & Gradation
Lacerations & avulsions Burns Severed tendons Tenosynovitis		Woodwork—curved sanding —flexion & extension Block printing—flexion & extension; abduction & adduction Hand press—for hyperex- tension Weighted checkers
	Work tolerance	As in **SHOULDER**
FINGERS *Diagnoses* Fractures Amputations Contusions Lacerations & avulsions Severed tendons Burns Median nerve injuries Ulnar nerve in- juries & other flaccid paralyses Radial nerve injuries Arthritis	Increase of range of motion and muscle strength Desensitizing stumps and scarred areas Work tolerance	Braid weaving & cord knot- ting Games Dr. I.Q. Checkers—grasp & oppo- sition Caroms—extension Silk screen Clay modeling Woodwork—grasping tools & sand blocks adapted to need Leather punching As in **SHOULDER**
THUMB *Diagnoses* Avulsions Fractures Partial amputa- tions Contusions Lacerations Burns Median nerve injuries Radial nerve injuries Ulnar nerve in- juries & other flaccid paralyses	Increase of range of motion Development of strength Work tolerance	Braid weaving Games Dr. I.Q. Hand checkers Chinese checkers Marbles Silk screen Woodwork—holding tools and sand blocks Leather punching Cutting with scissors Cutting with shears As in **SHOULDER**

ANALYSIS OF ACTIVITIES

The degree to which physical restoration is attained depends upon the proper selection, application and gradation of activities. Individuals vary in technic in the performance of an activity without thought of the exercise which it gives. One person may work in a position entirely different from that of another person, thus giving considerable variation in the actual motions or muscle groups used. The height of the individual affects the exercise obtained in some activities. The type of equipment, the relative height of the workbench, the stool or the chair or the position of the individual, the weight or the design of the tool or the equipment all may produce differences in actions. Therefore, when activities are being used for specific exercise, the therapist must analyze the exact results in joint and muscle action obtained by doing an activity in a specific way. Lacking this analysis, proper application and, therefore, the best results may not be attained.

In order to analyze an activity it is necessary to perform each motion a number of times, noting carefully the actions obtained and the muscle groups used. It is also helpful in making an analysis to observe another person working at the same task. Then the activity is divided into a series of actions, and a chart is made giving the results of the analysis. The chart may show (1) all activities providing a specific exercise grouped together or (2) it may contain the analysis of only one activity. An index-card system may be preferred to a chart. The analysis may be made for activities used for treating limitations of joint motion and also for flaccid paralysis, a distinct difference being noted in the two.

The following analysis of woodwork for the treatment of limitation of motion of a joint may be compared with that of braid weaving for the treatment of flaccid paralysis. These show two different methods of listing the findings. No motion is listed unless it is achieved easily, with sufficient repetition during the procedure for it to be regarded as exercise. For example, there is obviously occasional flexion and extension of the fingers in picking up and laying down tools. However, these actions occur too infrequently to be considered as exercise. It is also possible to obtain opposition of the thumb and the fingers in picking up nails, but this likewise does not occur often enough for woodwork to be prescribed for the purpose of obtaining opposition. Maintained contraction of the flexor muscles of the fingers used in grasping tools is not listed as active finger flexion but as grasp, because it does not give alternate contraction and relaxation of the muscles.

ANALYSIS OF WOODWORK FOR THE TREATMENT OF LIMITATION OF MOTION OF HAND AND WRIST JOINTS

The following analysis is presented only as an example. As technics and equipment vary, so will the results of the analysis of a given activity. For this reason an analysis is primarily useful to the therapist who made it. It is of value in helping to discover just what motions are obtained normally and how they may be adapted to meet each patient's needs.

General Considerations

Does the activity have a majority of the required characteristics?

1. Action rather than position?...Yes, except for the hand, in which grasping tools gives maintained contraction
2. Repetition? ....Yes
3. Adaptability to grading—
Range of motion? ....Yes
Resistance? ....Yes
Coordination? ....Yes

In analyzing the activity it is also important to determine what type of exercise is obtained in performing each motion. As woodwork requires the use of tools, most actions provide resistive exercise.

Specific Exercise Involved

Fingers and Thumb

Flexion: No active flexion is obtained, but there is maintained contraction in grasping the tool. Some forcing of motion of the joints is obtained in grasping tools or sandblocks.

Extension: No active extension is obtained, but passive extension with stretching of the flexor tendons can be obtained in holding down the wood when sawing or with sandblocks.

Abduction and Adduction: None obtained.

Opposition: None obtained, except as required in grasping.

Grasp: Obtained by holding tools.

Wrist

Flexion and Extension: Sanding a curved surface, with both hands holding a dowel sander. The handle should be large enough to prevent a tight grasp, as this will limit motion of the wrist. In limitation of motion of the fingers due to contractures of the long flexor and extensor muscles of the fingers, motion of the wrist may aid in stretching these.

AN ANALYSIS OF BRAID WEAVING FOR THE TREATMENT OF PATIENTS WITH FLACCID PARALYSIS OF HAND AND WRIST

General Considerations

Does the activity have a majority of the required characteristics?

1. Action rather than position?...Yes
2. Repetition? ....Yes
3. Adaptability to grading—
Range of motion? ....Yes

Resistance? ....Only in part. Many of the actions
in the classification of motions
used "against gravity and resistance" from tools or equipment cannot be graded.

Coordination? ....Yes

Specific Exercise Involved

Fingers and Thumb

Flexion

Distal Joints: In beating weaving. Against resistance.

Position: Frame flat on table, forearm pronated, proximal joints extended.

Localization: By return motion.

Muscles: Flexor digitorum profundus and superficialis.

Proximal Joints: In beating weaving. Against resistance.

Position: Frame flat on table, forearm pronated, distal joints extended.

Localization: By return motion.

Muscles: Lumbricales and interossei.

Extension

Distal Joints: In beating weaving. Against resistance.

Position: Frame flat on table, upside down so that the weaving is
beaten up, forearm pronated, proximal joints extended.

Localization: By return motion.

Muscles: Lumbricales and interossei.

Proximal Joints: In beating weaving. Against gravity and resistance.

Position: Frame flat but raised 3 inches from the table and upside
down so that the weaving is beaten up. Distal joints extended.

Localization: By return motion.

Muscles: Extensor digitorum communis, extensor indicis proprius,
extensor digiti quinti proprius.

Opposition: (thumb and fingers): Grasping weft or shuttle. Against
gravity.

Position: Any.

Localization: By return motion.

Muscles: Opponens pollicis and flexor muscles of the fingers.

Flexion and Extension of the distal and proximal joints of the thumb
may be obtained in the same manner as for the fingers.

Muscles: Flexor pollicis longus and brevis; distal joints.

Extensor pollicis longus and brevis; distal joints.

Abductor pollicis longus; metacarpal joint.

Opponens pollicis; abductor brevis pollicis; opposition of
metacarpal joint.

Note: When the patient is working for flexion of the fingers, the wrist should be in a position of slight extension; for extension of the fingers, in a position of slight flexion. If there is a paralysis of the muscles of the wrist, it may be advisable to stabilize the wrist with a light splint because motion of the fingers is dependent on the synergistic action of the muscles of the wrist.

Wrist

Flexion: In pulling through weft thread. May be with gravity eliminated or against gravity, depending upon the position.

Position: (1) With gravity eliminated, frame flat on table, polished piece of plywood laid over weaving to eliminate friction. Hand and forearm in neutral position. Weft thread is pulled through, flexing wrist, forearm not moving. (2) Against gravity, frame flat on table, forearm supinated. Pull weft through, flexing the wrist, and allow wrist to return slowly to its original position of lying flat on the weaving.

Localization: Return motion when gravity is eliminated. Eccentric contraction when action is against gravity.

Muscles: Flexor carpi ulnaris, flexor carpi radialis and palmaris longus.

Extension: In pulling through weft thread. May be (1) with gravity eliminated or (2) against gravity.

Position: (1) With gravity eliminated, the movement is the same as in flexion, only the wrist is extended. (2) Against gravity, frame flat on table, forearm pronated, weft thread is pulled through, extending the wrist, which is allowed to return slowly to original position of lying flat on the weaving.

Localization: Return motion when gravity is eliminated. Eccentric contraction when action is against gravity.

Muscles: Extensor carpi radialis longus and brevis and extensor carpi ulnaris.

Abduction: In pulling through weft thread. Action may be with gravity eliminated or against gravity.

Position: (1) Frame same as for wrist flexion. When gravity is eliminated, the forearm is supinated or pronated. Weft is pulled through, abducting wrist. (2) When action is against gravity, forearm in neutral position, weft is pulled through, abducting wrist.

Localization: Return motion when gravity is eliminated. Eccentric contraction when action is against gravity.

Muscles: Flexor carpi radialis, extensor carpi radialis longus and brevis, abductor pollicis longus.

Adduction: In pulling weft thread through. With gravity eliminated.
　　Position: Frame same as for flexion. Weft thread is pulled through,
　　　adducting the wrist, with forearm supinated or pronated.
　　Localization: Return motion.
　　Muscles: Flexor carpi ulnaris, extensor carpi ulnaris.
　　Note: Abduction and adduction should not be used for exercise of
weakened wrist muscles, unless both the flexor and the extensor muscle are affected.
　　In paralysis of the flexor or the extensor muscles of the wrist, there may be a greater weakness of one of the muscles. This will result in either radial or ulnar deviation. If this is the case, the wrist should be flexed with effort to deviate it in the opposite direction.

Another form combining both of the previous forms may be found more convenient.

Activity – Woodwork

Motion	Position of Patient and/or of Work	Direction of Resistance	Muscles Used	Muscle Strength Required	Method of Localization of Exercise
Hand grasp and flexion of fingers	Grasping tool	Flexion—maintained contraction	Flexors of thumb and hand	Good unless tool is strapped to hand	None required
Extension of fingers	Standing or sitting Utilization of special sand blocks Holding down wood in sanding	Passive stretching of finger flexors	None	None	None
Wrist flexion-extension	Standing or sitting Sanding curved surface— Sander built up to avoid tendon action	Resistance equal in both actions	Flexors of wrist Extensors of wrist	Good Good	Return motion Return motion

SPECIAL CONSIDERATIONS IN PLANNING PROGRAMS FOR DIFFERENT DIAGNOSTIC GROUPS

In actuality the therapist treats the residual disability and thus is interested in the findings of the evaluation of this disability and the prognosis. A patient may have limitation of motion in the ankle joint. The cause or diagnosis is in many instances immaterial. In other cases it may be of vital importance because it alerts the therapist to possible complications which may occur. However, there is too great a tendency to believe that the treatment should be outlined for each diagnosis. This is somewhat unrealistic when, for instance, such a common diagnosis as "low back pain" is considered. There are some 30 causes for this condition, and more often than not the patient recovers without anyone's knowing the real cause, although contributory factors such as bad posture may be recognized. For this reason specific diagnoses are not going to be discussed nor treatment outlined. A few will be indicated as examples of the residual disability being considered. The bibliography contains valuable reference material on specific diagnoses and their treatment.

Limitation of Motion of a Joint

The occupational therapy program should consist of graded activity which carries the part through the greatest possible range of motion with other activities which require the use of the part normally but do not necessitate use of the full range. Complicating conditions which occur are edema and acute pain. Edema, if not caused by a cardiac condition, a lymphatic disturbance or a circulatory condition such as phlebitis or Buerger's disease, usually may be reduced by graded exercise. An Ace bandage or elastic stocking may be worn by the patient to aid in controlling the edema. The patient's physician always should be consulted if marked swelling occurs or continues after treatment. Arthritis of all types, fibrositis and bursitis are conditions which are complicated by pain. Pain in itself limits motion because the patient subconsciously splints the painful joint by restricting motion, which in turn may cause changes in the joint structure.

Arthritis, especially of the rheumatoid type, is basically a medical condition rather than an orthopedic one. However, the residual deformity or loss of motion due to changes in the joint structure brings such cases under the care of the orthopedist. In treating the arthritic patient for maintenance or restoration of function, the therapist must be aware of the medical aspects and the psychological complications which may occur, as well as the orthopedic problem. For these cases a program of home exercise and care to prevent or to lessen deformity is essential, as treatment 2 or 3 times a week does little good. Many of these patients will need assistance in learning activities of daily living and in utilizing special devices. The constant pain, debility and gradually developing deformity frequently result in mental depression. Thus the occupational therapy program makes an important psychological contribution as well as a physical one. If the rheumatoid arthritis is in an acute phase, great care must be taken to avoid overfatigue or overexercise which may cause a set-back.

Other types of arthritis, osteoarthritis, due to the wearing out of the cartilaginous surfaces of the joint, and traumatic arthritis do not have the systemic complications of rheumatoid arthritis and tend to be primarily orthopedic problems.

MUSCLE WEAKNESS

Flaccid Paralysis

Two main types of flaccid paralysis most frequently seen have been anterior poliomyelitis and peripheral nerve injuries. Since the development of vaccine for poliomyelitis the acute phase is rapidly disappearing in some countries. Peripheral nerve injuries occur relatively rarely except in times of war. The therapist should be aware of indicated treatment procedures because of the resultant severe disability. The same procedures are applicable in the treatment of flaccid paralyses due to other causes.

Application and Adaptation of Activities for Patients with Flaccid Paralyses. In the treatment of patients with flaccid paralyses it is frequently necessary to make changes in the technics and the adaptations in the equipment in order to get the exact exercise desired. In the case of arm injuries, the patient may use the uninjured hand to assist the affected hand, thus eliminating undesired motions; for example, a patient with an injury to the radial nerve needs to regain extension of the wrist, extension of the proximal phalanges of the fingers and extension of the thumb. If the patient is given braid weaving to develop these motions, only the beating of the weaving with the frame upside down and the pulling through of the weft is done with the affected hand, the other hand being used to pick up the weft and make the weave. Sling suspension may be of value in obtaining shoulder and elbow motions with gravity eliminated.

In patients having both nerve injuries and limitation of joint motion, many complications occur in planning an occupational therapy program. An injury to the radial nerve may result from a bad fracture of the shaft of the humerus which results in stiffness of the shoulder and elbow and paralysis of the supinator muscles, with the exception of the biceps, the extensor muscles of the wrist, the extensor digitorum communis, the special extensor muscles of the fingers and the extensor muscles of the thumb. Such a patient usually is referred to occupational therapy for active and fairly heavy exercise for the shoulder and elbow at a time when the muscles of the wrist and the fingers are rated poor. This presents a problem because most activities that give adequate shoulder exercise require the use of tools which necessitate grasping. However, the necessary exercise may be obtained by making adaptations in the equipment used. For example, long sanding or furniture refinishing may be used for shoulder exercise by changing the sandblock so that it can be fastened to a cockup splint, thus maintaining the position of the wrist joint. Then the patient may exercise his shoulder freely without use of the muscles of the wrist and the fingers. Braid weaving also may be used to obtain shoulder motion if another person does the actual weaving and if the patient is allowed merely to lift his arm with the weft thread. This type of assisted activity is used particularly in working with small children.

Differentiation Between Anterior Horn Cell and Peripheral Nerve Lesions. There is a marked difference between the type of muscle weakness resulting from an injury to the anterior horn cell and an injury to the peripheral nerve outside of the spinal cord, such as an ulnar nerve injury. When the anterior horn is affected, the injury affects the actual cell body, which does not have the power of regeneration in the same manner as the axon. In a peripheral nerve injury the lesion occurs in the axon, which does have the power to regenerate if given proper medical care. When the lesion is in the anterior horn cells, it may involve one or more spinal nerves. Thus the distribution of the muscles paralyzed may be varied, sometimes affecting only one muscle in a muscle group, as, for example, a case in which only the extensor communis is paralyzed. In more severe cases when a large part of the limb is affected, the distribution may follow a more regular pattern, such as the frequently seen paralysis of the deltoid and the biceps, or it may be varied, with one finger flexor, a wrist extensor and an elbow flexor paralyzed. For this reason the occupational therapy for a flaccid paralysis due to conditions affecting the cord presents problems that differ from those which occur in peripheral nerve injuries. In lesions of the peripheral nerve the distribution is regular, all muscles which are supplied by the nerve below the site of the lesion being affected, and there is a sensory loss.

Peripheral Nerve Injuries. Injuries to the peripheral nerves outside of the spinal column, such as radial or median nerve injuries, result, as has been stated, in a more regular distribution of paralysis than injuries to the anterior horn cell. Usually all muscles whose innervation occurs below the point of injury to the nerve will be affected. Thus an injury to the radial nerve at the shoulder affects all those muscles supplied by the radial nerve below the point of trauma: namely, the triceps and the anconeus, extending the elbow; the brachioradialis and the supinator, supinating the forearm; the extensor carpi radialis longus and brevis and the extensor carpi ulnaris, extending the wrist and aiding in abduction and adduction; the extensor digitorum communis, extending the proximal phalanges of the fingers; the extensor quinti proprius digiti and the extensor indicis proprius, extending the little finger and the index finger respectively; and the extensor pollicis longus and brevis and the abductor pollicis longus, extending the thumb. If the injury occurs to the radial nerve at the level of the elbow then only the extensor muscles of the wrist and of the proximal joints of the fingers and the special extensor muscles of the finger and of the thumb are affected. The supinator muscles may or may not be affected, depending upon whether the injury occurred above or below the point at which they receive their innervation. Since innervation of a muscle usually occurs at the upper part of the belly of the muscle, an injury to the median and the ulnar nerves at the wrist paralyzes the intrinsic muscles of the palm of the hand but does not affect the long flexor muscles of the fingers or of the wrist, all of which receive their innervation well above the wrist. For this reason it is easier to determine the muscles affected in this type of injury than when the anterior horn cells are affected.

These cases should be observed carefully, as there tends to be a marked variation in the muscle strength; this is due to the gradual regeneration of the nerve, the proximal muscles receiving innervation first. A patient with an injury to the radial nerve in the upper arm may be referred for occupational therapy 6 months after the injury, at which time the strength of the extensor muscles of the elbow is rated as *good*, the supinators as *good*, the extensors of the wrist as *fair*, the extensors of the fingers as *fair* and the extensors of the thumb as *poor*.

In planning the occupational therapy for a patient with an injury of the type described in the preceding paragraph, the exercise for extension of the elbow and supination of the forearm should be against gravity and resistance but it should not require resisted contraction of the flexor muscles of the wrist and the fingers in performing the activity. The exercise for the extension of the wrist and the extensor digitorum communis should be against gravity but with no resistance. In the exercise of the extensor muscles of the thumb, gravity should be eliminated. In treating this patient, emphasis should be placed upon the use of the wrist and the fingers, as the function of the elbow and the forearm already has returned.

In treating patients with peripheral nerve damage, the amount of precaution exercised to prevent untoward effects and of attention directed to careful localization of the exercise varies in accordance with the condition of the individual patient. When no precautions are specified by the physician and the affected part is not maintained in a position of rest, there is no need to observe such precautions. When there is doubt as to the procedure indicated, the patient's physician should be consulted.

Loss of sensation must be noted lest further injury occur. In ulnar and median nerve injuries, the loss of sensation in the hand materially affects the treatment. Precautions must be taken to prevent injury to the hand, as the patient cannot feel abrasions, cuts or burns. This lack of sensation also affects the patient's ability to relearn certain motions because of the loss of tactile sense and proprioceptive impulses.

A weakened muscle never should be overstretched. A muscle which is stretched continuously loses its elasticity and may be damaged permanently. In the treatment of muscles rated as *poor* or *fair* in strength, the part should not be allowed to remain in a position that stretches the weakened muscle; for example, in treating a patient with paralysis of the extensor muscles of the wrist, the wrist never should be permitted to remain in a position of extreme flexion.

In treatment of flaccid paralysis, overfatigue may cause serious damage. For this reason the greatest care must be taken in the treatment of the patient, and frequent rest periods should be given.

Resistance never should be increased until the muscle test shows sufficient improvement in muscle strength to warrant the change. However, it should be remembered in grading the treatment that certain fibers of the muscles are used only when heavy resistance is given. Therefore, it is necessary to give maximal resistance for short periods.

Substitution of other muscles to perform the action of the affected muscles or the use of tendon action must be guarded against. It is necessary to know the muscles that perform a given motion and the substitutions likely to occur. For example, flexion of the wrist may be accomplished by substituting the action of the long flexor muscles of the fingers for the flexor muscles of the wrist. The substitution of the action of the long flexor muscles of the fingers may be detected by the flexing of the distal phalanges of the fingers when an attempt is made to flex the wrist. Normally, the fingers extend when the wrist is flexed. Another form of substitution may occur in occupational therapy when the part is moved by the mechanical action of the joint above. For example, flexion of the elbow is obtained in pulling the beater of a loom. Unless adaptations are made in the equipment so that the arm is stabilized, the flexion of the elbow that occurs is a passive motion performed by the extensor muscles of the shoulder. Tendon action also must be guarded against; for example, passive flexion of the distal phalanges of the fingers is obtained by extension of the wrist. If the long flexor muscles of the fingers are paralyzed, the patient will extend his wrist when attempting to flex his fingers, because of the synergistic action of the extensor muscles of the wrist. This will in turn result in passive flexion of the distal phalanges of the fingers because of tendon action. However, if the prognosis is poor and little or no further recovery is to be expected, such substitution should be encouraged.

In cases with involvement which affects activities of daily living, special instruction should be given and, if indicated, assistive devices should be provided.

Disabilities of the Back

In some occupational therapy departments patients with conditions affecting the back represent one fifth of the case load. Their disability may be caused by herniated nucleus pulposus (slipped disc), arthritic changes, strains, contusions, fractures of the vertebrae, muscle spasm, congenital deformities or poor posture, to name a few possibilities. Usually the patient has had or is having physical therapy and is referred for occupational therapy to develop work tolerance and to learn to maintain correct posture while working or lifting. There may be weakness or flaccid paralysis of one leg or acute pain, such as sciatica. Often, the patient is wearing a special brace or corset.

The occupational therapy program should begin with activities such as bicycle sawing, which improves the tone of the leg and trunk muscles; activities requiring the use of the upper back muscles, as the use of the hand press with bilateral handles, or cord knotting for cervical extension; and activities to develop standing and/or sitting tolerance. As the patient's condition improves, the length of work periods should be increased. When medical permission is given he should be trained in methods of correct weight-lifting. This is usually started in physical therapy, and, as the patient learns the correct technic, practice is given in occupational therapy. Floor checkers are often used for this purpose. If weight-lifting is a part of the patient's job, then actual practice is given in lifting similar weights.

The patient should be instructed as to the correct working height for different types of work. This one thing can do much to relieve strain. This is especially true of the housewife who often irons or washes dishes at equipment either too high or too low.

LOSS OF COORDINATION

Progressive Conditions Affecting Motor Function

There are a number of degenerative diseases of the central nervous system for which occupational therapy may offer a palliative program to prevent disuse disability, to give assistance in activities of daily living, to advise on adapted equipment and to serve as a supportive measure.

Multiple Sclerosis

Multiple sclerosis is defined as a degenerative disease of the central nervous system in which there are diffuse irregular patches of degeneration which occur in the white matter of the brain and the spinal cord.

The etiology of the disease is unknown. The symptoms vary, depending on the area affected. Some of the common symptoms of multiple sclerosis are nystagmus — usually involving one eye, slurred speech, ataxia (shuffling gait), intention tremor, spastic paralysis, euphoria and incontinence of urine and/or feces. The patient usually experiences periods of remission and exacerbation during the course of the disease. Acute or fulminating multiple sclerosis, in which the onset is sudden and the progression of the disease rapid, is an unusual, although recognized, entity.

At the present time there is no specific medical treatment for multiple sclerosis. The prognosis is variable, as the patient may live a very useful life for an indefinite period of time. However, eventually he may become totally incapacitated.

Occupational therapy often presents a useful and hopeful approach in the care and the management of the patient with multiple sclerosis. Its aims are:

1. Physical rehabilitation. Activities of daily living, maintenance of coordination and strength, prevention of disuse disability.
2. Psychological rehabilitation. Increased independence, outlet for feelings of anxiety and euphoria.
3. Redirection of recreational activities.
4. Redirection of vocational interests. Prevocational tryout.

The present development of research on multiple sclerosis has laid emphasis on the importance of a rehabilitation program for those patients who have become increasingly helpless or for a program of prevention of disuse disability for those cases where an early diagnosis has been made. Occupational therapy may play an important role in both instances.

For those cases with severe incoordination, weakness and eye involvement, a carefully graded treatment program may produce surprising results, not from any actual physical improvement in the disease but through the patient's discovering that he still can accomplish much that he thought was impossible. With these cases, training in activities of daily living are of prime importance. Constructive activities are of value in maintaining existing coordination. Two types should be used: one which requires the patient to use maximum coordination and skill, thus helping to maintain his present level, and another which requires considerably less coordination, so that as degeneration occurs the patient knows an activity which is within his increasing limitations.

With those cases for whom a preventive sustaining program is indicated, occupational therapy can be used on a consultative basis to assist the patient in overcoming difficulties as they arise.

Parkinson's Disease

Parkinson's disease is another progressive neurologic condition for which occupational therapy may be used. It is characterized by tremor, incoordination, loss of facial expression, volume of voice, rigidity and typical gait. The patient is self-conscious and gradually tends to become a recluse, with resulting psychological reactions. Drugs offer help to some patients.

The occupational therapy program should be directed toward maintenance of existing coordination, activities of daily living, redirection of recreational interests and maintenance of morale.

Muscular Dystrophies

Muscular dystrophy, unlike the two previously described diseases, is a progressive condition which affects the actual muscle itself. There are several different types, but it can be divided into two groups: one affecting young children, the other young adults or late adolescents. The condition is one that results in increasing loss of muscle power.

The treatment program should be supportive both to the parents and to the child. As the condition is one of progressive deterioration of muscle strength and of physical independence, every effort should be made to provide interesting and stimulating activities which will utilize as much of the patient's physical and mental abilities as possible. Two activities should be given concurrently—one requiring less strength and coordination than the other. As the patient regresses and can no longer do the more taxing activity, another requiring less strength should be given.

The program of activities of daily living becomes increasingly important as the condition progresses and special devices are needed.

The occupational therapist may often serve as a consultant, seeing only one of the parents and the child at clinic or visiting the home periodically.

TREATMENT OF PATIENTS INJURED IN INDUSTRIAL ACCIDENTS

In the treatment of patients with injuries sustained at work, the objective of occupational therapy is to aid in the return of the worker to his job in the shortest possible time. In addition to the restoration of motion of the injured part, work tolerance and special skills also must be regained. A metalworker disabled by a fracture of his ankle may recover normal motion of the joint but be unable to return to his job because he cannot stand at his lathe for from 6 to 8 hours a day. A disabled man whose work requires special manual skills may receive the best of surgery and physical therapy for his injured hand and still be unable to return to his job. In occupational therapy special skills and speed can be developed while normal motion and strength are being restored; this helps to make it possible for the worker to return to employment with less loss of time and money.

Special Considerations in Planning Occupational Therapy

Job Requirements. In the treatment of industrial accident cases and of all patients who return to a specific type of employment, the therapist should determine the motions, the special skills and the amount of strength required. The following should be given consideration:

1. The nature of the patient's job (e.g., truck driver, longshoreman, typist, punch press operator).
2. What the job entails.
   A. The position in which the person works (e.g., standing, sitting).
   B. The type of activity required (e.g., walking, stair climbing, ladder climbing).
   C. The tools used — such as hammers, pliers, wrenches, drills, — and the length of time they must be used.
   D. If weight must be lifted, how heavy, how often and in what way?
   E. Any special motions used, such as constant supination of the forearm, flexion of the shoulder, strong grasp or a combination of motions.
   F. Special skills required (e.g., finger dexterity in secretarial work or in the textile trades).
   G. The speed required on the job for the worker to be able to keep up with production.
   H. The number of daily and weekly hours of work.
   I. The climatic requirement of the job (e.g., outside work in all kinds of weather or inside work).

Selection and Gradation of an Activity for Use in Treatment. In the selection of the activity to be used for treatment of industrial accident cases, the analysis of the job should be used as a guide in the choice of the activity through which the necessary skills and strength may be developed most rapidly.

The activity selected must permit grading from short to long periods of time and from light to heavy work in order to develop work tolerance. If the patient must perform a given motion for 3 hours on his job, he should be graded up to this level in occupational therapy. If he must lift 25 or 125 pounds on his job, the treatment has not achieved its aim unless the patient has been graded up to equivalent heavy work in occupational therapy.

The following cases are illustrative of the points discussed.

1. A ladder man from the fire department was referred for occupational therapy because of a fractured right ankle. The essential part

of his job was ladder climbing. At first he was given specific exercise on the treadle saw for ankle dorsiflexion and plantarflexion and general exercize on the bicycle saw for strengthening his legs. As soon as he was permitted to bear weight for any length of time, he was given periods of standing, during which he assembled the pieces cut out on the saws. Stair-climbing and walking were given as home exercise, and as these were increased, the use of the bicycle saw was discontinued. When sufficient strength and motion of the ankle joint had been regained, ladder climbing was added. The patient was given only short periods at first, but as his ability returned, these intervals were increased until he could climb an 85-foot ladder in 1 minute, as his job required.

2. A hide washer from a leather company was referred for occupational therapy 6 weeks after fracturing his wrist. He had good motion in the joint but he could not do his work, which involved lifting wet hides weighing from 15 to 25 pounds from a vat and hanging them on hooks above his head. This required flexion of the shoulder, extension of the wrist and a strong grasp. He was given woodwork on a project requiring ripsawing and longsanding. The sawing was done above shoulder level, which requires flexion of the shoulder with considerable resistance. The sanding was done with the wood placed in such a position that it was at the same height as the hooks on which the patient had to hang the hides. Thus the exercises for flexion of the shoulder and extension of the wrist were combined. The sander was made with a length of lead pipe, which required a firm grasp with both hands. As the patient's strength improved, the weight of the sander was increased gradually from 1 to 15 pounds by putting lead weights in the pipe.

In this way the activity of woodwork was adapted to give the same motions as those needed by the patient on his job, and it was graded to meet the lifting requirements of his job. The length of treatment was increased from 2 to 6 hours a day during a period of 3 weeks, at the end of which time the patient returned to his former employment.

The Redevelopment of Special Skills or Speed. Many jobs entail the use of special skills or speed in the performance of given processes. Often after recovery from an injury the worker is unable to keep up with the speed required, and as a result the efficiency of the entire production line is disorganized. If the worker is paid on a piece basis, he may be unable to earn at his previous rate of pay and, therefore, may be unwilling to return to his job.

Occupational therapy must be planned to help to develop speed and skill, as well as motion, and work tolerance. For instance, if the patient must be able to screw 40 nuts a minute on an assembly job, his acquiring that speed becomes the aim of the treatment. When the patient has achieved a sufficient degree of motion and strength to attempt this, he should be given an activity using the same skills, which can be graded to the needed rate of speed. He should be timed on his performance, and a chart should be kept showing his improvement.

The more nearly the activity resembles the real job, the better the result, but it is often difficult to provide activities that are like those done on the job, since patients come from every conceivable type of occupation. Every effort should be made to simulate the job as closely as possible.

Psychological Problems. In addition to the usual types of psychological problems that arise in the treatment of patients with residual physical disabilities, certain ones are peculiar to industrial accident cases.

Fear of Further Injury. Patients seriously injured on a machine or while engaged in a hazardous occupation often fear to return to the job. Some consciously express their dread. A bridge painter who was injured seriously and whose companion was killed when a bridge scaffolding broke, insisted that no one could get him back on that job. However, other patients seem to be unaware that they have fear that may result in a marked delay in their recovery, especially in the later phases of recuperation. Their self-confidence must be restored through proof to themselves of their ability to do the job safely.

Fear of Loss of Prestige. Some patients who have been highly skilled workers may be afraid to return to their jobs because they fear that they will lose the respect of their fellow workers if they no longer can keep up with the speed and the standards of production. If such a patient can be shown that he can do his job in spite of his accident, this fear may be overcome.

Industrial Compensation and Complications

Some patients suffer from complications relative to their compensation. The trouble occurs in instances when it is not profitable financially for the patient to return to work. An example is the case of a power sewing machine operator 48 years of age, married, husband working. Her compensation was $40 a week, the minimum allowed by law. Her weekly wage was $60. She could live almost as comfortably on the $40 which was tax free with no labor involved; therefore, she was uninterested in returning to work. The solution to such a problem is to require a full day's treatment and to make the occupational therapy more unpleasant and harder work than the patient's job.

The amount of the patient's compensation, his weekly wage, the number of dependents he has, whether or not he is receiving additional compensation from another organization, whether or not his family is fully able and willing to support him and whether he has filed a suit should be ascertained, for these facts often will help to distinguish between a case of "compensationitis" and a true traumatic neurosis.

RECORDS OF PATIENTS WITH PHYSICAL DISABILITIES

In the treatment of patients with physical disabilities, specific records of their occupational therapy and the final disposition of the case are of great importance. How detailed these records should be depends upon the type of case and the circumstances of the department of occupational therapy. An ordinary record would differ greatly from that kept for a research project. Also, there is a marked difference between the type of record made for a patient whose disability is neither serious nor permanently disabling and that made for a badly handicapped individual. As has been pointed out, records for industrial accident cases must be far more detailed than those for ordinary cases because of the legal importance of the record.

In all records the material should be factual and should not express opinion. The record should be kept regularly; it should be written legibly, and correct grammar and spelling should be used. The first person pronoun should not be used. Subjective symptoms of the patient should be qualified in the record by the words, "appeared to be." In all instances careful selection of the information needed is advisable, and extraneous material should be omitted. All daily treatment records should be signed, or, if legal, initialed.

Record keeping can be facilitated by the use of forms and charts such as those for referral; they should contain information on medical history, joint measurement, muscle test, and activities of daily living. Social case histories and psychological reports usually are kept on the form on which they are received.

Report to Referring Physician. The types of report requested by the referring physician may vary greatly. Some desire to know only that the patient is or is not coming for treatment, while others wish to receive a more detailed report. Whatever the type of report, it should be brief and clear.

When working in a hospital or an outpatient clinic, brief notations may be made on the patient's chart. These should indicate frequency and length of treatment, regularity of attendance, improvement shown and any change in the method of treatment.

If a report on a case from a community workshop is made to a private physician or to a clinic, a postcard, such as the one illustrated, which is given to the patient to give to his physician, is most helpful.

Record forms that have proved to be useful in various departments of occupational therapy are given on the following pages.

Date

is coming to Occupational

Therapy   Hours a day,   days

a week

His treatment includes.

Please complete the following and return.

   Patient to continue treatment   _____

      Put on heavier work   _____

         lighter work   _____

   Patient to return to clinic on   _____

   Patient discharged date   _____

      He is to return to work   _____

      Case settled   _____

   Additional remarks:

Physician's signature

Chart 7–2

```
┌─────────────────────────────────────────────────────────────────────┐
│                                                                       │
│        MEDICAL REFERRAL FOR OCCUPATIONAL THERAPY                      │
│                                                                       │
│   Name                    Address             Age      Sex            │
│                                                                       │
│   Diagnosis                                                           │
│                                                                       │
│   History                                                             │
│                                                                       │
│                                                                       │
│   Present Conditions                                                  │
│                                                                       │
│                                                                       │
│   Prognosis                                                           │
│                                                                       │
│   Results desired from Occupational Therapy                          │
│                                                                       │
│      Psychological Adjustment      Development of Work Habit          │
│      Prevocational Tryout          Development of Work Tolerance      │
│                                                                       │
│      Physical Function                                                │
│                                          Graded Activity              │
│          Fingers      Flexion              Program                    │
│      R   Forearm      Extension          Light work                   │
│          Wrist        Abduction          Heavy work                   │
│          Elbow        Adduction          Standing tolerance           │
│      L   Shoulder     Pronation                                       │
│          Back         Supination       Activities of Daily            │
│          Hip          Rotation            Living                      │
│          Knee         Circumduction     Dressing                      │
│          Ankle        Opposition        Eating                        │
│          Foot                           Writing                       │
│                                         Typing                        │
│                                         Household                     │
│                                                                       │
│   Frequency and Duration of Treatments                               │
│                                                                       │
│   Precautions (braces to be left on or removed for treatment, lack of │
│     bony union, etc.)                                                 │
│                                                                       │
│   Remarks                                                             │
│                                                                       │
│                                                                       │
│   Date                                                                │
│                       Physician's Signature                          │
│                           Address                                     │
│                                                                       │
└─────────────────────────────────────────────────────────────────────┘
```

Chart 7–3

HISTORY

Treatment Schedule

Injury

Admission

Return to Work

Name   No.

Address   Sex   Age

Telephone   M S W D Sp.

Dependents

Employer   Occupation

Insurance Company

Industrial Accident   Compensation

Fee   Bill   Wages

Diagnosis

History

Referring Physician   Agency

Address

For

Physical Therapy

Home Treatment

General Health   Dominant Hand   ADL

Remarks

Progress & Disposition

Normal	Employed	Transferred
Maximum Imp.	Employable	Illness
Improved	School	Unable to Come
Unimproved	Normal Activities	Uncooperative
	Training	Case Settled

Date of Discharge   Total Treatments

Chart 7-4

CONDITION ON ADMISSION

Using Support:

Presence of Pain:

Sensation:

Range of Motion (Anatomical Position-0): Strength:

Side	Part	Motion	Dates							

X-ray Reports

Dates Seen by Dr.:

JOB REQUIREMENTS

Lifting:

Standing: Machines Used:

Climbing: Tools Used:

Other Motions:

OCCUPATIONAL THERAPY

Activities: Motions:

Grade to:

Chart 7-5

DISCHARGE SUMMARY

Name:

Date Patient Referred:

By Dr.:

For:

Statement of Regularity of Attendance:

Statement of Cooperation:

Activities Used In First Treatment:

Activities Used In Last Treatment:

Condition On Admission:

Condition On Discharge:

Any Persistent or Unusual Symptoms:

Date Patient Discharged: Number of Treatments:

By Dr.:

Conditions:

Additional Remarks:

CHART 7-6. REPORTS OF MUSCLE TEST

Case No. ....

Name .... Age .... Onset Date .... Date ....

Characteristic Gait ....

Contractures and Deformities ....

Left Leg			MUSCLES	Right Leg		Left Arm			MUSCLES	Right Arm		
			Hip						Shoulder			
			Hip extensors						Anterior deltoid			
			Hip flexors						Posterior deltoid			
			Hip abductors						Upper trapezius			
			Tensor fascia lata						Lower trapezius			
			Hip adductors						Serratus magnus			
			Hip outward rotators						Rhomboids			
			Hip inward rotators						Latissimus dorsi			
			Knee						Pectoralis major			
			Quadriceps						Outward rotators			
			Inner hamstrings						Elbow			
			Outer hamstrings						Biceps			
			Foot						Triceps			
			Gastrocnemius						Supinator brevis			
			Anterior tibial						Pronators			
			Posterior tibial						Wrist			
			Peroneals						Flex. carpi radialis			
			Ext. prop. hallucis						Flex. carpi ulnaris			
			Ext. longus dig.						Ext. carpi radialis			
			Flex. prop. hallucis						Ext. carpi ulnaris			
			Flexor brevis hallucis						Fingers			
			Flex. long. dig.						Flex. sublimis dig.			
			Flex. brevis dig.						Flex. profundis dig.			
			Measurements						Finger extensors			
			Length						Lumbricales			
			Thigh						Dorsal interossei			
			Calf						Palmar interossei			
									Opponens pollicis			
			Ant. abdominals						Thumb flexors			
			Lat. abdominals						Thumb extensors			
			Ant. neck						Measurements			
			Lat. neck						Upper arm			
			Back						Lower arm			

Anterior—Posterior

Shoulder High   Shoulder Back

Displacement

Deviation

Rotation

Flexibility

             ⎰ Full Insp   Height ⎰ Normal

Chest ⎨ Normal   ⎩ Corrected

             ⎱ Full Exp.   Weight

CHART 7-7. FIRST JOINT MEASUREMENT REPORT

Name

Diagnosis

FINGERS		INDEX		MIDDLE		RING		LITTLE		THUMB	
		Flex.	Ext.	Flex.	Ext.	Flex.	Ext.	Flex.	Ext.	Flex.	Ext.
1st J.	R										
	L										
2nd J.	R										
	L										
3rd J.	R										
	L										

WRIST		Flexion	Extension	Abduction	Adduction			Pronation	Supination
	R					Forearm	R		
	L						L		

ELBOW		Flexion	Extension				
	R						
	L						

SHOULDER		Abduction	Flexion	Adduction	Extension	Rotation In	Rotation Out
	R						
	L						

ANKLE		Flexion	Extension	Inversion	Eversion		
	R						
	L						

KNEE		Flexion	Extension				
	R						
	L						

HIP		Flexion	Extension	Abduction	Adduction	Rotation In	Rotation Out
	R						
	L						

CHART 7–8.   JOINT MEASUREMENT CHART

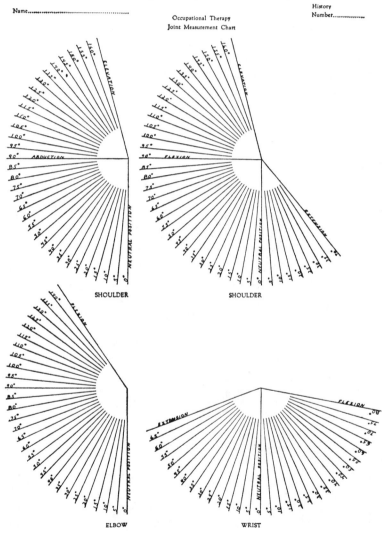

JOINT MOTIONS AND PRINCIPLES OF MEASUREMENT AND RECORDING

Although the following system is in use in most parts of the country, it is not accepted universally. Therefore, it is necessary for clarity and uniformity of records to check the definitions of joint motions and the system of measuring and recording in each hospital.

1. **Definitions of Joint Motions.** Taken from the anatomic position — body erect, face toward observer, palms turned forward.
   A. Flexion — the bending of a joint forward in the anteroposterior plane (except knee and toes).
   B. Extension — the straightening of a joint in the anteroposterior plane. The return from flexion to the anatomic position or beyond.
   C. Abduction — movement away from the body in the lateral plane. Fingers and toes — movement away from midline of hand or foot.
      Horizontal abduction — movement of the arm from front to side in the horizontal plane from position of 90° flexion to 90° abduction.
      Horizontal retraction — a continuation of horizontal abduction beyond the midline.
   D. Adduction — movement toward the body in the lateral plane. Fingers and toes — movement toward midline of hand or foot.
      Horizontal adduction — movement of arm from side to front in horizontal plane from position of 90° abduction to 90° flexion.
      Horizontal protraction — movement across front of body in horizontal plane.
   E. Pronation — movement of the *forearm* in turning the palm back or down. As applied to the *foot* — a combination of abduction at the midtarsal joint and eversion of the heel (valgus).
   F. Supination — movement of the *forearm* in turning the palm forward or up. As applied to the *foot* — a combination of adduction at the midtarsal joint and inversion at the heel (varus).
   G. Circumduction — complete circular or swinging motion around the axis.
   H. Rotation — turning or twisting of a bone on an axis without undergoing any displacement from the axis.

2. **Types of Joints with Which Occupational Therapy Is Concerned** — Diarthroses or Freely Movable
   A. Uniaxial — or movement around one axis only
      1. *Hinge Joints* (Ginglymus)
         Motions — flexion and extension
         Example — elbow

  2. *Pivot Joints* (Trochoid)
   Motion — rotation
   Example — radio-ulnar articulations in pronation and
   supination
 B. Biaxial — or movement around two axes
  1. *Condyloid* — ovoid surface received into elliptical cavity
   Motions — flexion, extension, abduction, adduction, cir-
   cumduction
   Example — wrist
  2. *Saddle Joint* — correspondingly concavoconvex surfaces —
   much the same as above
   Motions — as above
   Example — carpometacarpal joint of the thumb
 C. Polyaxial
  Ball and Socket Joints (Enarthroses)
   Motions — in all directions
   Examples — hip and shoulder
 D. Arthrodial — gliding joints
   Example — carpal bones

3. General Rules for Measuring Joint Motions
 A. One person should take measurements, as variations in method
  will cause difference in degrees of motion obtained.
 B. Placement of arthrometer: See below* Place hinge on axis of joint
  to be measured; put stationary bar in line with stationary bone;
  place movable bar in line with bone to be moved.
 C. Have patient put injured part through greatest possible range of
  motion, or, if it is difficult to hold instrument in place while patient makes motion, it may be placed after the motion is made.
  Use same method each time. Compare with average, or to be
  more exact, compare with same motion of uninjured part.
 D. To differentiate between muscle weakness and joint limitation
  take the part through the range of motion passively. If the passive range of motion is greater than the active range there is
  muscle weakness.

4. System of Recording Measurement
 Using an Arc (180°)
  Anatomic position — 0 (except when otherwise stated)
 The following directions apply to any *System*, using the two instru-
 ments shown.

---

* Also called goniometer

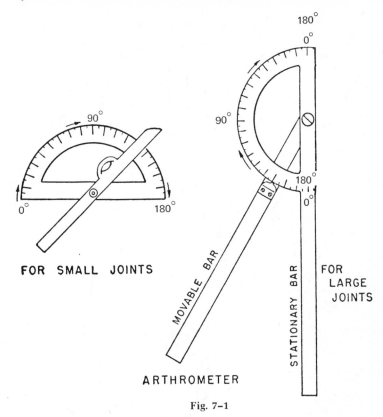

Fig. 7–1

5. Specific Directions for Measuring Each Joint

Hand: Fingers — *All Joints — Flexion and Extension*

Position — wrist in slight extension.

Placement — use small instrument, placing it on posterior surface of bones with angle apex directly over joint.

Support — give support just below joint being measured.

Proximal Joints — Abduction and Adduction. Can be taken for comparison best by laying hand flat on paper and drawing outline.

Thumb

Middle and Distal Joints — Flexion and Extension (as for flexion and extension of fingers).

Proximal Joints — Abduction in plane of hand (as for abduction of fingers). *Extension . or Diagonal Abduction* (not measured).

Adduction — return from abduction in either direction, toward base of middle finger (not measured).

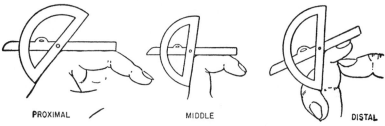

PROXIMAL   MIDDLE   DISTAL

Fig. 7-2   Measurement of finger joints.

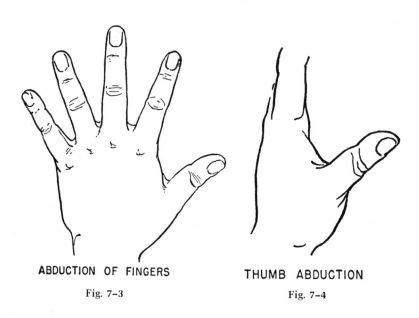

ABDUCTION OF FINGERS   THUMB ABDUCTION

Fig. 7-3   Fig. 7-4

Opposition — useful function of thumb is judged by its ability to oppose itself to the tips of all fingers without being adducted toward palm (not measured).

Averages of Motion

Fingers:	Flexion	Extension
Proximal joint	90°	0°
Middle joint	110°	0°
Distal joint	40°	0°
Thumb:		
Middle joint	70°	0°
Distal joint	90°	0°

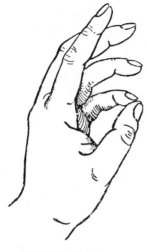

OPPOSITION

Fig. 7–5

Wrist—*Flexion and Extension*
   Position—hand and forearm resting on table in midposition (on
      fifth finger).
   Placement—stationary bar in line with radius. Movable bar in line
      with second metacarpal.
   Precautions—allow fingers to flex in wrist extension and allow
      fingers to extend in wrist flexion, to prevent restriction by 2-joint
      muscles.

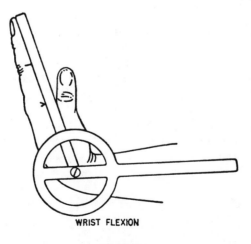

WRIST FLEXION

Fig. 7–6

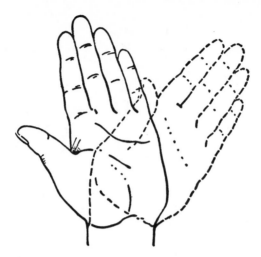

WRIST ABDUCTION AND ADDUCTION

Fig. 7–7

Abduction and Adduction
Position—hand and forearm on table in pronation.
Placement—immovable bar in line with mid-line of fore-arm.
   Movable bar in line with third metacarpal.

Averages of Motion

Flexion—80°
Extension—65°
Abduction—20°
Adduction—30°

Forearm—*Pronation and Supination*
   Usually done by comparison, testing both arms at once.
   Position—arms close to sides (to rule out substitution at shoulder
      joint); elbows flexed at 90° (to rule out rotation substitution at
      shoulder joint).
   Pronation—palm completely down.
   Supination—palm completely up.
      Possible Method of Measurement.
   Construct apparatus consisting of a handle which turns like a knob,
      with an arrow indicator which points to a degree-marked circle.

Averages of Motion

Pronation—90°
Supination—90°
Mid-position—0°

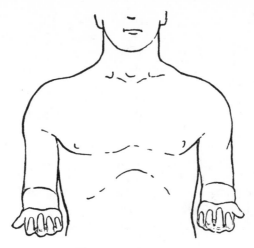

Fig. 7-8   Supination.

Elbow — *Flexion and Extension*
Placement — stationary bar in line with humerus. Hinge on lateral
  condyle of humerus. Movable bar — choice of following:
    Forearm in supination — bar in line with radius.
    Forearm in pronation — bar in line with ulna.
    Forearm in midposition — bar following center of arm.
    (Use same position every time.)

Averages of Motion

Flexion — 140°
Extension — 0°

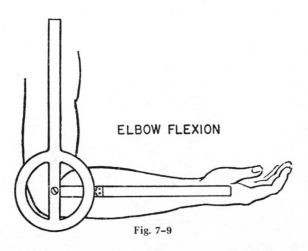

ELBOW FLEXION

Fig. 7-9

Shoulder—*Flexion, Extension, Abduction, Adduction*
  Position—have patient sit erect in chair with lumbar spine and
    shoulder against chair.
  Placement—hold stationary bar in line with side of body (perpen-
    dicular to floor). Movable bar in line with humerus.
  Precautions—in flexion—look for arching of back. In extension—
    look for forward thrust of shoulder. In abduction—look for side-
    ward body swing.
  Horizontal Abduction and Retraction } By comparison with
  Horizontal Adduction and Protraction ∫   normal part
      Rotation—Inward and Outward
  Usually done by comparison—testing both arms at once.
  Position—Inward Rotation—arms behind back as in tying apron
    strings. Outward Rotation—arms behind neck as in fixing hair.

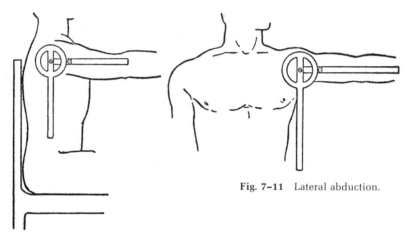

Fig. 7–11   Lateral abduction.

Fig. 7–10   Shoulder flexion.

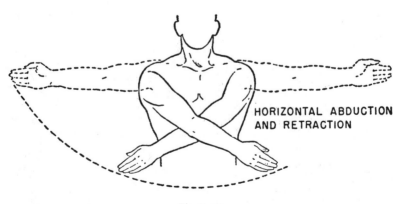

HORIZONTAL ABDUCTION
AND RETRACTION

Fig. 7–12

Or—arms at side, elbows flexed to 90°, have patient move hands from front to side.

Precautions—elbows are bent to rule out forearm motion. Both sides are tested together to rule out body substitution.

Possible Method of Measurement

Position—elbow flexed to 90°. Shoulder abducted to 90°.

Placement—stationary bar hangs down following line of body. Movable bar follows midline of forearm. Hinge at elbow.

Outward Rotation—forearm raised forward and up. Upper arm kept in position. Inward rotation—forearm lowered.

Averages of Motion

Flexion—160°
Extension—0°
Abduction—160°
Adduction—0°

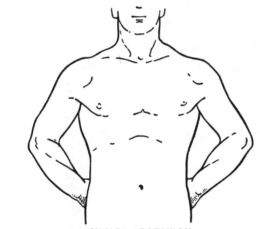

INWARD ROTATION

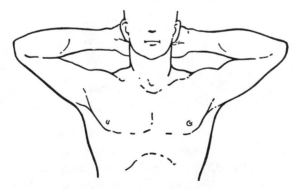

OUTWARD ROTATION

Fig. 7–13

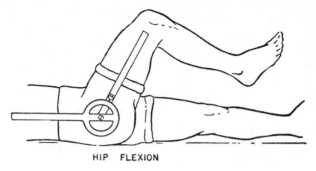

HIP   FLEXION

Fig. 7-14

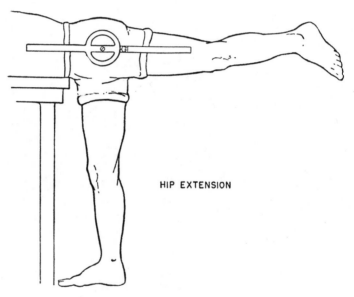

HIP EXTENSION

Fig. 7-15

Hip—*Flexion and Extension.*

Position—flexion—supine—lumbar spine flat on table opposite leg *in extension to fix pelvis.* Extension—prone—opposite thigh over end of table at *90° angle to fix pelvis.*

Placement—stationary bar parallel with body from under arm to hip. Movable bar in line with femur. Hinge at hip joint.

Precautions—allow knee to flex on measuring hip flexion. Allow knee to extend on measuring hip extension to prevent restrictions by two-joint muscles.

Abduction and Adduction (often not measured)

Position — supine.

Placement — stationary bar horizontal across body at crests of ilium. Movable bar in line with femur.

Averages of Motion

Flexion — 120°
Extension — 0°

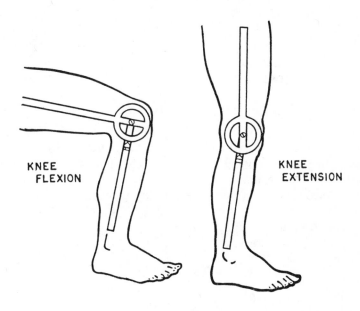

KNEE
FLEXION

KNEE
EXTENSION

Fig. 7–16

Knee — *Flexion and Extension*

Position — flexion — seated or sidelying. Extension — supine, prone, sidelying, or standing.

Placement — follow line of upper and lower leg with instrument at side of knee.

Precautions — measure knee flexion with hip flexed. Measure knee extension with hip extended, to prevent restriction by 2-joint muscles.

Averages of Motion

Flexion — 135°
Extension — 0°

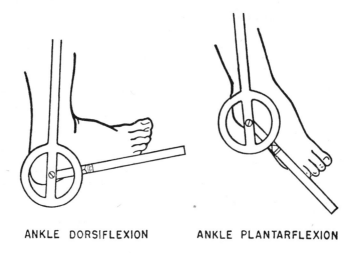

ANKLE DORSIFLEXION   ANKLE PLANTARFLEXION

Fig. 7-17

Ankle — *Plantarflexion and Dorsiflexion* (Ankle extension and flexion)
  Placement — stationary bar in line with leg. Movable bar along lateral
  border of plantar surface of foot.
  Precaution — relax gastrocnemius at knee when measuring dorsi-
  flexion.
    Pronation and Supination
  Judged by comparison only.

Averages of Motion

Anatomic position — 0°
Dorsiflexion — 25°
Plantarflexion — 35°

BIBLIOGRAPHY

Aids & Adaptations. O.T. Dept., Canadian Arthritis & Rheumatism Society,
    Vancouver, B. C., Canada. (Purchased from Canadian Arthritis & Rheuma-
    tism Society, 45 Charles Street East, Toronto 5, Ontario, Canada, 1967.)
Arthritis Special Issues. Am. J. Occup. Therapy, 19:125, 1965.
Eyler, R.: Treatment of flexion contractures. Am. J. Occup. Therapy, 19:86,
    1965.
Hall, D. S., et al.: Clothing adaptations. Am. J. Occup. Therapy, 18:108, 1964.
Heck, C. V., Hendryson, I. E., and Roe, C. R.: Joint Motion — Method of Measur-
    ing and Recording. Published by American Academy of Orthopaedic
    Surgeons, 1965.
Holmlund, V. A., and Kavanagh, R. N.: Communication aids for the handi-
    capped. Am. J. Occup. Therapy, 21:357, 1967.

Ishmael, W. K., and Shorbe, H. B.: Care of the Back. Philadelphia, J. B. Lippincott, 1963.

Ishmael, W. K., and Shorbe, B.: Care of the Back, Industrial Edition. Philadelphia, J. B. Lippincott, 1962.

Licht, S. (ed.): Therapeutic Exercise. ed. 2, Licht, New Haven, 1965.

Licht, S., Orthotics Etcetera. ed. 9, Licht, New Haven, 1966.

Lowman, E. W.: Rehabilitation Monograph VI, Self-Help Devices for the Arthritic. The Institute of Phys. Med. & Rehab., New York Univ. Bellevue Medical Center, 400 E. 34th St., New York, N. Y. 10016, 1954.

Lowman, E. W., and Rusk, H. A.: Rehabilitation Monograph XXI, Parts I & II combined, Self-Help Devices, Institute of Phys. Med. & Rehab., New York Univ. Medical Center, 1957.

Lowman, E. W. (ed.): Arthritis—General Principles Physical Medicine and Rehabilitation. Boston, Little, Brown, 1959.

McConnell, S.: The neurophysical effects of immobilization. Am. J. Occup. Therapy, 20:236, 1966.

MacDonald, E. M., MacCaul, G., and Mirrey, L.: Occupational Therapy in Rehabilitation. ed. 3, Baltimore, Williams & Wilkins, 1970.

Moskowitz, E. (ed.): Rehabilitation in Extremity Fractures. Springfield, Illinois, Charles C Thomas, 1968.

Rusk, H. A., Kristeller, E., Judson, J. S., Hunt, G. M., and Zimmerman, M. E.: Rehabilitation Monograph VIII, A Manual for Training the Disabled Homemaker. ed. 2, The Institute of Rehabilitation Medicine, New York Univ. Medical Center, 400 E. 34th St., New York, New York. 1961.

Spackman, C. S.: A history of the practice of occupational therapy for restoration of physical function: 1917–1967. Am. J. Occup. Therapy, 22:67, 1968.

Sullivan, R. A., Frieden, F. H., and Cordery, J.: Rehabilitation Monograph XXXVII, Telephone Services for the Handicapped. The Institute of Rehabilitation Medicine, New York Univ. Medical Center, 1969.

Wynn-Parry, C. B. (ed.): The Rehabilitation of the Hand. ed. 2, London, Butterworths, 1966.

Zamir, L. J. (ed.): Expanding Dimensions in Rehabilitation. Springfield, Illinois, Charles C Thomas, 1969.

World Federation of Occupational Therapists Study Courses 1962: Rehabilitation of the Injured Workman. Study Course I, 3rd International Congress of the World Federation of Occupational Therapists, Dubuque, Iowa, W. C. Brown, 1962.

———: Dynamic Living for the Long Term Patient. Study Course III, 3rd International Congress of the World Federation of Occupational Therapists, Dubuque, Iowa, W. C. Brown, 1962.

———: Approaches to Independent Living. Study Course IV, 3rd International Congress of the World Federation of Occupational Therapists, Dubuque, Iowa, W. C. Brown, 1962.

———: Approaches to the Treatment of Patients with Neuromuscular Dysfunction. Study Course VI, 3rd International Congress of the World Federation of Occupational Therapists, Dubuque, Iowa, W. C. Brown, 1962. (These may be obtained from Kendall/Hunt Publishing Co., 131 So. Locust, Dubuque, Iowa 52001.)

8

Activities of Daily Living

MURIEL E. ZIMMERMAN, M.S., O.T.R.

DEVELOPMENT AND SCOPE OF PROGRAM

With the total concept of rehabilitation the practice of medicine and concurrent therapy has expanded. Continued scientific research and observation of practice has necessitated further expansion, elimination, combining or complete revision of services. Change is normal, inevitable, and should be desirable if viewed with insight and not hindsight.

Occupational therapy must maintain a continuing evaluation of its role with program revisions as indicated. Basic principles remain constant although the verbal expression of these may be rewritten for coherency, completeness or detail. However, methods and technics may be completely altered.

With the advent of rehabilitation, the formal concept of Activities of Daily Living (ADL) became an accepted aspect of Occupational Therapy. It has always been acknowledged as a goal, especially with those persons with permanently limited functioning such as the cerebral palsied or severely affected poliomeylitics where a cure was impossible. The original experimentation was done with these patients. With the increase of traumatic injuries resulting in permanent disability, occupational therapy was broadened to include actual practice in ADL for most persons in a rehabilitation program. This could follow maximum restoration of muscle and joint function, or could be simultaneous, depending on the individual need and prognosis, always remembering the final goal to which all treatments are directed — maximum physical, psychosocial and vocational independence. Where all are indicated, it is best that they be integrated for more efficient and effective programming, for they are interdependent on each other.

The term ADL itself must be properly defined, for its usage can be as limited or as broad as one's knowledge or imagination. Originally the emphasis was upon self-care, but now it includes any activity necessary or desirable for each individual. Communications and travel are indispensable in today's social interaction and basic to so many suitable vocations. Various hand skills are relevant to both work and leisure activities, the latter of growing importance with increase of the life span. Some areas such as homemaking and clothing have received special attention and have become specialty areas within the ADL program.

A natural expansion of the ADL program has been the increased use of specialized equipment or self-help devices. Without such aids, independence for many would be impossible. For some, treatment would be less effective or prolonged.

Certain recognized procedures and technics have developed. A condensed overall view of them is presented in the following discussion.

ADL PROGRAM

Depending upon experience, the organization of hospital programs and the division of responsibility, the number of paramedical team members available and trained to participate, and the size and need of patient population, the occupational therapist may contribute to this program in several ways:

1. Testing and training in activities in total ADL program.
2. Testing and/or training in activities assigned to the occupational therapist (as a member of an ADL unit or as an assigned segment of the occupational therapy service).
3. Testing, providing and/or fabricating assistive equipment such as self-help devices or simple splints and braces.
4. Homemaking and housing evaluation and training.
5. Home visiting as it affects any of the above areas.

ADL check lists are in common usage now (see Chart 8-1). The patient is actually asked to perform each task, if feasible, and is rated according to performance. Most test forms list the activities in a normal sequence of achievement, starting with bed activities, then eating, dressing, grooming, and finally transfer and traveling in a wheelchair. There is also a corollary between these and the progression of the various physical and occupational therapy activities. Mat exercises, for instance, precede or coincide with sitting up in bed and transferring from the bed to the wheelchair. However, the needs and interest of the individual patients should always be considered. Independent eating

CHART 8–1

Institute of Rehabilitation Medicine

New York University Medical Center

TEST
ACTIVITIES OF DAILY LIVING

Mr.

Miss

Name: Mrs. _____ Age: _____ Room # _____ M.D. _____

Address: _____ Vocation: _____

Onset Date: _____ Lesion: _____ flaccid spastic   Admission Date _____

Disability: _____

Cause: _____

Decubiti: _____

Surgery: _____

Date of Initial Test _____ Patient In Out

METHOD OF RECORDING TEST AND PROGRESS

SYMBOLS for GRADE

✓ — patient can perform activity independently

S — patient needs supervision

A — patient needs assistance

L — patient has to be lifted

X — activity is not indicated

1. *At initial testing:* use *BLUE PENCIL:*
   Enter grade symbol in column G/1 and your initials in column 1.
   The initial date appears at top of page.

2. *Progress* is recorded with *RED PENCIL:*
   Enter grade symbol in column G/2 and your initials in column 1.
   Date in column "Date".

If there is more than one method or item listed with an activity, circle which indicated

BED ACTIVITIES	G/1	G/2	Date	1
Moving in bed: lying, sitting				
Roll to right: to left				
Turn on abdomen				
Manage: pillows, blankets				
Sit up				
Reach objects on night table				
Operate signal light				

CHART 8–1 (continued)

WHEELCHAIR ACTIVITIES	G/1	G/2	Date	1
Propel: forward, backward, turn				
Open, through, and close door				
Up, down ramp				
Bed to wheelchair				
Wheelchair to bed				
Wheelchair to straight chair				
Straight chair to wheelchair				
Wheelchair to easy chair, couch				
Easy chair, couch to wheelchair				
Wheelchair to toilet (high toilet seat, regular seat)				
Toilet to wheelchair				
Adjust clothing				
Wheelchair to tub				
Tub to wheelchair				
Wheelchair to shower (chair in stall shower, or tub)				
Shower to wheelchair				
TRAVEL: Wheelchair to car — on curb				
Car to wheelchair — on curb				
Wheelchair to car — no curb				
Car to wheelchair — no curb				
Place wheelchair in car — on street				

SELF-CARE ACTIVITIES

HYGIENE (TOILET ACTIVITIES)	G/1	G/2	Date	1
Comb, brush hair				
Brush teeth				
Shave (electric razor, safety razor), put on make up				
Turn faucet				
Wash, dry hands and face				
Wash, dry body and extremities				
Take bath (wheelchair, walking)				
Take shower (wheelchair, walking)				
Use urinal, bedpan				

EATING ACTIVITIES	G/1	G/2	Date	1
Eat with spoon				
Eat with fork				
Cut meat				
Handle: straw, cup, glass				

DRESSING ACTIVITIES	G/1	G/2	Date	1
Undershirt—bra				
Shorts—panties				
Slip-over garment				
Shirt—blouse				
Slacks—dress				
Tying neck tie—bow				
Socks—stockings				
Shoes (laces, buckles, slip-on)				
Coat, jacket				
Braces, prosthesis, corset				

CHART 8–1 (continued)

MISCELLANEOUS HAND-ACTIVITIES	G/1	G/2	Date	1
Write name and address				
Manage: watch				
match or cigarette lighter				
cigarette				
book, newspaper				
handkerchief				
lights; chain, switch, knob				
telephone: receiver, dial, coins				
handle: purse, coins, paper money				

WALKING ACTIVITIES	G/1	G/2	Date	1
Open, go through, and close door				
Walking outside				
Walking carrying				

STANDING UP AND SITTING DOWN	G/1	G/2	Date	1
Up from wheelchair				
Down on wheelchair				
Up from bed				
Down on bed				
Up from straight chair				
Down on straight chair				
Up from straight chair at table				
Down on straight chair at table				
Up from easy chair				
Down on easy chair				
Up from center of couch				
Down on center of couch				
Up from toilet				
Down on toilet				
Adjust clothing				
Into car, on curb, up curb				
Out of car				
Down on floor				
Up from floor				

CLIMBING AND TRAVELING ACTIVITIES	G/1	G/2	Date	1
Up flight of stairs (railing, no railing)				
Down flight of stairs (railing, no railing)				
Into and out of car, taxi				
Walk one block and back				
Down curb, cross street, on curb				
Into bus				
Sit down, get up from bus seat				
Out of bus				

CHART 8–1 (continued)

HOME SITUATION

Note suggestions for adaptation next to each line or check when so indicated. In special instances, diagram of lay-out will be advisable.

Location: Urban _____ Suburban _____ Rural _____

APARTMENT: Floor _____ Rooms _____ Elevator _____ (self-service _____)   None _____
Walk up _____

PRIVATE HOUSE: Floors _____ Rooms _____ Elevator _____ (self-service _____)   None _____

ENTRANCE: Door _____ # steps _____ Railing: right _____ left _____ none _____ ramp _____

Note floor if in private Home: bedroom _____ living-room _____ kitchen _____
bathroom _____

BATHROOM: _____
Door: width _____ Tub _____ Shower over tub _____ Stall shower _____

Information uncertain: (explain) _____

Information unavailable: (explain) _____

APPLIANCES

Column 1 — Initial Summary check blue ° - °   Column 2 — Discharge Summary check red

WHEELCHAIR

	1	2			1	2
8″ casters			Footrests:	removable		
Wheels: knobs, tape				adjustable		
Pneumatic tires				stationary		
Cushion: seat ___ back			Armrests:	removable		
Board: seat ___ back				desk		
Back — snap				stationary		
reclining			Brakes ___ extension			

BRACES	1	2	CRUTCHES	1	2	GAIT	1	2	DEVICES	1	2
Short leg			Axillary			Swing to					
double			Lofstrand			Swing through					
Long leg			Canes			4 point					
double			None			Other					
Pelvic band			Other			Hemi					
Knight spinal											

-4-

CHART 8–1 (continued)

INITIAL SUMMARY:

_____

_____

_____

_____

_____

_____

_____

_____

_____

_____

_____

Date: _____   Signature: _____

DISCHARGE SUMMARY:

_____

_____

_____

_____

_____

_____

_____

_____

_____

_____

_____

_____

_____

Date: _____   Signature: _____

CHART 8–1 (continued)

Discharge Summary (continued)

1. *RECOMMENDATIONS:*   (circle)

Patient is Independent
Patient needs: Supervision   Assistance   Lifting

Patient uses wheelchair: Exclusively   Partly
Patient is ambulatory: Exclusively   Partly

2. *ENDURANCE AND SPEED:*

Endurance:
Propelling   wheelchair: State number of feet _____ Time_____
            walking: State number of feet _____ Time_____
            climbing: State number of steps_____ Time_____

Speed:
Propelling   wheelchair: State time for 60 feet _____
            walking: State time for 60 feet _____
            climbing: State time for 10 steps_____

3. *ACTIVITIES:*
<u>Grade</u> in column G as follows: —Independence; S—Supervision; A—Assistance; L—Lifting
<u>Time</u> in column T

	G	T
GETTING READY IN THE MORNING: _____ Total		
Toilet-needs: From wheelchair:		
Standing:		
Complete dressing:		
Eating: Breakfast:		
Lunch:		
GETTING OUT OF THE HOUSE: Stairs, ramp, entrance door: ____ Total		
TRAVEL TO WORK: Own car (hand controls) taxi ____ Total		
Car: From wheelchair (including placing wheelchair):		
From standing		
Bus: Walk to station, cross street:		
Date:_____ Signature:_____		

may be started as soon as a patient can sit comfortably in bed or in a wheelchair, and in some instances it may be started while the patient is being tilted on tilt-bed or tilt-board.

After the initial test, the patient is scheduled for training sessions in activities in which he is deficient and which are deemed suitable. He may merely need a few practice periods, with or without special guidance or equipment, or he may need carefully planned and supervised methods of procedure, such as sequence of performance, and the placement of the body or the hands, with repeated practice. The following is an illustration of teaching a patient with weakness of all four extremities and trunk to put on her shoes while sitting in her wheelchair. She had to learn to do this with one hand, since she needed the other hand for balance. She also had difficulty in raising her leg off the floor.

First the patient was instructed to move forward in her wheelchair, so that she was sitting nearer to the edge of the seat. Then, hooking her right forearm under the armrest for balance, she placed her left hand under her left knee, thereby raising the left leg off the floor, until she could place her toe in the shoe and thus pull it back to just under the edge of the seat. Leaning forward, using body weight to stabilize the shoe, she could thrust her foot completely into it.

Much has already been done and written regarding ADL technic. Edith Buchwald Lawton has written two of the most outstanding references (see Book Bibliography, 2, 6).

Motor deficiences may be increased by sensitivity losses, perceptual deficits and loss of inhibition. The therapist may also be faced with problems of motivation or difficulties of speech, sight, hearing, fatigue or reaction to disability. Along with medical supervision, it is helpful to have the advice and recommendation of other personnel, such as a psychologist or psychiatrist, and a speech and hearing pathologist.

ASSISTIVE DEVICES

Indication and Purpose

Often a patient is unable to manage an activity without special equipment or even to start without such aid. While every attempt should be made to do without extra equipment, or at least to keep it at a minimum, it should be recognized that devices, if wisely selected, may not only provide independence for some, but may increase speed and safety. They may also make it suitable to initiate an activity much earlier in the treatment program than would otherwise be possible, and thereby increase therapeutic benefits.

Role of the Occupational Therapist

The area of devices has advanced rapidly, but it is still a field in which participation is open to many persons. Not only doctors, occupational therapists, physical therapists, nurses and patients may become involved, but orthotists and special technicians have been added to the team in many places. Interested volunteers and manufacturers have made many contributions, and today, more and more designers and engineers are devoting their skills to help solve these problems.

Here again, the occupational therapists may still participate on many levels. With their skill in the use of certain tools and materials, their knowledge and understanding of the various physical functions and disabilities and the facilities of an available workshop, they may frequently be called on to fabricate devices, even if only temporary or experimental ones. Many highly motivated occupational therapists have already made outstanding contributions. Today, because of the increasing supply of commercial devices and the gradual interest and training of orthotists, the need for occupational therapists to make devices is gradually lessening. However, in the role of evaluation, testing and training, the occupational therapist is and probably always will be the key performer. Although he should continue to give assistance wherever needed, according to development in his locality or institution, the main emphasis of the role described here will be on evaluation, testing and training.

Evaluation of Devices

Devices, just as any other aspect of rehabilitation, have certain fundamental requirements. The approach to them is similar to the approach to rehabilitation itself, for a *total approach* is required for the best results.

General Requirements

Devices should not be adopted on the basis of physical disability per se, but on the basis of the patient's functional need, depending on the total physical, social, psychological and vocational aspects of the problem.

The doctor will make the prescription, or referral, depending on physical need and progress. If devices are not used initially in a program, the prescription may result from a therapist's treatment report made from day to day observation of activity and resulting performance.

The reports and information obtained from the different rehabilitation specialists who are working with the patient are necessary to provide data required for prescription of devices. The attitudes and social and financial situations as well as community and cultural background may dictate such factors as the cost, the type, or even the suitability of any device. Electrical equipment, for instance, is not indicated for all parts of the world or even for all communities in the United States. Neither are complicated devices which may need servicing by specialized persons. In some places, personal service is cheap and more socially acceptable than special equipment.

The psychologist gives us data as to patient's intellectual capacity and functioning and his personality or emotional needs. Sometimes depending on another person is unavoidable. A husband or wife may need a sense of dependence on the non-disabled spouse, or vice versa. As one woman expressed it, she preferred to have her husband help her in dressing so she could help him prepare breakfast, thus spending together their short time before he left for his work.

There are other general considerations which will be discussed later under psychological factors.

Specific Requirements

Once it has been determined that a device is necessary and desirable, it is important to select and provide the most effective one possible. Using both a general and an individual approach, the relationship between human and mechanical construction and operation must be studied. In contrast with some other types of engineering and construction in which the emphasis is placed most often on the machine and its product, here the product—the device—will become an integral part of the activities of the man. Therefore, the human function—of both the normal person, and the disabled individual—must be considered. We must adapt the basic principles of physics to human function, both normal and abnormal.

Many tools have also been devised to extend man's powers beyond what he might accomplish with his hands, feet or body, and we have been concerned more and more with machines or apparatus that replace human function. Science has made rapid strides along this line. For example, the computer calculates in a few minutes the answers that a statistician could find by himself only after months or years of work. For the person who is almost totally dependent, this provides a significant contribution (The Possum is one such machine). Otherwise it is preferable to provide equipment to assist and permit him to use what little muscle power or control he has left to perform some functional activity himself.

To obtain these ends, three factors for special analysis are:

1. The patient's physical performance in various activities.
2. His psychological reactions to devices.
3. The construction and/or manufacturing aspects of the devices themselves.

CHART 8-2 ANALYSIS OF MOTIONS USED IN EATING
(One Arm Only)

Body Part	Motion	Purpose	Substitution	Loss	Device used to Compensate
Hand	Pick-up palmar prehension Holding lateral prehension to middle finger (modified lateral pinch)	Pick up and hold utensil	1. Lacing spoon between fingers 2. Adduction of fingers 3. Hook grasp	Minimal Moderate Severe Complete	1. Utensil interlaced in fingers (some shaping may be necessary) 2. Moleskin or tape over handle to prevent slipping 3. Built-up handle (wood, sponge or other material) 4. Grip-shaped handles 5. Handle with horizontal and vertical dowels (pegged handle) 6. Handle with finger rings 7. Warm Springs type short opponens with C-bar and utensil attachment 8. Plastic and metal holder 9. ADL (universal) cuff 10. Prehension orthosis – manually operated – power operated
Wrist	Stabilization (slight flexion and extension or radial and ulnar deviation normally used depending on whether grasp is hook or pinch)	Positioning of hand for optimal function (to prevent wrist flexion)	1. Use of finger or thumb extensors	Partial stability Complete	1. ADL wrist support, dorsal (leather with spring steel insert) 2. Flexible, adjustable nylon wrist support or Klenzac joints 3. Tubular spring-clip (ADL) orthosis 4. Cock-up splint, rigid, palmar 5. Warm Springs type long opponens
Forearm	Pronation Supination	Pick up food on utensil Keep utensil level while putting food in mouth to avoid spill	1. Shoulder abduction and internal rotation 2. Raise forearm to vertical position and then rotate 1. Shoulder adduction and external rotation	Partial or complete	1. Swivel spoon 2. Bent fork or spoon 1. Swivel spoon 2. Placing fork or spoon over thumb, use thumb extensors
Elbow	Flexion of forearm Extension	Raising hand to mouth Lowering hand to plate	1. Use of knee 2. Shoulder abduction 3. Trunk flexion 4. Rock forearm on edge of table	Partial or complete	1. Balanced Forearm Orthosis (ball bearing feeder) 2. Overhead sling with 'feeder' attachment 3. Overhead sling with built-up lapboard 4. Long handled utensil 5. Functional arm orthosis
Shoulder	Stabilization against hyperextension and internal rotation in position of – Slight flexion – Slight abduction	Provides positioning and assists in raising hand to level of mouth	1. Trunk flexion 2. Prop elbow on table	Partial or complete	1. Pillow behind upper arm 2. Overhead sling 3. Balanced Forearm Orthosis (BFO) 4. Functional arm orthosis with hyperextension stop

CHART 8–3 ANALYSIS OF MOTIONS FOR WRITING
(Right Hand Only)

Method and Position	Body Part	Motion	Purpose	Devices Used to Compensate
Commonly used method Sitting with arm on writing surface	Hand	Opposition of thumb to index finger and lateral opposition to middle finger (modified palmar prehension) and/or Flexion and extension of middle phalangeal joints	Provides grasp Moves pencil	1. Built-up pencils, diameter increased 2. Spring-clip holder (used in ADL cuff) 3. Leather holding device 4. Clothespin holder with pegs 5. Holder with finger rings or finger bands 6. Adjustable holder (used with ADL cuff) 7. Fiberglas cuff 8. Prehension orthosis – manually operated – power operated
	Wrist	Slight flexion and extension . . . . or . . . . . . stabilization in neutral or slight cock-up position	Moves pencil Provides positioning	1. ADL wrist support, dorsal (leather with spring steel insert) – flexible 1. Anterior cock-up, rigid 2. Long opponens orthosis 3. ADL orthosis
	Forearm	Stabilization in approximate mid-position	Provides positioning	1. Supination assist
	Elbow	Stabilization in approximately 90° flexion Alternating action of – flexors – extensors Slight flexion and extension with →	Provides positioning Lifts weight of arm from writing surface Provides pressure during writing Moves hand across paper	1. Overhead sling 2. Balanced Forearm Orthosis 3. Functional arm orthosis 1. Overhead sling 2. Foot operated cable control to elbow of functional arm orthosis 1. Soft lead pencil (needs less pressure) 2. Certain pens, ball point pens, felt-tip pens 3. Elastic strap from hand to forearm on anterior surface (substituting wrist flexors for elbow extensors) 1. Ball caster support 2. Powder on board, formica surface or teflon covered arm (elbow) cuffs
	Shoulder	Slight internal and external rotation Stabilization in position of slight flexion and abduction Minimal synergistic action of shoulder girdle muscles	Moves hand across paper Provides positioning and Minimum motion and pressure	1. Overhead slings 2. Rotation mechanism on functional arm orthosis 1. Overhead slings 2. Balanced Forearm Orthosis (BFO) 3. Functional arm orthosis

The Patient

Physical Aspects. To understand appropriately the physical functioning of a disabled person, one must first take a look at normal function. Much study has been done in this area by Gilbreth and others. Time and motion study is an invaluable technic to learn and to be guided by. It presents a total concept, including the use of sight, decision making, work area (height and placement of tools) and other environmental factors. However, it does not involve any specific analysis of the actual movements of an extremity during the actual phase of work.

To better understand the functioning of the disabled person, one must do more detailed analysis of the various phases of the work processes themselves, such as the act of eating or writing once the tool is selected and held. This has been done and examples of such studies are illustrated in Charts 8–2 and 8–3. Each work activity involves various phases. Eating involves not only the eating process, but also cutting food, applying butter, salt and pepper (and other condiments), and using cups or glasses for drinking. Writing requires positioning and stabilizing the paper or pad. Using the telephone requires picking up and holding the receiver and dialing. Frequently one may need to write while using the phone.

If the results of several activities are correlated and further analyzed as to frequency and type of motion (Chart 8–4), certain fundamental guidelines for function are revealed. Noting that some motions are aided by gravity, we are left with three primary arm motions most necessary for any activity. These are shoulder flexion, elbow flexion, and wrist extension (dorsiflexion). The wrist is almost always a stabilizing joint. The position depends on the hand moving toward the body or away from it, and also on the height of the work surface in relation to trunk. The shoulder is primarily a stabilizer against the influences of gravity to hyperextend it, but more active when reaching above the level of the chin or any distance from the body. The elbow uses a more active range of motion than stabilization. Two other motions are next frequently needed. Whenever both shoulder and elbow flexion are used simultaneously and the forearm moves into the frontal plane, external rotators are necessary to prevent shoulder abduction. Supination is used more frequently when the hand is engaged near or around the head.

Experience in observing activities is essential in quick recognition of the above guidelines.

The *Functional Motion Test* (Chart 8–5) is a practical application of the motion analysis of activities. A quick test of each motion reveals the area, extent and type of deficiency. The therapist is then in a position to summarize the results in terms of potential function for *any activity*,

CHART 8-4   FINDINGS AND SUMMARY OF ANALYSIS OF MOTION
(Eating, Combing Hair, Writing, Typing, Turning Pages)

		Active motion	Holding motion	TOTAL
Shoulder	−abduction	0	0	0
	−adduction		5	5*
	−flexion	3	2	5##
	−extension	3		3*
	−external rotation	4		4#
	−internal rotation	4		4*
Elbow	−flexion	3	2	5##
	−extension	3		3*
Forearm	−supination	3		3#
	−pronation	3	2	5*
Wrist	−flexion	1		1*
	−extension	1	4	5##
Hand pinch	−palmar	1		1
	−lateral		3	3**
	−hook	1		1

*   Gravity aided
**   It has been found that palmar can be substituted for lateral
\#\#   The most frequently used arm motions not aided by gravity are:
          (1) Shoulder flexion
          (2) Elbow flexion
          (3) Wrist extension
\#   Next important are: (1) Shoulder external rotation
                         (2) Forearm supination
Some type of hand function (with or without splints) is mandatory

providing motivation, endurance, or other general factors such as intellectual capacity are not additional deterrents.

At the same time, one must also interpret the results in terms of the
type of resultant disability and the treatment rationale for a particular
disease or injury. Disabilities may be generally described by an arbitrary listing as follows:

1. Loss of strength: partial or complete, temporary or permanent.
2. Loss of range of motion: partial or complete, temporary or permanent.
3. Loss of coordination: minimal, moderate or severe.
4. Spasticity or spasm: minimal, moderate or severe.
5. Sensory deficiencies (touch, temperature, pain).

CHART 8–5

Institute of Rehabilitation Medicine

New York University Medical Center

OCCUPATIONAL THERAPY

FUNCTIONAL MOTION TEST REPORT

Date:_____

Name:_____

Address:_____

Age:_____Chart No._____

Disability:_____

Occupation:_____

Summary of Findings

Activity Limitations or Problems

GOALS

Immediate

Long Range

Recommended Program

Recommended Devices (if any)

LEFT (dominant)										RIGHT (dominant)								
									Examiner's Initials									
									Date									
lack of control		loss of R.O.M.		active strength						active strength		loss of R.O.M.		lack of control				
									SHOULDER									
									Abduction									
									Adduction									
									Flexion									
									Extension									
									Int. Rotation									
									Ext. Rotation									
									ELBOW									
									Flexion									
									Extension									
									FOREARM									
									Supination									
									Pronation									
									WRIST									
									Flexion									
									Extension									
									Radial Deviation									
									Ulnar Deviation									
									HAND									
									Flexion MCP									
									Flexion PIP									
									Flexion DIP									
									Extension MCP									
									Extension PIP									
									Extension DIP									
									Finger Abduction									
									Finger Adduction									
									Thumb Abduction									
									Thumb Adduction									
									Thumb Flexion									
									Thumb Extension									
									Thumb Opposition									
									Grasp — palmar									
									— lateral									
									— hook									

Trunk Balance_____

Sitting Posture_____

Fatigue_____

Sensory Losses_____

Visual Problems_____

Auditory Problems_____

Temperature or Pain_____

Motivation_____

Coding Keys:

0 = zero	1 = minimal		
T = trace	2 = moderate		
P = poor	3 = severe		
F = fair			
G = good	red = 0 to F−		
N = normal	black = F to N		

Activities Performed	*potential*	*actual*
Eating		
Bathing		
Grooming — shaving		
— teeth		
— cosmetics		
Dressing		
Communications — writing		
— typing		
— telephone		
— reading		
Wheelchair Manipulation		

Sample of

Patient's Signature_____

It is now possible to predict the need for and to suggest the type of suitable device that may be necessary. If, for example, all motions are *fair* to *normal* strength and there is no loss of range of motion or co-ordination (except from disuse), and fatigue is not a problem, then no assistive equipment is necessary and one can proceed with any ADL or treatment to increase strength, adding resistance gradually after a grade of *good* is reached. However, when *any* anti-gravity motion is below a grade of *fair* the moving part must be either protected through stabilization or given adequate assistance.

By knowing the particular loss and what is necessary for performance in different activities such as eating or writing, one has a rationale for selection of equipment. It may, for instance, aid weak grasp, compensate for loss of range of motion of supination and pronation, or control incoordination. In the charts mentioned before, the devices listed are mainly used to assist or compensate for weakness or loss of range of motion, but some could also apply to other disability problems.

Psychological Aspects. Of special importance is the consideration of the psychological reactions of the patient in relation to the use of mechanical aids or devices. Some of the factors found to influence their satisfactory acceptance and use are:

Interest. It may be influenced by any of the other reactions or by the patient's feeling that he is "sick" and ought to be waited on.

Duration and Extent of Disability. The newly disabled person often expects complete recovery and, therefore, feels no need for devices, especially when he thinks they emphasize rather than minimize a handicap. While avoiding the creation of false hopes or assurances of recovery, one should encourage their use even on a temporary basis by arousing an interest in independence at all times. A careful evaluation of physical functioning with good selection of proper devices will foster use rather than cause discouragement.

Age. May be a liability or an asset, or may not be important.

Reaction to the New or Different. Some individuals are inspired by new ideas. The majority tend to favor accustomed and previously accepted methods of doing things.

Cosmetic Factors. One of the goals of rehabilitation is to give the greatest possible appearance of normality whenever it can be done. Avoid the "Rube Goldberg" as much as possible, except when it is the patient's own creation. Some ways to accomplish this are inherent in the mechanical considerations which are described later.

Social or Cultural Factors. It is unfortunate that we cannot completely accept the disabled. Since the earliest ages our assumptions have tended to present the ideal man as the physically perfect person, excelling in all things physical. At the same time, we have created a mechanical world for all men, and have striven to increase our normal powers by all manner of complex machinery. It is strange that not one person who uses such modern equipment thinks of himself as disabled! Yet today few of us could function as we do without automobiles, telephones, elevators and other electrical devices.

Knowing why patients react to devices as they do is only part of the need. Knowing how to relieve or minimize such reactions is equally important. Although some of them are not within our power to eliminate or change, there are certain procedures that do help. Here are a few that have been proved.

1. Introduce devices early in a treatment program. Then they do not have the stigma of being a last resort. They are more apt to be considered as treatment and, if used properly, can be made to augment any program, inasmuch as they encourage or make possible earlier active participation of the patient in the practice of those skills which are the end goal. They may provide the opportunity, through skill or improvement, to reduce the amount of equipment, or even to discard it completely before discharge. If needed permanently, there is opportunity to perfect the use and adjustment of equipment to better insure continued use after leaving the hospital. They help restore confidence to the disabled patient by helping him achieve independence.
2. Provide the best device possible, carefully selecting for suitability and excellence of construction.
3. Let the patient participate in selecting and approving his own devices. Offer him a choice, if possible. It is, after all, his problem that he is experiencing. Frequently we learn about devices ourselves through the patient's own observation and reports. Listen to him. He will have more confidence in you if you respect his ideas, and if he is in error he will be much more willing to take advice.

The Device

Mechanical aspects. Design or fabrication of a device may not be the responsibility of the occupational therapist. However, knowledge of the essential factors enhances his own understanding of devices fabricated by others. This does not mean that the occupational therapist should add mechanical engineering to his own present training, or that he use any of his knowledge to infringe upon responsibilities of other team members. It suggests only that, if he makes devices, the occupational therapist be equipped with as much "knowhow" as possible. Even if he only participates in testing and training, understanding the fitness or limits of materials and their methods of fabrication is invaluable in setting expectations of performance of the device itself and in knowing where to look for true trouble spots.

Today we have an ever-increasing variety of materials, tools and scientific knowledge to assist us in any mechanical construction efforts. Below are listed some of the more helpful factors to use as criteria.

Time. Patient's *need* versus *time* for construction. If a patient's interest is elicited, maintain that enthusiasm by supplying a device as quickly as possible. Waiting diminishes his receptiveness. But beware of poor construction and unsuitable materials which reduce durability and ease of operation. Breakdowns are frustrating. The goal should always be the best possible device within the limits of time allowed.

Materials. Select the material according to needs, evaluating factors such as weight, strength, flexibility, durability, washability, life expectancy and color—evaluating them against cost, method of fabrication and facilities for construction. Most of the new plastics and many metals can be handled successfully in the small shop with a minimum amount of experience. However, shaping spring steel is a job for the expert.

Construction. The keynote here is simplification and durability. The less complicated the construction, the more quickly and easily one can meet the demand. Durability results in fewer repairs and visits to the shop. Both these requirements are best answered through better knowledge of materials.

Operation. This factor goes hand-in-hand with the construction. Usually simplification of construction means ease of use. This, however, may not be true in regard to sliding parts, where friction may have to be eliminated. And we must here again refer to the individual needs—patient's disability, intellectual functioning, manual dexterity and environment.

Design. Depends upon all the other factors (time, construction, operation) plus the cosmetic needs. Good design usually has as its foundation the basic principles of good construction. Good architecture offers many fine examples. Beauty of construction and function can go hand-in-hand.

Manufacturing aspects. While manufacture of devices on a production basis is not generally our concern, it is probably from our efforts and the efforts of other individuals that many such endeavors will originate. Therefore, by being aware of the essentials and of the needs for this approach and by considering them as much as possible, one can increase the potentials for supply of devices. The following are the most important factors to be considered:

1. *Extent* or *Amount of Use.* To manufacture most items practically and to place them within the financial reach of the average individual, quantity production is necessary. The first question by an interested manufacturer probably will be, "For how many of

such items is there a demand?" As yet we have no specific answer to this question. We know the proportionate number of disabled persons in the total population. We know approximately how many of certain disabilities exist, especially among those caused by contagious diseases and war casualties, but we have no statistics concerning the specific disabilities of these persons and their particular needs. We know the possibilities that exist and we know the rapidly increasing interest and the demand for such appliances, but that is all we can offer. Therefore, it is important to emphasize the need to design a universal device suited to many types of disability but quickly and easily adjustable and adaptable to individual differences. Production methods, even applied in the small shop, will save time and effort.

2. *Availability and Cost of Materials.* Commonly available and inexpensive materials should be considered first. Here, production methods may produce different design requirements than methods of individual construction. On a production basis, plastics may be relatively cheap but not necessarily so for individual models. Contact with production engineers and a knowledge of production requirements will be extremely helpful.

3. *Interpretation of Requirements of the Device for Production.* Since most business construction is set up on a basis of specific requirements, it is well to be able to make a complete analysis of detailed needs. Plans for such will include:

   a. Functional requirements (by all its users and for all potential uses), purpose and operational needs.

   b. Construction requirements: weight, size, type of operation, positioning (maximum and minimum requirements).

   c. Manufacturing goals: flexibility, simplicity, designing for mass production.

   d. Estimate of potential market and buying: universal usage and cost.

ORTHOSES FOR UPPER EXTREMITIES

Although orthoses are not considered adapted equipment and are not necessarily a part of ADL, still, because the average orthosis is functional and is used to accomplish ADL activities, a short discussion is almost imperative here.

The primary difference between an assistive or self-help device and a functional orthosis is that in the device standard objects of daily use are adapted or redesigned for ease of handling, while the orthosis enables the patient to handle standard objects without adaptation. Also basic in the use of any orthoses are factors such as prevention of deformity by proper positioning, support of weakened segments, control or stabilization of joints proximally to those activated, or prevention of substitution. Orthoses may also be used to correct present deformities. They are both therapeutic and functional.

While their design, especially for therapeutic purposes, is largely the concern of the physician, the provisions for function are the concern of the therapist, since it is he who will supervise the training and use. Many of the same fundamental principles and factors previously discussed in connection with assistive equipment will apply to orthoses as well. The disability problems are the same, the activities to be accomplished are the same, similar materials may be used, and the patient's reactions will not differ, except that perhaps they may be even more intensified. Some of this is due to the complexity of the orthosis, its possible "mechanical-man-like" appearance and the need to wear it constantly.

Other factors are those of limited function as compared with normal function. Since the upper extremity is a very complex mechanism and it would be impossible to duplicate every motion, it is necessary to se-

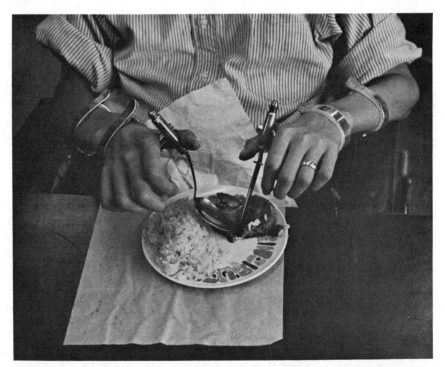

Fig. 8–1 Wrist orthoses with ADL unit and adapted utensils enables a C-5 Quadraplegic to feed himself and cut his food.

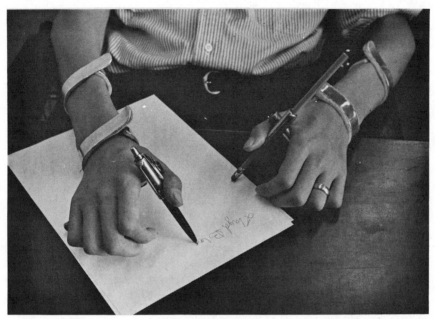

Fig. 8–2 Wrist orthoses with ADL unit used for writing, erasures and stabilization of paper.

lect those seeming basic and most commonly used. Such an approach has already been made through scientific study connected with the design of prosthetic appliances. Data obtained from these studies have also been applied to orthotic devices. Thus the type of pinch most commonly provided is palmar prehension. However, most activities in the study were done in a standing position and some were not necessarily suitable for the more severely disabled wheelchair-bound person. Also, the analysis did not include action of the shoulder – presuming this would be present and normal in the amputee subject, except for the high disarticulation which was not included in requirements of study. Therefore, it is possible that further investigation directed towards the needs of the patient with neurological impairment would, for instance, alter selection of the type of grasp most frequently used. Observation of hand function reveals that the more basic activities use lateral prehension (eating, combing hair, brushing teeth), while palmar is used in more skilled activities. Many times a combination of the two is used; for example, in writing.

Wrist flexion and extension is easily obtained, but will require special design considerations when it occurs only in either radial or ulnar deviation. Units that allow or assist pronation and supination are still being attempted but to date with little success. Elbow function is easy to provide, but again, provision for shoulder movements is either limited or requires complex design. Add to this, operation by external forces and the orthosis does indeed become either a miracle or a nightmare.

Even though all apparatus should be given thoughtful and serious attention, it is especially so with orthoses. Certainly, considerably more study of function seems to be indicated. Careful training, as well as orientation of the patient to his need for the device, is paramount.

Special problems—stabilizing the device on the patient using three points of attachment or "anchoring," alleviating the pressure points due to the change of the contour of body parts during movement or spasticity or spasm—are ever present and require special attention.

TRAINING

Just as a person cannot be expected to drive a car without learning, or perform an acrobatic feat without repeated practice, so the person with a new device or orthosis needs a period of training in its use. A patient never should be discharged without having the opportunity first to perform successfully whatever activity he has undertaken. There are some cardinal rules:

1. Learning something may require time. It is a process, not an end result, so allow adequate time for practice.
2. Mistakes are part of learning. If not repeated too often, they may even be helpful. They remind us of precautions and suggest that there may be a better way.
3. The patient may have valuable suggestions to offer. Listen carefully and objectively before rejecting ideas different from your own.
4. Keep alert to better and more effective methods of training. Enthusiasm properly controlled is always essential.
5. Even though careful planning has been given to designing a device, in actual use one may find that certain adjustments or modifications are necessary.

The need for specific, routine procedures of training depends on the type and complexity of equipment. Often the activity is performed adequately on the first or next few attempts. Sometimes, however, the equipment may need checking for use on a "dry run" before actually attempting the desired goal. This is habitually done in prosthetic training. It is also desirable in functional splinting, for underarm or overhead slings or supports and in more complex devices. One may practice portions of motions, then combine these separate motions in a formalized pattern, and finally progress to complex, free, unlimited motions. Things handled may range from simple blocks and pegs to the actual object, such as a spoon or cup (see Chart 8–6).

CHART 8-6

HAND SPLINT CHECK-OUT

Patient's name_____ (R)_____(L)_____Date: initial _____

final _____

MODIFIED ADL SPLINT

Initial		Final		Fit and Comfort
Yes	No	Yes	No	
				Does palmar piece lie angularly across palm, proximal to ulnar crease and above thenar eminence?
				Is ulnar deviation of wrist controlled?
				Is wrist held in extension between $10°$ and $30°$?
				Does distal arm clip fit snugly enough to prevent wrist flexion?
				Is ulnar styloid free from pressure?
				Is proximal arm band loose enough to allow forearm rotation?
				Function
				Can patient put splint on independently?
				Does patient pinch himself when closing spring clips?
				Do ends of spring clip interfere with resting of arm on work surface?
				Can patient rotate forearm (if motion is available)?
				Does the proximal arm clip stay closed during use?
				Does patient use splint in unilateral activities only?
				Does patient use splint in bilateral activities only?

Comments:

Institute of Physical Medicine and Rehabilitation, New York University Medical Center
Occupational Therapy Service

1964/MEZ

CHART 8-6 (continued)

COMBINED ADL-LONG OPPONENS SPLINT

Purpose — support weak wrist and hold thumb in abduction
   prevent deformity
   — provide function for ADL activities

Indications for Use — O to P hand function
   — O to F—wrist motion

Fitting Principles

   — opponens bar should lie over metacarpal of thumb
   — metacarpal of thumb should be rotated and held in line with metacarpal of index finger
   — C-bar — posterior (top) end should lie PROXIMALLY to MCP joint of index finger
      — anterior (bottom) end should lie just PROXIMALLY to IP joint of thumb
         should maintain maximum web space opening
   — palmar band should be curved to palmar arch and should lie PROXIMALLY (below)
      distal ulnar crease (transverse palmar crease)
   — wrist strap should fit SNUGLY at base of metacarpals and distal to the wrist joint
   — longitudinal bar should be arched over wrist joint to avoid pressure and should be free
      of ulnar styloid
   — proximal arm band should fit LOOSELY about 2/3 of the way up the forearm.

Training in Use of Splint

   Unilateral activities

   Eating
   — place adapted utensil in spring-clip holder to provide 'normal' positioning
   — check rotation of utensil for pick-up of food and correct angle to place food in mouth
   — if patient has loss of forearm pronation, practice rotating forearm while hand is in the
      UP position before lowering to plate

   Playing checkers
   — place pencil (eraser and down) in spring-clip holder
   — position checker board within patient's reach; if range is limited, adjust board from time
      to time to increase range in deficient areas

   Painting
   — same as for checkers
   — paper may be placed in vertical position to increase function of hand in all planes of motion

   Bilateral activities

   Typing
   — use pencils in spring-clip holders bilaterally
   — position height and distance of typewriter for optimum use and comfort
   — if trunk balance is poor, position forearm in mid-supination; remove spring-clip holders and
      place pencil directly in palmar leather pocket with end extending out ulnar side of hand.

   Mosaic tiles
   — use spring-clip holders with glue brush in one and pencil or stick in other
   — start with large pieces and symmetrical pattern
   — increase co-ordination by using small pieces and intricate pattern

Remembering progression of skills is important. Gross activities should be started first. Writing, for example, is best preceded by typing, to build up coordination, trunk balance and control, since frequently writing is done largely through shoulder movements. Even typing may be preceded by craft activities such as sanding.

SPECIAL ACTIVITIES

Clothing

The management of clothing is an activity that has always been a part of the ADL program and special attention has been given to solving this problem. For the most part, the results have been directed toward handling standard garments and the use of some assistive devices. Although these methods have been helpful, they have not been sufficient.

Studies made several years ago showed that of 51 random cases treated at the Institute of Physical Medicine and Rehabilitation at least one half still had clothing problems upon discharge. It was felt that the design of clothing itself must be the basis for study, with adjustment, alteration or new design as a goal. With the enlistment of such designers as Helen Cookman and Clarice Scott, who are among the first to devote full-time effort to clothing problems of the disabled, more rapid strides are being made.

As in other areas, analysis of the activity of dressing proved fruitful. Observing how a person moves, what happens in regard to the article of clothing under study, what obstacles it presents, has been most helpful. Some of these observations are illustrated in Chart 8–7. Further reports on such studies are available in the booklet *Functional Fashions for the Physically Handicapped.*

Some of the problems regarding dresses are caused by armholes and sleeves that restrict movement and which tear too easily, by long sleeves interfering with the movement of wheelchairs, by fastenings in difficult places which are hard to manage with weak hands or only one hand, and by too full or too tight skirts.

Solutions to these problems were such features as high-cut armholes with gussets or inverted pleats, side-back blouse fullness, three-quarter length sleeves wide enough not to be binding, gored or slightly flared skirts, wrap-around styles with large hook-and-eye fasteners, side-front 14 in. length zipper closures on skirts, and Velcro or cleat closings in place of buttons or snaps.

In men's clothing, the first garments to receive attention were trousers. The main problems involved getting trouser legs over shoes when attached to braces with 90° stops, preventing wear and tear at the

CHART 8–7   CLOTHING ANALYSIS (One Garment Only)

Type of Garment	Problem Involved	Disability	Suggested Solutions
Blouse short sleeved and cardigan	1) Putting on 2) Taking off	Loss of motion of shoulder and elbow	1) Loose arm holes, such as raglan, kimono or dolman 2) Action-back pleats 3) Vertical style dress (divided into 2 pieces) 4) Stick with closet hook on end (to remove garment from shoulders)
	3) Fastening front	Weakness of both hands Use of only one hand	1) Vertical rather than horizontal buttonholes 2) Flat buttons 3) Larger buttons, size at least $3/8$ inch 4) Snaps instead of buttons 5) Slip-over blouse or sweater 6) Buttonhook (regular or wire hook)
Blouse long sleeved and shirts	Same as other with addition of 4) Fastening cuffs	Use of only one hand	1) Large enough cuff to let hand pass through 2) Elasticized or knit cuff 3) Elasticized thread on button 4) Elasticized loop over button
Both of above	5) Keeping shirt or blouse tucked in	Weakness of hands and arms	1) Long tails 2) Latex gripper inside skirt or trousers band 3) Tape from shirt tail to sock tops (for men)
	6) Wear underarm from crutches	Weakness or loss of use	1) Knitted gusset piece under arms 2) Action pleat at armhole in blouse back
	7) Tear or binding when wheeling chair	Weakness or loss of use	1) Material with stretch (such as jersey) 2) Action-back pleats (center back or at arm-hole) 3) Three-quarter length sleeves (to prevent soiling cuffs)

knees due to brace joints, keeping the trousers from dropping to the floor when the person used the toilet and providing easy access into side or hip pockets.

One solution to trousers (or women's slacks) problem was double-cam-lock, full-length zippers in both side seams which permitted opening from either top or bottom. Bottom openings not only permit easier donning over braces, but also allow for putting on and removing either a short or long leg brace without removing the trousers. A nylon lining inside the trouser leg at the knee prevents wear. A half-belt provides for either a drop seat or a drop front. Half-hitch pockets and front pleats make pockets more accessible.

All types of garments, including underclothing and outerwear, are being studied. Of the underclothing, bras and girdles are probably the most challenging. Fastening of these garments requires manipulation of closures, simultaneously maintaining stretch of the fabric. When grasp is weak or when there is use of only one hand, this is usually impossible with the present types of design.

Children's clothing presents problems similar to those of adults and also includes growth problems. Perceptual losses may result in difficulties in putting on garments. For babies who must be dressed, problems may arise when mothers are physically disabled.

Footwear presents problems for all ages. Shoe fastenings cause one problem. Some of the answers are the use of one-buckle closings or of Shu-Lok or Velcro as closures. Putting on stockings or socks usually requires the aid of special devices. Easy-to-manage garters for persons with hand difficulties are still not available, but certain adaptations have made their use possible for some disabilities.

Another matter of general concern is suitable fabrics, easy to care for and long wearing. Good grooming is quite as essential as fashion, if not considerably more so. Simple classic designs are usually longer in style, although skirt lengths may vary and should be kept somewhat near the trend, regardless of whether leg orthoses may or may not be covered. Looking dowdy only accentuates an appliance. It does not minimize it.

HOMEMAKING

When emphasis was given to training the disabled in various vocational needs, little concern was evinced for the housewife. Although it is usually a full-time job, only in 1956 was homemaking recognized as a vocation by the Social Rehabilitation Services (SRS) and funds made available for training in this field. Despite this, some persons saw the need before and spent time studying the problems. Attention was first centered on the cardiac disabilities and is now extended to all disabilities. From the 10 to 12 years or more of specialized study of home economists, physical therapists, occupational therapists, and time and motion study engineers and physicians, some basic principles have been derived and laid down for our guidance. There are many publications worthy of our study. One of the foremost of these is the manual *Training the Disabled Homemaker.*

Energy Saving in Housework

Regardless of the disability, there is one general principle which can be applied for all, that of *saving energy.* Here again, the work of Gilbreth, with guidelines known as "therblings," has a specific application. The following work simplification technics have been adapted from the studies:

1. Use both hands in opposite and symmetrical, smooth flowing motions.
2. Arrange work areas within normal reach.
3. Slide objects; don't lift or carry them.
4. Arrange work areas and tools for different tasks, such as preparation and clean-up areas, mixing and baking center, etc.
5. Eliminate any unnecessary motions or processes.
6. Avoid holding — use clamps, stationary equipment.
7. Use assistance of gravity where possible.
8. Preposition tools, ready for easy grasp or pickup.
9. Locate switches and controls within easy reach.
10. Sit whenever possible; don't stand.
11. Use proper work heights, according to the job and the individual.
12. Good working conditions, proper light and ventilation, pleasing colors, comfortable clothing, etc.

Each of these technics can be applied to various tasks. Two hands (if possible) are helpful, not only in dishwashing but also in ironing, dusting and many cleaning jobs. Arrange work centers with necessary tools and equipment located at each area and within normal reach and in a position easy to handle. For instance, the refrigerator should be placed next to the preparation area with the door opening at the side next to the work counter. If the sink is located on the other side, continuous with or adjoining the counter surface, little moving about or lifting of objects is necessary. It is also advisable to have the sink and stove located close together, with counter surface in the middle, as trips between these two pieces of equipment are made more frequently than between any other areas. Use of time and motion study charts are helpful with some patients for demonstrating the needs in arrangements of work areas and appliances. Wheeled tables and laundry carts show how lifting and carrying can be minimized, also how fewer trips save both time and energy.

Proper work heights, either for standing, sitting on a stool or in a wheelchair or in a regular chair will improve posture and lessen fatigue. One can sit to wash dishes, iron or bake. Even laundry, housecleaning and bedmaking can be managed from a wheelchair.

Sufficient lighting with switches that are easy-to-reach and operate should not be neglected. Appliance controls, if located at the front, require less reaching and are just as suitable as if located at back, unless there are small children in the house.

Another area of work simplification is organization of work, such as scheduling of jobs for most convenient times and allowing for rest periods. Allocating tasks to other members of the family may be helpful. Sometimes standards should be checked to determine if certain tasks are really necessary. These approaches are often the most difficult to achieve, but they can be as important as other methods of energy saving, and should not be overlooked.

Retraining of Physical Disabilities

In addition to general techniques such as work simplification, when certain problems are present, such as weakness of upper extremities or ability to use one hand only, adjustments of certain specific tasks or of equipment may be necessary; for example:

1. Stabilization of tools and appliances.
2. Selection of tools which require only one hand to operate.
3. Selection of tools or utensils for type of handle easiest to grasp.
4. Consideration of type of motion used to operate equipment— whether up and down, push and pull, rotary.
5. Use of electrical equipment to eliminate manual operation.
6. Selection of utensils according to weight, shape, durability, ease of care.
7. Selection of containers (jars, packages) for ease of opening.
8. Use of special adapted equipment.

Stabilization can be obtained through use of suction-cup bases, plastic or rubber mats, cut-out boards or wall or table-attached appliances (can openers and grinders). There are many tools requiring only one-handed operation, such as whisks, one-handed egg beaters, long handled dustpan and broom and clip-around aprons. While lightweight bowls may help those with arm weakness, it is more important to consider the shape of the bowl. Select one with a good flat bottom and either or both a rim and good handles (or extended lips). For the per-

CHART 8–8

INSTITUTE OF REHABILITATION MEDICINE
NEW YORK UNIVERSITY MEDICAL CENTER

OCCUPATIONAL THERAPY SERVICE

Homemaking Evaluation

Name _____ Room No. _____ Date _____

Diagnosis_____ Onset _____

Disability_____ Admitted to I.R.M._____
R & L U.E.'s_____ Social Worker_____
w/c or Amb. _____ Sponsorship (DVR)_____

Home Address_____

Apt. or House_____

No. in Family_____

Comment _____
_____
_____
_____

Previous Responsibilities (cooking, child care, management, cleaning, etc.) _____
_____
_____
_____

Type of Cooking (Ethnic, Top of stove, Oven-casseroles, Broil, etc.)_____
_____
_____
_____

Description of Kitchen & Housing Situation (including rough sketch of floor plan)

CHART 8-8 (continued)

Report on Patient's Performance in Homemaking Kitchen

Activity (such as: cake mix, tuna salad, meat loaf) ————————————————
——

Gathering Ingredients (from w/c or walking with table — reach high & low shelves, open refrigerator — etc.)————————————————————————————————
——
——
——
——

Work Set-Up (Standard Kitchen — lowered counter — w/c or high chair)————————
——
——
——

Equipment Used (can opener, mixer, etc.)————————————————————————
——
——

Communication and Ability to Follow Written and Verbal Directions————————————
——
——
——

Mental and Emotional Reliability (confusion — judgement)————————————————
——
——
——

Visual and/or Perceptual Deficits————————————————————————————————
——
——

Safety——
——
——

Comment and/or Recommendations:

CHART 8–8 (continued)

INSTITUTE OF REHABILITATION MEDICINE
NEW YORK UNIVERSITY MEDICAL CENTER

OCCUPATIONAL THERAPY SERVICE

Outline of Homemaking Evaluation

I   *Brief* medical history

II   Description of family living patterns

III   Specific duties that will be required of the homemaker

IV   Possibilities for outside help or assistance from other members of the family with

        1)   heavy cleaning
        2)   laundry
        3)   shopping
        4)   child care, etc.

V   Report on patient's performance in homemaking kitchen

        1)   physical functioning
        2)   mental and emotional reliability
        3)   motivation
        4)   safety

VI   Recommended Program

    Immediate goals
        Training in homemaking kitchen.

    Future goals
        Plans for return to home and follow-up program.

VII   List of appliances and special utensils (with sources and approximate prices) that would be useful.

son with incoordination, pottery or even iron ware may be the most practical. The new Teflon-covered utensils are easier to clean than ordinary surfaces.

Dish wiping can be eliminated by rinsing with hot water and allowing dishes to be air-dried. Eggs, if held properly can be broken and separated with one hand. Where dexterity for separating the shell is not possible (as with the quadraplegic), a tenodesis grasp may be used to hold the egg, which can then be "dropped" into bowl to break the shell. Cutting can be managed by using a sharp knife (French chef's knife), placing the tip on the cutting surface and pressing down (instead of using push and pull method) or by using a cutting board with nails. For the person with incoordination, stabilization for cutting is best done by holding the food with a fork and then cutting, or peeling with a floating blade peeler.

For those with involvement of the lower extremities only, who usually are wheelchair-bound, suggestions discussed under work simplification will be helpful — using lower work surfaces and rearranging work areas and equipment to save extra moving of chair. Storage areas can be arranged within limits of reach, using vertical filing, narrow shelves, pull-out bins and revolving corner cupboards. Built-in vacuum cleaning systems and ironing boards save lifting and carrying.

Treatment Programming and Teaching

When a patient is first seen for evaluation in the homemaking area, a special check of household and family routines is helpful in determining the areas of proficiency and/or limitation (Chart 8–8). Depending then, on management planning, energy saving, or skill retraining through techniques or special equipment, a program can be planned around various household tasks. If cooking skills need practice, a list of certain kinds of dishes or recipes are helpful for checking on ability to mix, chop, cut, peel, pour, measure, use surface burners or ovens, and so on.

Although cooking as an activity is seldom needed for training in "cooking" per se, except perhaps for the adolescent or the very young housewife, its value in confidence building and in the nutritional aspects should not be overlooked. The latter should not be confused with dieting, which should not be engaged in unless specifically recommended and prescribed by the physician.

When a therapist is instructing or demonstrating, it is helpful if she is skilled in the various activities, particularly in one-handed tasks. It is also wise to have several methods or technics and to let the patient test for herself which seems easiest to manage.

HOUSING

One of the most disheartening of experiences is to receive training in a rehabilitation center and through proficiency in skills achieve independence only to return home to an environment totally unsuitable because of architectural barriers. Because of these experiences, most rehabilitation centers now understand that inquiry into the housing situation itself, as well as into family and financial problems, is necessary. When unsuitable housing is recognized, assistance must be given in planning of alterations or adjustments. Features commonly found in homes, that often present barriers to independence, are too narrow halls and doorways, door sills and entrance steps, high windows with out-of-reach or difficult type of opening. Other problems may stem from floor composition and covering, placement of electrical outlets and switches, arrangement of fixtures in bathroom, inaccessible closets and poor furniture arrangement allowing little maneuvering space. Two-story houses or apartment buildings with no elevators add difficulties. This may mean either relocating or replanning rooms, and/or adding a bathroom on the first floor.

Although ideal housing should be used as a guide, adjustments need not necessarily be elaborate. This is very often true in the kitchen. Where extensive alterations are called for, the help of a builder or architect should be enlisted, especially when eliminating walls or changing plumbing installations.

Recommendations regarding special features, whether in old or new housing are as follows:

1. Ramps should be no more than a 5 to 6° (1 to 12 in.) incline if possible and at least 36 to 40 in. wide. Rails are advisable, extending beyond both top and bottom with ends curving out of the way.
2. All inside sills should be eliminated. Outside sills should be confined to a minimum.
3. All doorways should be from 32 to 36 in. wide. (Sometimes 30 in. width is possible, but there should be adequate hall or turning space at entrance.)
4. The door to the bathroom may need to slide or fold to allow closing behind a chair. Closet doors are best when sliding or folding.
5. Floors should be non-skid. Suggested materials are terrazzo with carborundum chips, or vinyl tile. *No wax.*
6. Floor coverings should be eliminated; when used, they should be firm surfaces such as woven mats or vinyl tile.
7. Wall switches should be no more than 36 in. high; electrical outlets no less than 24 in. high.
8. Grab bars over the tub and beside the toilet should be added.

9. Kitchen area. Look for counter surface space, height of same, possibility of open areas under counters and beneath sink, storage accessibility, placement and type of control fixtures on equipment, direction of door opening on refrigerator, oven and cupboards. For further details, refer to section on Homemaking or special publications listed in bibliography.

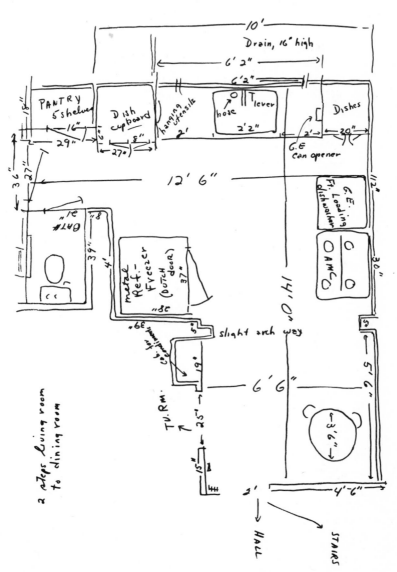

Fig. 8–3. Rough sketch of floor plan.

In addition to recognizing architectural barriers and the requirements for their elimination, a method is needed to attain these objectives. The following procedure is set forth as a guide:

1. Timing for introducing patient to home alterations (start as soon as patient is motivated or accepting).
2. Obtaining information of current housing situations (an on-the-site visit is preferable, if possible, to take measurements and rough sketchs of floor plan and equipment lay-out (Fig. 8–3).
3. Assessment of necessary changes (correlate with patients performance in homemaking training and ADL).
4. Provision of scale drawing of alterations (should be suitable for conveying details necessary for builder or architect (Fig. 8–4).
5. Agency contacts for financial aid.

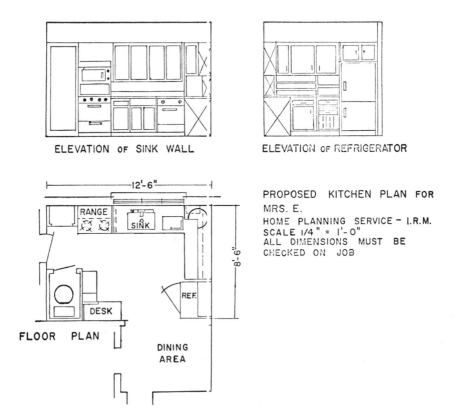

ELEVATION OF SINK WALL   ELEVATION OF REFRIGERATOR

PROPOSED KITCHEN PLAN FOR MRS. E.
HOME PLANNING SERVICE – I.R.M.
SCALE 1/4 " = 1'-0"
ALL DIMENSIONS MUST BE CHECKED ON JOB

Scaled drawings of home revisions

Fig. 8–4   Scaled drawings of home revisions.

Whenever possible, after alterations are completed and the patient has returned home, a follow-up visit is desirable. Even the best of plans may be subject to some oversight or misjudgment.

BIBLIOGRAPHY

Books

Anderson, M. H.: Upper Extremity Orthotics. Springfield, Ill., Charles C Thomas, 1965.

Buchwald, E., et al.: Physical Rehabilitation for Daily Living. New York, McGraw-Hill, 1952.

Gilbreth, L., Thomas, O. M., and Clymer, E.: Management in the Home. New York, Dodd Mead, revised 1959.

Institute of Physical Medicine and Rehabilitation: Self-Help Devices for Rehabilitation. Dubuque, Iowa, Wm. C. Brown, 1958.

Klinger, J. L., Frieden, F. H., and Sullivan R. M.: Mealtime Manual for the Aged and Handicapped. New York, Essandess Special Editions, a division of Simon & Shuster, Inc. 1970.

Lawton, E. B.: Activities of Daily Living for Physical Rehabilitation. New York, McGraw-Hill, 1963.

Lowman, E. W., and Klinger, J. L.: Aids To Independent Living. New York, McGraw-Hill, 1970.

Lowman, E. W., et al.: Arthritis: General Principles. Physical Medicine and Rehabilitation, Boston, Little, Brown, 1959.

May, E. E., Waggoner, N. R., and Boettke, E. M.: Homemaking for the Handicapped. New York, Dodd Mead, 1966.

Rusk, H. A., et al.: Rehabilitation Medicine. ed. 3, St. Louis, C. V. Mosby, 1964.

Brochures and Pamphlets

Clothes for the Physically Handicapped Homemaker with Features Suitable for All Women. Home Economics Research Report No. 12, Washington, D.C., U.S. Dept. of Agriculture, 1961.

Cookman, H., and Zimmerman, M. E.: Functional Fashions for the Physically Handicapped. New York I.P.M.R., 1961.

Institute of Physical Medicine and Rehabilitation: Rx for the Disabled Housewife. I.P.M.R., New York, reprinted 1961.

Institute of Rehabilitation Medicine: Bibliography on Self-Help Devices and Orthotics 1950–1967. New York, N.Y.U. Medical Center, Institute of Rehabilitation Medicine, 1967.

Homemaking & Homeplanning Service. O. T. Dept.: Training the Young Hemiplegic Homemaker—A Picture Study In Rehabilitation. New York, Institute of Rehabilitation Medicine, 1968.

Judson, J. S., Wagner, E. M., and Zimmerman, M. E.: Rehabilitation Monograph XX: Homemaking and Housing for the Disabled in the United States of America, New York, I.P.M.R., 1962.

Lawton, E. B.: Rehabilitation Monograph X: A.D.L. Activities of Daily Living, Testing, Training and Equipment. New York, Institute of Physical Medicine and Rehabilitation, 1956.

McCullough, H. E., and Farnham, M. B.: Space and Design Requirement for Wheel Chair Kitchens. Agricultural Experiment Station, Bulletin 661, Urbana, University of Illinois, November 1961.

Rusk, H. A., and Associates: A Functional Home for Easier Living. New York, I.P.M.R., 1960.

Rusk, H. A., Kristeller, E. L., Judson, J. S., Hunt, G. M., and Zimmerman, M. E.: Rehabilitation Monograph VIII: A Manual for Training the Disabled Homemaker. ed. 2, New York, I.P.M.R., 1961.

Wheeler, V. H.: Planning Kitchens for Handicapped Homemakers. Rehabilitation Monograph XXVII: New York, Institute of Rehabilitation Medicine, 1965.

Journals

Bennett, R. L., and Stevens, H. R.: Orthetics: part I: prescription, part II: patient training. Phys. Therapy Rev. 36:11, 721-745, 1956.

Smith, C. R.: Home planning for the severely disabled. Med. Clin. N. Am. 53, pp. 703-711, 1969.

Zimmerman, M. E.: The functional motion test as an evaluation tool for patients with lower motor neuron disturbance, Am. J. Occup. Therapy, 23 pp. 49-56, 1969.

9

Amputations

ELINOR ANNE SPENCER, B.A., O.T.R.

UPPER EXTREMITY AMPUTATIONS

To be an amputee is to be without a limb or limbs as a result of injury, disease, or congenital deformity. Bodily functions develop in the presence of anomalies in children with congenital deformities or early post-birth amputations, but post-adolescent amputees suffer the loss of a part of the body which had previously been integrated into the total body image. Function, sensation, and cosmesis of the involved extremity are affected, and the amputee must rely on a "strange" mechanical device as a replacement for his natural limb. Since the traumatic amputee has usually matured physically, the circumstances of the amputation, its meaning and its consequences are different from those of the congenital or very young amputee. This chapter will emphasize the rehabilitation team's work with a person who has suffered traumatic amputation after adolescence.

There are many causes of amputations: trauma, peripheral vascular disease, thrombosis, embolism, malignancy, and trophic changes, in addition to congenital absence or deformities. The most common cause of upper extremity (UE) amputations is trauma resulting from industrial accidents, which are usually connected with the use of high speed power tools. The most common cause of lower extremity (LE) amputations is peripheral vascular disease.

The physical therapy service is responsible for the largest amount of training of the LE amputee; but since LE amputees are frequently referred to the occupational therapy service for assistance in motivation, physical restoration, self-care independence (ADL), and prevocational assessment, this chapter will discuss some appropriate treatment objectives and modalities. However, because the occupational therapist participates actively in the prosthetic training program of the UE amputee, this will be the main focus of the chapter.

One must remember that a patient's reactions to the loss of a limb vary depending on his age when the amputation occurred, as well as his intelligence, physical development, sex, vocation, avocational interests, social status, and finances. He may also have problems in function because of the presence of phantom sensations, a phenomenon in which the amputee actually feels the presence of part of the limb which has been amputated. This can lead to difficulties in his accepting, tolerating, and learning to use the prosthesis (the artificial limb).

The amputee rehabilitation program begins with the decision to amputate and ends with the successful functional and cosmetic integration of the prosthesis into the body scheme. Whether the cause of the amputation is trauma or disease, the first step in the total program is the consideration of the type and level of surgery and the psychological and physical preparation of the patient.

SURGICAL CONSIDERATIONS

During the surgical procedure of amputation, the physicians try to save as much tissue as possible. The importance of structural length and support of the bone, length and strength of the cut or damaged muscles, and sensation through adequate skin coverage bear out the practicality and necessity of preserving tissue. Regardless of the level of the amputation, the muscles involved directly or indirectly in the function of the amputated part are affected by the loss.

Prior to the operation, the necessity of the amputation, the expected result, the post-operative conditioning program, the possibility of difficulties in adjustment, and the prosthetic training program are explained to the patient. He must be prepared both medically and psychologically for the problems which he may encounter as he prepares to use his prosthesis.

Both during and after surgery, effort is made to form the stump in such a way as to maintain maximum function of the remaining tissue and to provide maximum use of the prosthesis. Blood vessels and nerves are pulled down, cut, and allowed to retract so that they do not interfere with the amputee's use of the prosthesis by causing pain in the stump when he uses the device.

Either a *closed* or an *open* amputation may be done by the surgeon. The open amputation allows free drainage of affected material, minimizing the possibility of infection before closure. The immediate closed amputation may reduce the period of hospitalization, but also reduces free drainage and introduces the danger of bacterial growth. When the closed amputation is performed, either immediately or following sufficient drainage, the maximum amount of tissue is saved. However, regardless of the surgical method used, the stump must be

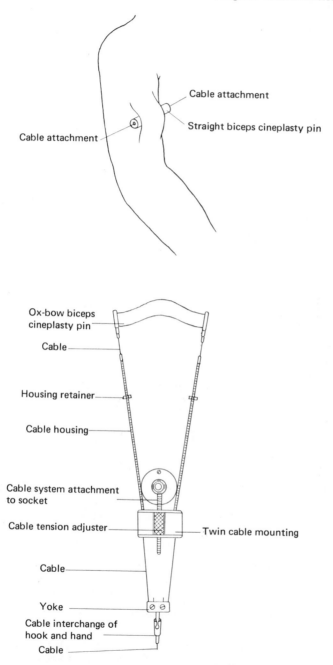

Fig. 9-1 (Top) Biceps cineplasty tunnel with straight cineplasty pin.
(Bottom) Biceps cineplasty cable control system.

strong and resilient and have a snug, comfortable contact with the socket of the prosthesis, for the amputee will exert much pressure on the stump while using the device.

Cineplasty

Under most circumstances, a conventional prosthesis, using shoulder harnessing for suspension and control of prosthetic function which is channeled through a control cable, is provided for the amputee.

However, if the rehabilitation team and the patient wish, a second surgical procedure can be done after the initial procedure is well-healed. The biceps or pectoral cineplasty is occasionally done in order to eliminate the shoulder harnessing and to increase sensory feedback from the terminal device. The more common of the two sites for cineplasty is the biceps muscle. A surgical tunnel is made through the muscle into which a plastic pin is inserted. The control cable is attached to both ends of this pin. The prosthesis is then controlled by the contraction and relaxation of the biceps muscle (Fig. 9–1).

Because the tunnel must be kept clean consistently, there is considerable chance of infection if the amputee does not take sufficient care of his hygiene. Additionally, the amputee who has had a cineplasty procedure must be able to accept the cosmetic effect of the tunnel through the biceps muscle (Fig. 9–1).

Levels of Amputations of the Upper Extremity

The higher the level of amputation, the more the amputee must depend on the prosthesis for replacement of bodily function and the more extensive the prosthesis must be. Generally accepted levels of amputation are indicated in Figure 9–2.

Amputations at the joints are referred to as *disarticulations* (i.e., finger, wrist, elbow, or shoulder disarticulation). Amputations below the wrist across the metacarpal bones are referred to as *transmetacarpal*. At this level and below, amputations are referred to as *partial hand*. Should the amputation occur between the wrist and the elbow, the level is referred to as *below elbow* (BE); and amputation between the elbow and the shoulder is referred to as *above elbow* (AE). Amputations at the surgical neck of the humerus (distal to the humeral head) to the shoulder articulation are referred to as *shoulder disarticulations*. Amputations above the shoulder joint involving the clavicle and scapula are referred to as *forequarter*.

Although there are general types of prostheses for each level of amputation, each prosthesis is medically prescribed for the person's individual needs, and the artificial limb is custom-made and individually fitted.

Special Considerations—Problems

There are several problems related to the amputation. One of the factors to be considered in the training program is the level of the amputation.

Physical problems may affect or hinder the prosthetic training program with either the UE or the LE amputee. Such problems are: the length of the stump, its skin coverage, its sensitivity (i.e., presence of hypersensitivity and/or edema), its healing, the condition of the skin,

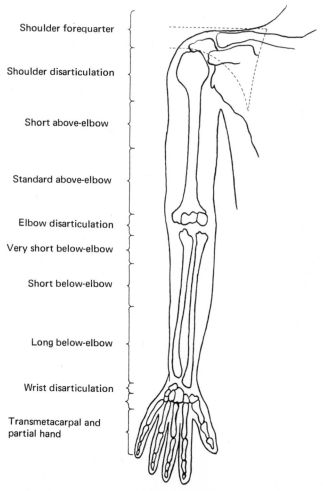

Shoulder forequarter

Shoulder disarticulation

Short above-elbow

Standard above-elbow

Elbow disarticulation

Very short below-elbow

Short below-elbow

Long below-elbow

Wrist disarticulation

Transmetacarpal and partial hand

Fig. 9–2 Amputation levels.

the presence of infection. For example, an amputee with either a very long stump or a very short one may find the design of the various components of his prosthesis unsatisfactory either cosmetically or functionally.

Perspiration, the natural result of physical effort, may result from excessive confinement of the stump in the prosthesis' socket, for the stump lacks ventilation. The occupational therapist must also be aware of the possibility of the amputee's being allergic to plastics and resins from which the socket is made.

The sensation of the stump is important to the rehabilitation of the amputee. If his hand has been amputated and he has been fitted with a prosthetic prehension device, he no longer experiences functional sensation in the area which has been amputated. Although he has sensation in his stump, it is functionally lost when he puts on his prosthesis. Therefore, he will have to depend on visual cues in order to use the terminal device to handle objects.

Sensation can also be a problem if the socket is ill-fitting or if the stump is not well-formed at the distal end. Therefore, the amputee must become adjusted to the pressure of the socket on the stump. He also must become used to the pressure of the harness on his shoulders and to the weight of the prosthesis.

Phantom Sensations

The presence of phantom sensations is common among amputees. Frequently, "crush injuries," with their accompanying sensations of burning or cramping, are the most prevalent causes of phantom sensations. The sensation is that the limb remains a part of the person in spite of the amputation. Although, in most cases, this awareness is painless, at times it can become intolerable to the patient, and actual pain may result. In such a case, a revision of the stump through surgical methods may be necessary.

The phantom sensations are usually felt as the distal parts of the extremity (i.e., the amputee "senses" the existence of a non-existent hand or foot). These phantom sensations seldom involve the total extremity.

Usually the patient will describe the feeling of a presence, perhaps a tingling sensation. In addition to supportive counselling, the most effective compensation for the phantom sensation is the early use of the stump combined with either a temporary or a permanent prosthesis. The distal contact of the stump with the socket can have a desensitizing effect on the stump and can thus minimize phantom or painful sensations.

The amputee may also have to accept a new body image, and for some amputees, this is difficult, as major changes in their body images will occur with the loss. Some amputees may be disturbed by this change in body concept and may have subsequent difficulties in prosthetic training. To be functionally useful, the prosthesis must be integrated into the body schema and become a part of the individual.

PSYCHOLOGICAL REACTIONS

In assisting the amputee in adjusting to his condition and in becoming motivated to learn the function and care of his prosthesis, the occupational therapist must recognize the amputee's psychological reactions to his situation. If the patient feels guilt or shame regarding the amputation, his relationships with his family and friends may be affected, presenting difficulties. He may be depressed and may refuse to cooperate with the training program. Or he may be interested in compensating for the loss by learning as much as he can about the prosthesis, by accepting change and by demonstrating eagerness to learn.

It is very important to consider the patient's feelings and attitudes. The prosthesis should be presented in a way that is meaningful to the amputee and that is useful to him. For some persons, function is most important; for others, cosmesis is the greatest concern. For either, prosthetic replacement can help the amputee by providing function and cosmesis.

PHYSICAL CONSIDERATIONS

Generally speaking, the longer the stump the more the amputee can do both in the pre-prosthetic program and in the prosthetic training program. With a well-healed, healthy stump, the amputee has a good purchase power on the socket and security in its fit. In the case of a BE amputation, the longer the stump the more active supination and pronation the patient is likely to have. This situation will assist him in positioning the hook for grasp and placement of objects. Also, if the stump is long, either AE or BE, it is more useful to the amputee; he has a tendency to use it more frequently, thus maintaining normal range of motion and strength.

During the postoperative and pre-prosthetic periods, the patient will usually automatically change his dominance to his sound extremity. If the dominant extremity has been amputated and the patient is forced to use his non-dominant extremity for grasp and placement of objects, he may have some incoordination. In this case, he can benefit from activities with the sound extremity to improve the fine coordination of his non-dominant arm. The amputee who has suffered loss of his non-dominant extremity may be less motivated to use the prosthesis, for he will depend on his dominant extremity to compensate for his other arm.

It is important to stress bilateral activities to help the patient adjust to his limitations in reach and in holding large objects, as well as to aid his bimanual coordination. Involvement in activities aids in the healing of the stump and in learning to use the prosthesis.

The bilateral amputee usually chooses the side with the longer stump to become his dominant side. Sometimes he is trained in the use of one prosthesis at a time. However, since the two prostheses have a common harness and the body must adjust to the weight and balance of the mechanical devices, he may start his training program with both limbs, concentrating on one at a time.

Early Fitting

It is commonly recognized that early fitting of the prosthesis or prostheses aids the training program. Some doctors and therapists think that it is more desirable to fit several temporary prostheses rather than to wait for several months for the arrival of the permanent one. This technic provides early prosthetic training while the permanent limb is being fabricated. There are four approaches to shortening the time between the amputation and the fitting of the permanent prosthesis.

1. In some cases, particularly if the patient has a long stump or stumps, utensils can be fitted into the Ace bandage, which is applied to the stump to facilitate shrinkage.
2. Utensils can be fitted into the pocket of a strap and wrapped around the stump with a Velcro fastening. A temporary prosthetic cuff can be devised from plaster or leather to which either utensils or the terminal device and controls can be attached.
3. Early fitting, several weeks postoperatively, has met with success. This temporary prosthesis consists of a plaster cuff with components and a control system similar to the ones the permanent prosthesis will have.
4. The immediate post-surgical fitting is also being done with upper extremity amputees. It has been found that immediate fitting, in addition to shortening the time between amputation and the wearing of the prosthesis, has hastened control of edema, lessened post-surgical pain, encouraged conditioning of the stump, and provided more rapid use of the controls and the prosthesis. The plaster dressing with conventional harness and controls is applied at the time of surgery or during the immediate postoperative period. The plaster casts are changed as the stump shrinks. Provision of this type of immediate prosthesis encourages a positive approach from the patient and early learning of prosthetic use; thus, when the amputee receives his permanent prosthesis, he has developed appropriate muscle use and has learned controls.

PREPARING THE PATIENT

In preparing the patient for prosthetic wear and in providing the prosthesis appropriate to his needs and expectations, the occupational therapist must consider several important questions. First, does the patient need it? This will depend on his limitations as a result of the amputation, his vocational and avocational needs and interests, and his attitude toward the value of the prosthesis for him. Another question relevant to the prescription is, what does he need it for, and will he wear it? This will depend largely upon his attitude toward the loss he has suffered and his attitude toward his loss of function and his relationships with other people. Does he need and want function or cosmesis or both? What is most important to him in his homelife, in his work, in his hobbies, and in his social life?

Following the pre-prosthetic program, or near its end, these questions are taken into serious consideration in order to prescribe the appropriate prosthetic components for the maximum benefit to the amputee. At this point the rehabilitation team comes together for consultation.

Prior to the prescription the physiatrist measures the stump and examines the patient. The parts and controls of the prosthesis are determined by many factors: range of motion, strength, length, skin coverage and appearance, incision site, shoulder strength, and job requirements.

The following pre-prosthetic evaluation form (Chart 9-1) can be used by the occupational therapist as a guide to determine what would be appropriate components (hook and hand) for the amputee. If the patient has not remained in the hospital during the postoperative, pre-prosthetic period, the evaluation form is helpful in determining his limitations and needs in terms of strengthening the extremity and trunk for prosthetic wear and use. Should an amputee return to the hospital's amputee clinic for prescription of a new prosthesis, this form would be helpful in evaluating whether he should be given the same type of prosthesis or if different components would be more helpful to him. The occupational therapist can also assess the amputee's needs for further training, especially if he has not used his prosthesis extensively in daily activities.

The Team Approach

A successful training program for an amputee requires the coordinated efforts of a rehabilitation team. This team includes the surgeon, nurse, physiatrist, physical therapist, occupational therapist, social worker, prosthetist, rehabilitation counsellor, and psychiatrist or psychologist. A coordinated effort of these persons is necessary for the provision of appropriate prosthetic replacement and training in the use of the prosthesis.

CHART 9-1   PRE-PROSTHETIC EVALUATION FORM

OCCUPATIONAL THERAPY

Pre-Prosthetic Evaluation

Name:_____ Date:_____

Address:_____ Telephone No. _____

Age:_____ Dominance:_____

Date, Cause, and Type of Amputation:_____

_____

Level of Amputation:_____ Length of Stump:_____

Prosthesis: #1_____ #2_____ #3_____ #4_____

Type of Present Prosthesis:_____

Occupation:_____

_____

Date last worked:_____

R.O.M. in shoulder:_____ elbow:_____ wrist:_____

supination-pronation:_____

Strength in shoulder:_____ elbow:_____

Pain in stump:_____

Phantom Sensations:_____

Current use of limb without prosthesis:_____

Use of previous prosthesis:_____

Attitude toward new prosthesis:_____

    a)   function:_____

    b)   cosmesis:_____

Additional remarks:_____

_____

_____

Prescription at Clinic:_____

_____

Prosthetist:_____ #Training sessions:_____

Signed:_____

Ideally, the physiatrist prescribes the prosthesis at the amputee clinic in the presence of the rehabilitation team and the patient and with the consultation of those who will be training the patient to adjust to and to use the prosthesis. At this time, if not before, the occupational therapist can acquaint the new amputee with the various components and harnessing which he is likely to have and perhaps can introduce him to another amputee who has completed the training program and is using his prosthesis successfully.

Pre-Prosthetic Period

The pre-prosthetic period is the time between the amputation and the fitting of the prosthesis. This is the period of "getting ready" for the prosthesis. Thus, the patient should be confronted with the importance of the pre-prosthetic program as preparation for prosthetic replacement. A successful pre-prosthetic program will hasten physical and psychological adjustment to the prosthesis and will minimize problems in wearing and using the permanent prosthesis. In this period it is important to counsel and guide the amputee regarding both the acceptance of his condition and the acceptance of the mechanical device which must substitute for natural motor power, sensation, and physical appearance. Counselling sessions with the amputee should also include his family and friends in order to involve them in his training program.

When medically approved, passive and active strengthening activities are started by the physical therapist and the occupational therapist to encourage maximum use of the stump, maximum range of motion (ROM), and maximum use of muscles, especially those of the arm and shoulder. A well-planned pre-prosthetic exercise program contributes to successful adaptation and provides strong muscles for the training in isolated motions for control and use of the prosthesis.

Following the amputation, the loss of the weight of the missing part causes a shift in the amputee's center of gravity. Atrophy of the musculature on the side of the amputation, scoliosis, and compensatory curves may occur if the patient does not have proper exercise. Therefore, the beginning exercise program is geared toward correcting faulty body mechanics and providing the amputee with sufficient ROM and strength to operate the prosthesis.

The first step, of course, is to establish good rapport with the patient so that it will be possible to help him in working through his necessary adjustments and in learning independence in daily living with the aid of an artificial limb. The relationship between the training therapist and the patient is a very important one, for the therapist must understand the patient's attitudes toward the prosthesis in order to help him accept and use it. He may have fears of being different; he may question the attitudes of others toward himself; he may even question himself and his possible inadequacies.

Before the amputee receives his prosthesis, he must develop strength and tolerance in his stump. As soon as possible following the amputation, exercises are begun to maintain and, if necessary, to regain normal passive and active ROM in the joints proximal to the amputation. Since the hospital stay may be short, these exercises are designed so that they can be done in out-patient situations in the clinic. Although this may be painful to the patient, it is important to maintain and encourage maximum movement and use of the extremity during the healing period in order to prepare the amputee for the prosthesis, to prevent weakening of muscles through disuse, and to encourage shrinkage of the stump.

After complete healing, the stump is massaged to encourage circulation, to prevent adhesions from scar tissue, to reduce swelling, to encourage desensitization, and to prevent the patient from fearing to handle the stump. Bandaging with an elastic Ace bandage or "shrinker" is done several times per day to encourage shrinkage and shaping. Wrapping should be done carefully with attention to tightness, unnecessary folds in the bandage, and complete, even coverage of the stump to insure comfort to the patient. Bandaging should be done from the distal to the proximal end. Care must be taken not to bandage so tightly as to produce muscle atrophy.

To encourage the use of the stump, the occupational therapist may strap utensils to it which are used in ADL. Such utensils may include a knife, a fork, or a toothbrush. The amputee should be encouraged to use the individual implements in his ADL.

The shrinking and shaping are also hastened by provision of a temporary prosthesis in the form of either a leather or a plaster cuff to which utensils can be attached for functional use of the extremity.

In this period, maximum use of the arms should be encouraged in both unilateral and bilateral exercise and functional activities. Additionally, since posture can be affected by the loss of a part, balance and posture exercises are necessary to prevent substitution patterns; these help to make the amputee aware of his new body image.

Although the pre-prosthetic program can be enhanced by the use of a temporary prosthesis, the amputee's tolerance determines when this may be applied. The temporary prosthesis aids the amputee in overcoming the initial psychological shock of amputation in the following ways: it provides a temporary replacement for the length of the missing arm; it provides him with a degree of independence, since a fork or a tool or other utensils may be attached to it to provide functional use of the amputated extremity. Additionally, a temporary prosthesis aids in cosmetic lengthening of the stump and, most significantly, is a device with which the amputee can perform bimanual and bilateral activities. One of the most important parts of the training program lies in the amputee's early involvement in activities which show results.

At this time, the amputee should be encouraged to use his sound arm in one-handed activities, even though he may not be naturally motivated to do so. If the amputated arm had been his dominant one, he may have temporary difficulties in accepting his loss and in using his non-dominant arm. In this case, he may need exercises to develop coordination patterns in the remaining limb. Activities such as eating, dressing, writing, and bathing may be difficult with the non-dominant hand. It is very important at this time to provide a program to encourage successful one-handed use in daily activities.

For the amputee with a cineplasty, the biceps muscle becomes the motor for the prosthesis, thus providing the link between the muscle and the prosthetic mechanism. Because the cineplasty provides increased arm ROM and the amputee is free of a harness, it allows him to hold the prosthesis in any position without affecting the operation of the terminal device. For maximum use of the cineplasty prosthesis, it is necessary to have a 1½ to 2-in. excursion of the surgical tunnel. Routine exercises to maintain this excursion include: isolated muscle exercise of the biceps, isometric contractions and holds, and sufficient relaxation for the excursion and the opening of the terminal device. The cineplasty prosthesis is reported to provide improved dexterity and sensitivity to the amputated limb by the physiological use of the stump muscles.

PARTS OF THE PROSTHESIS

The most significant component of the prosthesis is the terminal device (TD), which provides both function and cosmesis.

A *cosmetic terminal device* (cosmesis) may be as simple as a flesh-colored glove used to cover a partial hand. Aside from being used to hold light objects or to position objects by pushing or pulling, this glove has little functional value for the amputee. However, its psychological value is unquestioned.

A second type of cosmetic terminal device, the Army Prosthetics Research Laboratory (APRL) hand, is functional and can be attached to the wrist unit of most UE prostheses (Fig. 9–3). The APRL hand consists of a plastic spring-controlled device with fingers which are controlled in flexion and extension at the metacarpophalangeal joints by the control cable of the prosthesis. The thumb of the APRL hand can be placed in either of two positions: to grasp small objects or to grasp large ones. A plastic glove fits over the hand, presenting a "natural" appearance. The gloves are available in a variety of skin tones.

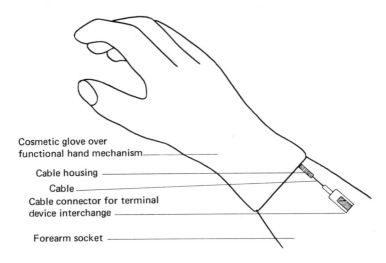

Cosmetic glove over
functional hand mechanism

Cable housing

Cable

Cable connector for terminal
device interchange

Forearm socket

Fig. 9–3 Functional hand with cosmetic glove and cable attachment.

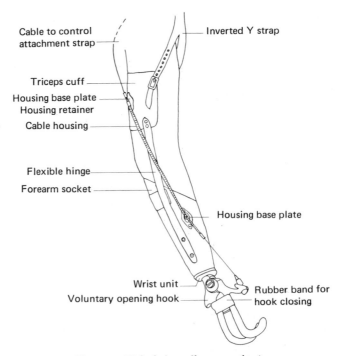

Cable to control
attachment strap

Inverted Y strap

Triceps cuff

Housing base plate
Housing retainer

Cable housing

Flexible hinge

Forearm socket

Housing base plate

Wrist unit

Rubber band for
hook closing

Voluntary opening hook

Fig. 9–4 Right below-elbow prosthesis.

The hook is the most functional of the terminal devices. It is made of either steel or aluminum and is canted or lyre-shaped. It is either locking or non-locking, with either voluntary opening or voluntary closing capacity (Figs. 9–4,5). The hook is usually lined with neoprene, which protects objects while the amputee is grasping them. The needs of the amputee determine the weight, length, design, and function of the hook device chosen by the rehabilitation team.

Wrist Unit

The terminal device (either cosmetic or functional) is connected to the forearm socket (or shell) by the wrist unit. The three basic wrist units are: (1) locking, (2) friction, and (3) oval.

The advantage of the locking unit is that it prevents the hook from rotating during heavy industrial work. By pushing a button on it, the amputee manually operates the wrist unit, which allows the position of the hook to be changed by rotation. The hook can be easily ejected for interchange of hook and hand.

The friction unit has threads and the hook must be screwed into the

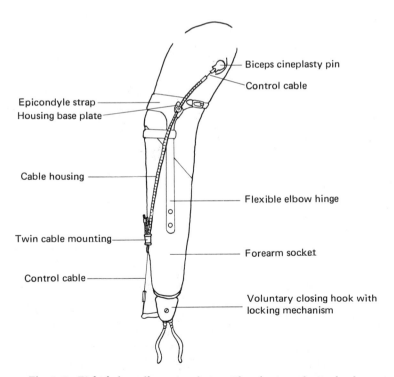

Fig. 9–5   Right below-elbow cineplasty with voluntary closing hook.

unit. Although this procedure is more time-consuming than that of the locking unit, the hook can be more easily positioned for specific tasks. Either the locking or the friction unit can be used with both BE and AE prostheses.

The oval unit is a special, thin unit for a wrist disarticulation prosthesis; it is used where the length of the components must be minimal in order to make the length of the amputated arm conform to that of the sound extremity.

Terminal devices and wrist units have standard connections. When the desired type of terminal device is chosen, one needs simply to determine the type and size of the wrist unit to accompany it. Usually the wrist unit is chosen according to the way in which the amputee will use his prosthesis in ADL and in his occupation.

The Socket

The plastic laminate socket may be either single or double-walled. Since overall weight and bulk must be minimized for the AE and shoulder disarticulation amputees, a single-walled forearm socket, or shell, is best for these prostheses. The socket provides length and contour to the forearm replacement. A double-walled socket is provided for the upper arm stump. A BE amputee has a double-walled socket consisting of an inner wall which conforms to his stump and an outer wall which provides length and contour to the forearm replacement.

The wrist unit is laminated onto the distal end of the forearm socket. Since the forearm socket can be used by both the AE and the BE amputee to carry objects (i.e., a coat, a handbag, or packages) as well as to push or to pull large or heavy objects, it is made of strong plastic resins which provide lightness and durability.

The Munster-Type Socket

The Munster-type socket was devised mainly for the short stump of the BE amputee to eliminate problems of fit, security, and poor leverage which were prevalent with the conventional split-sockets, difficult to fit on this type of amputee. It consists of a single double-walled forearm socket which extends just proximal to the olecranon process posteriorly and fits around the biceps tendon anteriorly. The "figure 9 harness" of the Munster-type prosthesis is not necessary for the suspension of the prosthesis; thus the "figure 9 harness" can be used with or without a triceps cuff. The socket is preflexed at approximately 35°, thus limiting complete flexion and extension of the elbow. However, even with this disadvantage in ROM, the fit is adequate for lifting and holding.

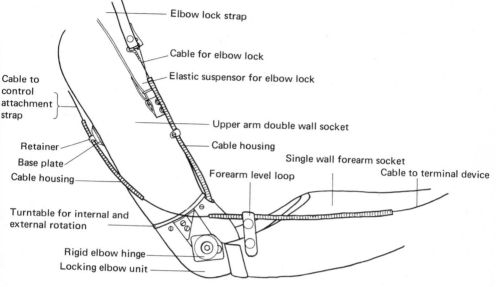

Elbow lock strap

Cable for elbow lock

Elastic suspensor for elbow lock

Cable to control attachment strap

Upper arm double wall socket

Retainer

Cable housing

Base plate

Single wall forearm socket

Cable housing

Forearm level loop

Cable to terminal device

Turntable for internal and external rotation

Rigid elbow hinge

Locking elbow unit

Fig. 9–6   Right above-elbow prosthesis with locking elbow unit.

The Upper-Arm Unit

The upper-arm unit of the AE prosthesis is a double-walled socket with the locking elbow unit laminated onto the socket. Since the AE amputee lacks independent elbow flexion and extension, these are provided mechanically by an elbow unit which is activated, locked, and unlocked by the cable control system. The forearm shell is attached to the locking elbow unit and the upper-arm socket (Fig. 9–6).

The Shoulder Disarticulation Prosthesis

The shoulder disarticulation prosthesis has a supporting socket portion which sometimes extends to the anterior and posterior aspects of the shoulder, depending on the level of the amputation. Frequently, a passive abduction hinge joint is added at the shoulder for ease in positioning and donning clothing.

Hinges

The hinges provide functional alignment and positioning between the forearm and the upper-arm socket or the harness. In addition, the flexible dacron or leather hinges used in the BE prosthesis allow active rotation of the forearm with a minimum of restriction. In the AE prosthesis the steel hinges provide rigidity to the mechanical elbow joint to insure strength, durability, and dependability.

The Harness

The function of the harness is to provide stable support of the prosthesis on the amputee to facilitate his wearing and using of it, to provide attachment for the control cables, and to assist the cables in the operation of the prosthesis. Basically, the dacron straps are formed in a figure 8 pattern with extra straps added as needed for better support or additional control function. For ease in use, the "figure 9 harness" is used with the Munster prosthesis. For the wrist disarticulation amputee, a simple cuff socket and a "figure 9 harness" may suffice.

The Stump Sock

A stump sock is worn by the amputee to aid in absorption of perspiration, to provide warmth to the stump, and padding for comfort and fit of the socket. An AE amputee frequently uses the short sleeve of a T-shirt in place of the stump sock. Use of an underblouse or T-shirt can alleviate discomfort from the harness straps in beginning training sessions.

The Control System

The control system is a very important part of the prosthesis. It determines the functional value of the prosthesis for the amputee. The control cable of the terminal device is attached to the device and to the harness. This cable is guided along the socket and cuff or the upper-arm socket by retainers which hold it in the most advantageous position for ease of function. Terminal device operation is generally accomplished by forward flexion of the shoulder. During the training period the amputee practices this isolated motion so that eventually he is able to operate the hook or hand with minimal physical strain (Fig. 9–7).

For the AE amputee this basic terminal device control cable also serves in flexion and extension of the mechanical elbow when the elbow unit is unlocked. It is activated by forward shoulder flexion. At times, additional joint motions are used in this cable operation: (1) because of limitation of shoulder control or strength; (2) to provide smooth operation of the prosthesis; (3) to enable the wearer to achieve maximum function of the mechanical arm and hand in reach, grasp, release, and hold. These motions may be shoulder abduction and adduction, scapular abduction and adduction, or shoulder flexion of the unamputated arm.

The second basic cable operates the elbow lock. It is attached internally or externally to the elbow unit and extends to the anterior deltoid-pectoral strap of the harness. A combination of shoulder elevation, depression, external rotation and extension is used both to lock and to unlock the elbow unit.

Control cables for the shoulder disarticulation and forequarter prostheses are attached to the humeral or scapular part of the upper-arm socket, and their exact design and function are determined by the needs of the individual amputee.

During the training period the amputee is carefully instructed to isolate the patterns of joint and muscle movement which control the operation of the prosthesis. (The instruction process will be discussed in the section on prosthetic training.) The extent to which the prosthesis provides the amputee with increased function depends on the quality of the fabrication of the prosthesis, its fit, the comfort of the wearer and his limitations, and the range of mechanical function. The amputee's limitations may be physical, psychological, and/or social. The range of mechanical function of the prosthesis includes grasp, release, hold, push, pull, and reach; which, depending upon the control by the wearer and the types of prescription components, can be extensive for the amputee.

THE CINEPLASTY PROSTHESIS

As was mentioned earlier, the cineplasty prosthesis is a special form of prosthetic device. In this case, the harness functions as additional support and comfort for the wearer, but it is not necessary for the actual function of the prosthesis. The same terminal devices, wrist units, and socket design can be used as those described earlier.

However, the control system is different because the surgical procedure consists of forming a tunnel through the biceps muscle (Fig. 9-1). This procedure is undertaken following the standard amputation. A plastic pin is inserted through this tunnel. At each end of the pin is a cable attachment from which a cable extends. These cables eventually join in a common adjustment plate and another cable extends from this point to the terminal device (Figs. 9-1, *bottom* and 9-6).

For added security, a triceps cuff may be strapped around the upper arm (Fig. 9-4). This cuff is attached to the forearm shell with flexible hinges.

In addition to eliminating the necessity of binding harnessing, the cineplasty control system approximates normal isolated muscle function. Rather than joint motion or muscle expansion for control, the cineplasty prosthesis is operated by the biceps muscle. With biceps control there is some simulation in sensation in the terminal device.

A person who has a cineplastic procedure generally has undergone pre-prosthetic training and has learned to use a harness-controlled prosthesis prior to cineplastic surgery. Thus, if necessary, he can revert to the use of a standard control system.

CHECK-OUT OF THE PROSTHESIS

Before the amputee begins his training program, members of the rehabilitation team examine the prosthesis to make sure that it conforms to the prescription and that it is mechanically sound. In performing the check-out of the prosthesis, the occupational therapist evaluates its fit and comfort for the wearer. He checks the motion and function of the components. Should adjustments need to be made in any part or parts of the prosthesis, the rehabilitation team makes recommendations to the prosthetist in order to insure that the amputee does not begin his training program with an uncomfortable or mechanically mediocre device. The physician makes the final approval of the prosthesis.

At the time of the check-out, which occurs during the first training session, the occupational therapist begins to acquaint the amputee with "prosthetic terminology." He learns the names of the parts and their functions. He learns the proper attachment of the harness and the components so that he can keep the prosthesis clean and can interchange the terminal devices efficiently.

In instructing the patient in the care of the prosthesis, the occupational therapist teaches the amputee the proper use of the hook, wrist unit, and cable system. He is instructed to use just enough motion to

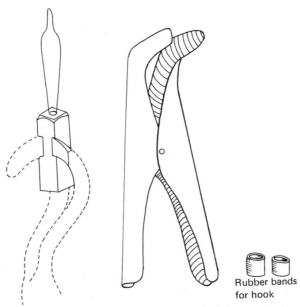

Rubber bands
for hook

Fig. 9–7 (Left)   Amputee button hook.

Fig. 9–8 (Right)   Band applier for voluntary opening hook.

open or to close the hook, to watch for worn rubber bands, to avoid putting unnecessary strain on the cable, and to watch for spreading of the housing and excessive friction between the cable and the housing.

The socket should be kept clean with soap and water; the stump socks should be washed daily; and the harness should be washed at least once per week. Leather parts can be cleaned with saddle soap. If the tips of the dacron harness straps begin to fray, they can be sealed at the edge by singeing with a match.

The amputee should be instructed to use only cable control to operate the APRL locking hooks and hands. Should he use his other hand, he might damage the mechanism. He should also be warned never to use the terminal device in such activities as hammering nails or removing screws.

The cosmetic gloves on the APRL hand are very perishable. It is important to guard the glove against tearing, since it functions as a protection of the hand mechanism from dirt and wetness. Also, these gloves soil easily, can be stained or marked if laid on dirty surfaces, and darken with age. Substances such as certain foods, ink, newsprint, and chemicals can damage the glove and hinder its cosmetic effect. The occupational therapist should recommend that the amputee keep the APRL hand in a plastic bag when he is not using it. The amputee should be warned against oiling parts of the prosthesis or removing the glove from the APRL hand. He should be counselled to return to the prosthetist for any assistance he may need.

CLOTHING

At the beginning of the training program, the prosthesis should be put on over a light-weight shirt so that the occupational therapist and the amputee can see the prosthesis function and so that it is not hindered by tight clothing. The amputee should become accustomed to using the mirror as a guide to learning the correct positioning of the harness straps in back and in learning the control motions.

Loose clothing is recommended for the amputee to facilitate putting on, wearing, and using the prosthesis. Clothing with front fastenings, velcro closures, and wide shirt cuffs are helpful. The use of a button hook designed especially for the amputee can assist him with the problem of fastening the sleeve button on his sound side (Fig. 9–7). Sewing the buttons on with elastic thread enables the amputee to leave the button fastened when removing the shirt, even if the cuffs are narrow, for the cuff will then stretch enough for him to remove his hand and arm from the sleeve. When he puts his shirt on, the amputee should remember to put it on the amputated side first. One-handed shoe tying and special closures can simplify dressing procedures.

THE TRAINING PROGRAM

There are two approaches commonly used in training amputees. In one, the training program can be directed toward developing the *potential* level of the amputee's performance. With this approach a unilateral amputee learns to develop fine coordination with his prosthesis, so that he can have maximum use of it even in case of an injury to the remaining extremity. The other approach varies from the potential approach in that the amputee is trained in the use of the prosthesis only as an aid in bimanual activities. Regardless of the approach, activities should be chosen which are suitable to the amputee's needs. The occupational therapist should encourage the amputee to indicate any additional and special training which he desires.

The training period serves as a "try out" period to check the efficiency of the prosthesis, the practicality of the components to suit the amputee's individual needs and to make adjustments of malfunctions of the device.

The length of the training sessions should be increased as the amputee's tolerance and adaptation increase. He must master its use in training before combining the prosthesis and remaining extremity in bimanual activities and before wearing the prosthesis outside the clinic. Wearing it outside the clinic for an overnight period is advised for the first out-of-clinic experience. This is preferable to having the amputee wear it at home for an entire weekend. Training with the APRL hand should be delayed until use of the hook has been mastered.

The general goals of training include: independence in self-care and ADL, return to former work or to a better job, improved appearance, return to hobbies and recreation, and learning new skills.

Certain factors affecting the amputee's capacity to learn may, unfortunately, be detrimental. They include: poor habits uncorrected in pre-prosthetic training, lack of motivation, lack of sensory feedback from the non-sensory prosthesis, time needed for training, age, inability to learn, and lack of a sense of accomplishment. The occupational therapist must attempt to minimize an amputee's negative attitude toward any or all of these factors.

The positive attitude of the amputee is very important; he must want to learn. The occupational therapist must encourage the amputee to have varying positive attitudes toward the prosthesis, such as considering it as a tool, a device to conceal his disability, an improvement of his body image, and/or a substitute for loss. Since it is important for the amputee to eventually integrate the prosthesis into his bodily function, he must become acquainted with it as a potential part of himself, both functionally and cosmetically. The amputee should have a feeling of success after each training session.

Early training in successful use of control motions can enable the amputee to feel that he will be successful in his future training activities. He should be cautioned against using the opposite shoulder to control the device and should be taught to operate the prosthesis with the amputated extremity as much as possible. His control motions should be minimal to save his strength and thus to extend the time during which he can wear and use the prosthesis.

In the first training session, the amputee should be taught the use and care of the stump sock (mentioned earlier).

Sensation is a natural guide to motor control. We recognize objects by shape, texture, size, and movement. But the amputee must often substitute vision for sensation (e.g., using visual cues in observing the amount of hook opening). He combines this with the sensation of cable tension to provide visual-sensory training, using the perception of both position and force. The proprioceptive sensation in the stump and the arm can aid here. He also uses auditory cues, such as the clicks in the elbow lock, APRL hand, and hook for efficient operation of the prosthesis.

During the first session it is important to acquaint the amputee with the actual function of the hook by teaching him exercises for opening and closing it. Since many Dorrance voluntary opening hooks are prescribed for amputees, let us use them as an example (Fig. 9–4).

Following the cable pull by shoulder flexion, the cable tension is released and the hook is pulled closed by its rubber bands, which yield 1 lb. of pressure each. The standard number of rubber bands employed is usually 3 or 4, although up to 8 and more may be used for added grip strength. (See Fig. 9–8 for an illustration of a device for applying rubber bands.) The amputee begins his training by learning to isolate the control motions needed to activate the hook. Then, using visual cues and sensing in his shoulder the resistance of the hook rubber bands, he learns how to control the exact opening of the hook. In order to minimize the energy expenditure needed to use the hook, the amputee should be encouraged to open the hook only slightly more than the size of the object he wishes to pick up — just enough to grasp the object. He should practice with objects of different sizes and weights in order to achieve control. Additionally, drills requiring the grasp of objects of different forms, textures, and materials are necessary for the amputee to learn the basic motions used in operating the hook. Since some materials are light, breakable, or easily crushed (i.e., a paper or plastic cup), it is important to teach the amputee to employ a minimum of pressure by maintaining tension on the cable during grasp. The amputee should also learn to operate the hook in different planes of arm movements, so that he will achieve maximum functional use.

These drills for grip control should be extended to other components of the prosthesis. The amputee must learn how to preposition the terminal device, how to operate the elbow unit, how to coordinate the elbow lock and elbow flexion and extension, and how to preposition his shoulder. In these drills the use of the terminal device is combined with a number of gross arm functions. The amputee learns the grasp, placement, and release of objects on shelves, tables, and the floor and learns to depend on the grip of the hook or functional hand.

During this early drill period, use of the sound extremity should be encouraged. During the rest periods the amputee should be encouraged to practice unilateral activities as well as bilateral ones. It is through these more complicated coordination activities that the prosthesis begins to be functionally integrated into the bilateral UE activities of the amputee. Although the unilateral amputee may already have become independent in ADL during the pre-prosthetic period, there are many things which we are accustomed to doing with two hands. For example, the amputee may find it difficult to cut meat, button his shirt sleeve, tie his shoes, or wrap a package with one hand. His prosthesis may help him to accomplish these things, or the occupational therapist may discover that he needs additional adaptive devices.

Whatever the problem, the occupational therapist should encourage the amputee to become skillful in the use of the hook and to devise ways to increase his independence in function. Participation in woodworking, sewing, weaving, or other avocational activities can be motivating for the amputee, can provide coordination and strength, can show him how his prosthesis can help him do things, and can aid him in integrating the prosthesis into his bodily function.

Using a worksheet checklist of activities accomplished can be helpful in recording the amputee's progress of training in both the clinic and the home. Since there are many activities that the patient will do at home that cannot be simulated in the clinic, the therapist should continue to encourage the amputee to do new things at home following each training session and to report successes or difficulties with new tasks. In this way, the therapist is able to assist the patient not only in controls, training drills, and activities, but also in his tasks and responsibilities in the routine of daily living. Thus, the program becomes relevant to each amputee's needs.

Activity categories on the worksheet should include: basic prehension activities, dressing and grooming (including putting on and taking off the prosthesis), eating and social skills (using keys and opening an umbrella), homemaking, clerical activities, and activities related to vocational and avocational interests.

Another training aid is a prosthetic training board with common objects (locks, light switches, pencil sharpener) attached to it.

Recreational activities during the pre-prosthetic and prosthetic training periods provide general body conditioning and development of a new image for the amputee.

EXTERNAL POWER

Currently the two common control systems used to operate the UE prosthesis are gross joint movements through the conventional shoulder harness and muscle contraction through the cineplasty. The principal disadvantages of the first system are the cumbersome and binding harness and the minimal sensory feedback the system provides. Among the disadvantages of the cineplasty are skin breakdown and minimal cosmesis. However, with the cineplasty prosthesis, amputees have commented on the presence of sensory feedback.

For some time there has been research into the area of biomechanical engineering to devise a prosthesis controlled by external rather than internal power. Physicians and engineers are cooperating in the effort to perfect externally powered control devices for persons with severe disabilities. The rationale behind providing a prosthesis controlled by external power is the development of a circuit system between the body and the prosthesis which insures sensory feedback and an integration of bodily and mechanical prosthetic function. This integration is necessary to prevent exaggerated concentration by the amputee on the operation and function of the prosthesis. Work is being done to determine control sites that are appropriate to the needs of the individual.

As parts of this type of prosthesis are experimental and not standardized, the cost of the externally powered prosthesis is prohibitive at this time. Also, the control sites must still be individualized.

In these experimental prostheses, power is supplied by motors, hydraulic devices, electrical systems, batteries, actuators, or pneumatic control. Electrodes placed on the skin surface near the muscle can be used as control signals. The advantages of the pneumatic control are the ease of supination and pronation and the powerful artificial hand.

In addition to research into more effective control systems and sites, work is continuing on the development of improved components to simulate natural movements and functions. Efforts are being made to lessen weight, to improve locking and grasping mechanisms in the APRL hand and the hook, to improve the glove material, and to increase the overall cosmesis of the prosthesis. Specific considerations are: development of a more efficient elbow unit, rerouting of the cables to the inside of the arm instead of the outside, improved cosmetic appearance, higher operating efficiencies, and decreased wear on clothing. There is also research interest in providing active wrist rotation.

The electric arm, a complex experimental mechanism, provides the amputee with an electric elbow and forearm rotation control. This mechanism is controlled by small batteries and a motor which are placed on the arm structure or in the amputee's pocket. The experimentation into electric control is an effort toward providing the mechanical extremity with a total coordination pattern and better integration into the body system. The aim is to provide a link between man and the mechanical device by using a stimulus from man's energy to activate the prosthesis.

Another idea is the use of phantom sensations to aid in the control of the BE prosthesis, using the signals from the forearm muscles for prehension and forearm rotation (pronation and supination). This method does not apply to the AE amputee, since the forearm muscles are gone and the power source muscles are removed from the terminal device.

In addition to the prohibitive cost of these experimental devices, another problem with an external power source is the replenishment of power. But efforts to produce designs which will simulate characteristics of normal muscle functions continue, to achieve the goal of successful integration of the device and the person.

With the continuing research into the use and application of external power, the concept of "man-machine," or the integration of the man and his assistive device, is often cited. Since the physician and the prosthetist recognize the need for an engineer who can provide devices operated with external power, the engineer or a specialist in bioengineering has become a new member of the rehabilitation team.

LOWER EXTREMITY AMPUTATIONS

Due to the high incidence of peripheral vascular disease and traumatic injuries affecting the lower limbs, amputations of the lower extremities are generally more common than those of the upper extremities. Since age, body build, physical and medical condition, vascular supply, and motivation are factors in the rehabilitation of the lower extremity amputee, there are some patients for whom provision of a prosthesis is contraindicated. These persons are encouraged to maintain maximum independence and mobility with the aid of a wheelchair, crutches, and other necessary assistive devices. The amputee for whom a prosthesis is appropriately prescribed can usually look forward to partial restoration of basic functions, independence in self-care, and the opportunity of returning to work of some kind.

Basically, the detailed study of lower extremity (LE) function, preprosthetic preparation, prosthetic prescription, check-out and training, and the management of problems encountered by the LE amputee are handled by the physician and the physical therapist. However, there are many ways in which the occupational therapist can also contribute to the functional rehabilitation of the LE amputee. In a general hospital or a rehabilitation center the occupational therapist may actually work with as many or more LE amputees as UE amputees.

The LE amputee may be referred to occupational therapy in the pre-prosthetic or the prosthetic phase of training or both. In either case, the occupational therapist should familiarize himself with the medical aspects of the patient's care and the goals of his rehabilitation program. Pertinent information the occupational therapist should learn from the chart or from the staff members should include:

1. Location, type, level, and cause of amputation.
2. Condition of the stump and amputated extremity.
3. General body condition.
4. Precautions.
5. Previous prosthetic replacement, if any.
6. Recommendations for passive and active positioning of the joints of the amputated extremity.
7. The appropriate amount of standing and walking to encourage and the degree of safe support needed by the amputee.
8. Complicating factors.

Throughout the pre-prosthetic and prosthetic stages of training the amputee may go through changes in attitude and behavior as he gradually realizes the extent of his loss and its effect on his life. Continual counselling is often necessary to help the amputee to adjust to the amputation, the change in body image, the wear and use of the mechanical device to substitute for natural function. He must also adjust to working with his arms, gearing himself to his abilities rather than disability, finding new interests, and socializing his new situation.

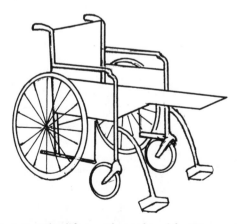

Fig. 9–9   Wheelchair with seat-board for LE amputee.

Pre-Prosthetic Period

During the early postoperative period of healing, passive and active exercises of the lower extremities are performed or supervised by the physical therapist. The amputee is taught by the nurse or physical therapist to bandage the stump to encourage shrinkage and forming of the stump for prosthetic fitting. Proper positioning of the body in the wheelchair is important to prevent contractures in the joints proximal to the amputation, scoliosis of the spinal column, and edema – all of which could hinder successful prosthetic function. In the case of below-knee (BK) amputation, the use of a seat-board (Fig. 9–9) adapted for the individual amputee can be used in a regular chair or a wheelchair to maintain the knee in passive extension with knee flexors stretched while the amputee is performing activities in a sitting position.

The seat-board can be made by the amputee as part of his upper extremity exercise program. It can be made of ½ or ¾ in. plywood which conforms to the measurement of the inside of the chair seat; one side extends to the end of the amputee's stump. The extended side should be narrow enough to prevent interference with the comfort of the sound leg in a sitting position, and at the same time should provide passive extension to the knee of the amputated leg. The seat-board should be padded sufficiently for comfort, and particular attention should be paid to such sensitive areas as the end of the stump.

In this pre-prosthetic phase the amputee may come to occupational therapy either in a wheelchair or walking with crutches. A variety of treatment technics can be used. Since balance and upper extremity and trunk strength will be very important in prosthetic use, maximum function of these areas is encouraged. Insofar as the amputee can tolerate the exercise, his sitting tolerance and balance is challenged by the use of upper extremity activities. Although at first an amputee with a high above-knee (AK) amputation or bilateral leg amputations may need to hold onto the chair with one hand to support himself in a sitting position while using the other hand, he should be encouraged to depend on his trunk for balance to leave both arms free for UE activities. As his upper extremity strength and confidence in his balance increase, ROM and resistance required in performing manual activities is increased to further challenge trunk balance. Activities such as woodworking, weaving and printing may be adapted to the amputee's individual needs. An activity in which the patient has a vocational or avocational interest may provide motivation in the activity so that he can increase tolerance of the given position and redirect energies from anxieties regarding his condition toward purposeful activity. Activities at this stage are directed toward the amputee's achieving independent function of his arms and trunk while he is seated in a wheelchair.

Another aspect of independence regards self-care tasks. These include bathing and care of the stump, transfers, and dressing. A unilateral amputee should have little or no difficulty in this area. However, aids such as grab bars for bath and toilet, a transfer board or tub seat for bathing, and a raised toilet seat can be helpful as the amputee adjusts to his new body image and copes with the problems of balance. Phantom limb sensations can be a complicating factor if the amputee suddenly moves to get up and forgets that he cannot stand on his amputated limb, even though he "feels" his foot. Continued physical and psychological support in these instances is necessary to minimize fear and to encourage confidence. Dressing is usually easier from a sitting position on the bed. Front fastenings and loose clothing also help to minimize frustrations.

Maximum independent function should be encouraged both with and without the prosthesis. For example, the amputee should be encouraged to stand on his sound leg in front of a table for short periods of time. This will encourage hip extension of the amputated side and will develop his balance. However, attention must be paid to the amount of standing time so as not to encourage scoliosis of the spine.

In England and France therapists have found that the use of a temporary pylon and the working prosthesis is beneficial to the LE amputee training program after the amputee's scar tissue has healed. The temporary pylon provides the amputee with early replacement of the amputated limb to encourage functional activity while the stump is being conditioned and the permanent prosthesis is being made.* The pylon consists of a plaster stump socket to which a pylon is attached to provide length and base support to the amputated leg. With the pylon the amputee can stand and ambulate soon after the amputation.

The working prosthesis is permanently attached to the machine that the amputee will use for exercise (i.e., to the foot-powered lathe or the bicycle jigsaw). It also consists of a stump cuff which is laced up the sides for ease in putting on and provides a comfortable fit for different persons. It is open at the distal end to eliminate pressure on the end of the stump.

When the patient has put the cuff on his stump, he fits the pylon shafts into the cuff. As the base is attached to the bicycle jigsaw or the lathe, the amputee is then able to operate these machines and thus engage in active LE exercise of the amputated limb. The working prosthesis could be used with a foot-powered floor press, treadle sewing machine, or loom, if properly adapted to the needs of the amputee. ROM and resistance can be graded, and the amputee can engage in an

---

* For specific designs of the pylon, see Mary S. Jones, Chapter 6, *An Approach to Occupational Therapy.*

activity challenging coordination, balance, and strength of all four extremities and the trunk.

It must be remembered that at first the amputee fatigues more rapidly, even in the activity of maintaining sitting and standing positions, and that until tolerance increases, energy is directed toward these basic functions.

Prosthetic Training Program

The LE amputee depends on the prosthesis for support of the body in standing and walking. It is important that the prosthesis be appropriately prescribed, that it fit comfortably, and that it provide adequate functional assistance. The prescription and mechanical function of the prosthesis are checked thoroughly by the physical therapist. Function of the parts, how the amputee should put the prosthesis on, and how he should use it are taught by the physical therapist.

Independent locomotion depends on the fit and comfort of the prosthesis as well as on the general condition and tolerance of the amputee. Some may be able to discard their wheelchairs fairly soon. However, the amputee with poor tolerance of the prosthesis or a poorly fitting one may need the security of the wheelchair for a long time. In either case, the occupational therapy program can benefit the amputee by encouraging him to work in the treatment room doing activities in a standing position when he can tolerate it. Even if the amputee is still dependent on the wheelchair early in his prosthetic training, he must eventually adjust to the mechanical, insensitive prosthesis by learning to judge where it is relative to the rest of his body, and he must learn how to function with it.

When the amputee receives his prosthesis, most of his attention will be on the fit and use of it. However, since he needs rest periods, both for his stump tolerance and for his strength, he continues in an occupational therapy program. The activities outlined in the pre-prosthetic period are continued. At this point, they are done with the prosthesis on unless the amputee is resting the stump or it is irritated by the prosthesis. His program is geared toward encouraging acceptance of the prosthesis (to function in activities challenging UE and LE coordination and function), prosthetic tolerance, development of ADL independence, UE and LE activity exercise program, realization of his capacities, and vocational and avocational guidance.

Wearing time of the prosthesis is gradually increased according to the comfort and tolerance of the socket in sitting and standing positions. As the amputee will be weight-bearing in the standing position, he must adjust to the sensation of bilateral weight-bearing and the sensitivity of his stump to the hard edges and base of the socket. According to the amputee's tolerance and balance, he can decrease the support he uses while standing. Engagement in UE activities in a standing position which provides a wide range of motion and resistance, helps to challenge and to increase standing balance. Walking to cabinets to get and replace materials or tools and walking around tables and machines should be encouraged to increase functional independence. Carrying articles from place to place also further challenges balance and independent function. Aids such as a cart with wheels or a tray can minimize the stress of carrying items.

In ADL, the patient now learns to incorporate the prosthesis into his bodily activities. He learns at what point in his dressing activities to put on the prosthesis so that it will aid, rather than interfere with, ease and speed in clothing himself.

An important part of the prosthetic training program is aiding the amputee to realize his capabilities. In the occupational therapy environment, both tasks to improve the amputee's tolerance and function with the prosthesis and those related to the requirements of his job may be set up.

Prevocational Exploration

Since the amputation may prevent the person from returning to his former line of work, it may be a great source of anxiety to him. Although the UE activities provided in occupational therapy may help psychologically and physically, it may be necessary to consider new vocational possibilities for the amputee.

Some occupational therapists may be qualified to provide evaluation and training in vocational areas. However, the usual goals of prevocational exploration are to provide the rehabilitation counsellor with information related to the interests, intelligence, physical abilities, work tolerance in both sitting and standing positions, and motivation of the amputee.

BIBLIOGRAPHY

Anderson, M. H., Bechtol, C. O., and Sollars, R. E.: Clinical Prosthetics for Physicians and Therapists. Springfield, Illinois, Charles C Thomas, 1959.

Amputees, Amputations, and Artificial Limbs. An Annotated Bibliography. Washington, D.C., Committee on Prosthetic-Orthotic Education, Division of Medical Sciences, National Academy of Sciences, National Research Council, 1969 (July).

Blakeslee, B.: The Limb-Deficient Child. Berkeley and Los Angeles, University of California Press, 1963.

Fishman, S., and Kay, H. W.: The munster-type below-elbow socket, an evaluation. Artif. Limbs, 8:4, 1964.

Garrett, J. F., and Levine, E. S. (eds.): Psychological Practice with the Physically Disabled. New York, Columbia University Press, 1961.

Gerhardt, J. J., et al.: Immediate post-surgical prosthetics: rehabilitation aspects. Am. J. Phys. Med., 49:3, 1970.

Hartman, H. H., et al.: A myoelectrically controlled powered elbow. Artif. Limbs, 12:61, 1968.

Jones, M. S.: An Approach to Occupational Therapy. London, Butterworth, 1964.

Kay, H. W., et al.: The munster-type below-elbow socket, a fabrication technique. Artif. Limbs, 9:4, 1965.

Klopsteg, P. E., and Wilson, P. D., et al.: Human Limbs and Their Substitutes. New York, Hafner, 1968.

Licht, S. (ed.): Rehabilitation Medicine. Baltimore, Maryland, Waverly, 1968.

Long, C., and Ebskov, B.: Research applications of myoelectric control. Arch. Phys. Med., 47:190, 1966.

Loughlin, E., Stanford, J. W., and Phelps, M.: Immediate postsurgical prosthetics fitting of a bilateral, below-elbow amputee, a report. Artif. Limbs, 12:17, 1968.

Mulhern, F. P.: Biceps cineplasty exercise. Am. J. Occup. Therapy, 11:322, 1957.

Reilly, G. V.: Pre-prosthetic exercises for upper extremity amputee with special reference to cineplasty. Phys. Therapy Rev., 31:183, 1951.

Review of Visual Aids for Prosthetics and Orthotics. Washington, D.C., Committee on Prosthetic-Orthotic Education, Division of Medical Sciences, National Academy of Sciences, National Research Council, 1969.

Santschi, W. R.: Manual of Upper Extremity Prosthetics. ed. 2, Los Angeles, Department of Engineering, UCLA, 1958.

Sarmiento, A., et al.: Immediate postsurgical prosthetics fitting in the management of upper-extremity amputees. Artif. Limbs, 12:14, 1968.

Scott, R. N.: Myoelectric control of prosthesis. Arch. Phys. Med., 47:174, 1966.

Shaperman, J. W.: Learning techniques applied to prehension. Am. J. Occup. Therapy, 14:70, 1960.

The Control of External Power in Upper-Extremity Rehabilitation, Washington, D.C., National Academy of Sciences, National Research Council, Publication #1352, 1966.

Tosberg, W. A.: Upper and Lower Extremity Prostheses. Springfield, Illinois, Charles C Thomas, 1962.

Wellerson, T. L.: A Manual for Occupational Therapists on the Rehabilitation of Upper Extremity Amputees. New York, published under the auspices of the American Occupational Therapy Association, 1958.

Willard, H. S., and Spackman, C. S.: Occupational Therapy, ed. 3, p. 308, Philadelphia, J. B. Lippincott, 1963.

The following journals are invaluable to the occupational therapist working with amputees.

Artificial Limbs: A Review of Current Developments. Washington, D.C., Committee on Prosthetics Research and Development, Division of Engineering and Committee on Prosthetic-Orthotic Education, Division of Medical Sciences of the National Research Council, National Academy of Sciences.

Bulletin of Prosthetics Research. Washington, D.C., Superintendent of Documents, U.S. Government Printing Office.

Orthotics and Prosthetics. Washington, D.C., American Orthotic and Prosthetic Association.

ACKNOWLEDGEMENTS

The author wishes to thank Patricia A. Curran for editorial and typing services and Barry W. Kaufmann for assistance in preparing the illustrations.

10

Occupational Therapy Management of Spinal Cord Injuries–Paraplegia and Quadriplegia

HELEN L. HOPKINS, M.A., O.T.R.

Spinal cord injuries have varying causes including vascular accidents (hemorrhage, thrombosis, embolus, hematoma), scarring (arachnoiditis), extrinsic cord compression (tumor, arthritic spurs, pyogenic abscess from tuberculosis) and trauma (fracture, fracture dislocation, gunshot or stab wound). The majority of patients who are treated by the occupational therapist are teenagers or young adults who have acquired their disability from trauma, war injuries, sports injuries or automobile accidents. Because of antibiotics, as well as improved emergency and medical care, life expectancy for persons with spinal cord injuries has increased to very near that of the general population. This means that the entire rehabilitation team is challenged to assist the patient to adjust to a new life pattern, redirect life goals and "provide emotional, physical and technical resources for accomplishment of these goals."[35]

When there is complete severance of the spinal cord, no functional control can be expected below the level of injury. If the severance is incomplete or has a lower motor neuron component (nerve damage at injury site, or cauda equina lesion), some nerve fibers may be intact or regenerate, resulting in the return of some function. Spinal cord injury, therefore, generally results in a permanent disability in which there is loss of sensation, as well as loss of motor power of extremities and internal organs below the level of the lesion. Physical complications, along with these losses in function, create additional problems relative to self-image and social function. This complex of problems requires understanding and support on the part of the entire rehabilitation team as well as the family and the community, in order to help the spinal cord injured person adjust to his disability and become a functioning member of society.

IMPACT OF SPINAL CORD INJURY ON THE HUMAN ORGANISM

Anatomical Considerations for Expected Function

The level of the lesion in the spinal cord should reflect the potential for function. However, there is anatomical variability among individuals in regard to exact segmental innervation,[4] and there may be variation of as much as one spinal cord level when assessing function. For this reason, exact anatomical location of the lesion may not give a true picture of functional ability unless this anatomical variability in innervation is considered (Chart 10–1). Trauma may cause a lower motoneuron or a peripheral nerve lesion, as well as damage to the spinal cord, thus changing the functional potential through regeneration of nerves. Prognostication of functional capacity, using only levels of lesions, [10,24,26] may underestimate the actual functional potential of the patient, and, therefore, can only be determined by assessment of actual physical capacity.

Physical Problems

Loss of motor power is the most obvious problem of the spinal cord injured patient. When the lesion is in the cervical area, there is paralysis or weakness in all four extremities and the trunk. This is referred to as quadriplegia or quadriparesis. When the lesion is in the thoracic or lumbar level, there is paralysis or weakness in both lower extremities and the trunk, depending upon the level. This is referred to as paraplegia or paraparesis.

Additional Physical Factors that Influence Rehabilitation of the Spinal Cord Person

Loss of sensation below the level of lesion creates the potential problem of decubiti from prolonged pressure to an area. Prolonged pressure causes loss of blood in the area and results in local necrosis. Pressure areas develop especially over bony prominences, such as the sacrum, ischium, trochanter, calcaneus, elbows or head of the second metacarpal (with hand splints). Prevention of pressure areas can only be accomplished through close, constant inspection and observation for signs of pressure (redness, blisters); first on the part of the nurse and

CHART 10–1

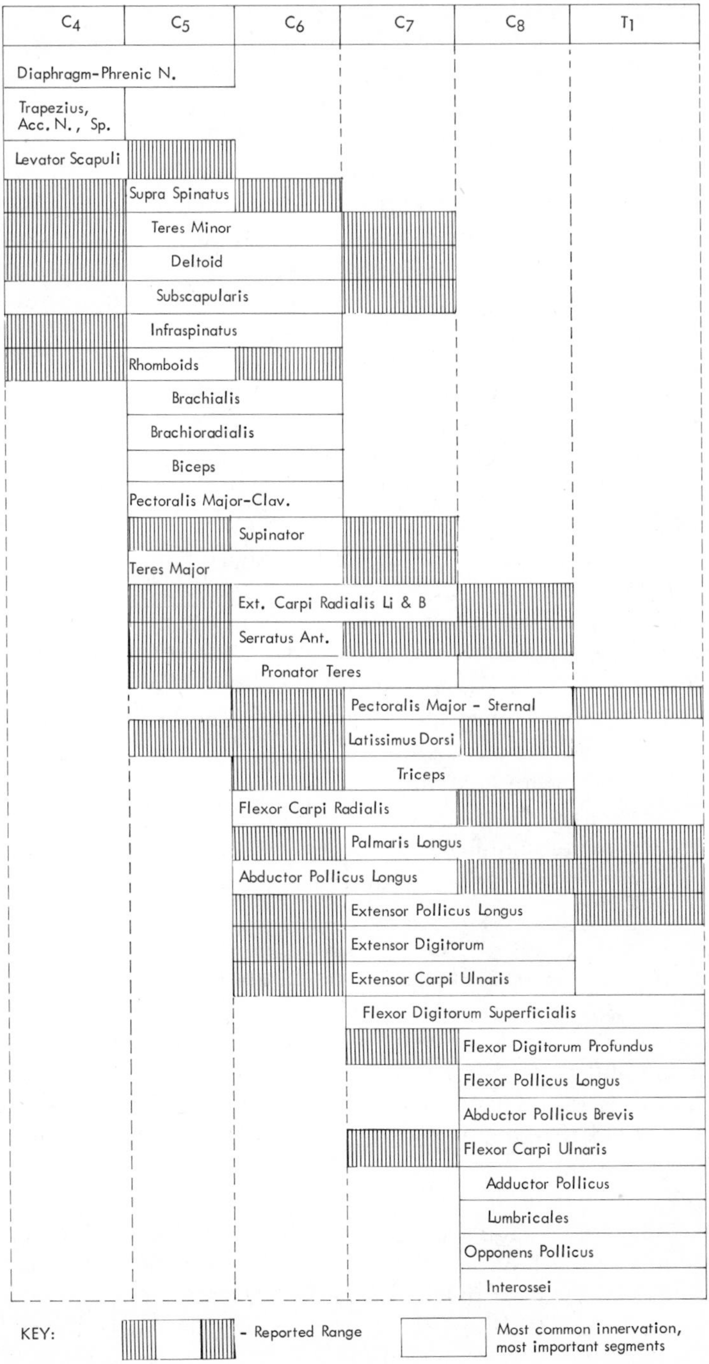

C$_4$	C$_5$	C$_6$	C$_7$	C$_8$	T$_1$

Diaphragm–Phrenic N.

Trapezius, Acc. N., Sp.

Levator Scapuli

Supra Spinatus

Teres Minor

Deltoid

Subscapularis

Infraspinatus

Rhomboids

Brachialis

Brachioradialis

Biceps

Pectoralis Major–Clav.

Supinator

Teres Major

Ext. Carpi Radialis Li & B

Serratus Ant.

Pronator Teres

Pectoralis Major – Sternal

Latissimus Dorsi

Triceps

Flexor Carpi Radialis

Palmaris Longus

Abductor Pollicus Longus

Extensor Pollicus Longus

Extensor Digitorum

Extensor Carpi Ulnaris

Flexor Digitorum Superficialis

Flexor Digitorum Profundus

Flexor Pollicus Longus

Abductor Pollicus Brevis

Flexor Carpi Ulnaris

Adductor Pollicus

Lumbricales

Opponens Pollicus

Interossei

KEY: ▦ ▦ – Reported Range   ▢ Most common innervation, most important segments other personnel, then on the part of the patient (using a mirror when necessary). Special equipment such as Stryker cushions, water beds and alternating pressure pads, are excellent for relieving pressure and assisting in healing decubiti, but they cannot take the place of frequent position change in preventing breakdown. Patients should be turned at least every 2 hours while they are in bed and must be taught to shift position in the chair even more frequently when sitting.

Loss of sensation also increases the danger of skin breakdown in the anesthetized areas through burns (cigarettes, hot dishes, radiators) and trauma (bumps). The skin breakdowns from trauma, burns or pressure heal very slowly and may cause delay in rehabilitation for from 2 to 6 months.

With loss of all sensation below the injury site, kinesthetic as well as tactile perception is involved. The patient, therefore, must locate his body parts and orient himself to space through visual cues. The lack of kinesthesia and tactile cues may lead to perceptual problems, particularly those relating to body image.

Loss of bowel and bladder control create both physical and psychological problems. Due to the danger of urinary retention, a catheter is frequently necessary for bladder management which introduces the danger of urinary tract infection and calculi formation. A catheter-free existence often results in frequent accidents causing social embarrassment and the resultant danger of skin breakdown. If a catheter is needed, it is important that aseptic technics be used in insertion of the catheter, that there be periodic irrigation of the catheter, and that antibiotic drugs be used to reduce infection. When the patient can become catheter-free through reflex action, or surgical procedures (transurethral resection, pudental neurectomy), he must continue to use antibiotic drugs to reduce infection and he should have periodic urological examinations.[2,7]

Lack of bowel control and irregularity may create bowel impaction. Bowel control may be managed by using enemas, laxatives or suppository routines. For satisfactory management of the bowel and the bladder, strict routines must be established and be adhered to so that they become a habit pattern. To avoid complications, a high fluid intake is recommended to lower the concentration of urine and a high protein diet is needed to compensate for increased protein breakdown and metabolic demands.

Disturbances in autonomic nervous system function may be evidenced in patients with lesions above T_2 by their inability to control body temperature. Bladder distention also affects the autonomic nervous system and causes patchy sweating above or below the lesion or both. An autonomic rise in blood pressure may be caused by irritation in the bowel or the bladder. This may be relieved by unclamping the catheter or tapping over the bladder to encourage it to empty. This is an emergency situation and death may occur if blood pressure is not controlled promptly. In this case, immediate medical attention should be sought.[29]

Pain and Spasticity cause additional problems for the spinal cord injured person. Although sensory function is lost in spinal cord lesions, the patient may experience sharp, burning pain and abnormal sensations, especially paraesthesias and phantom impressions similar to those of amputees. Most patients learn to live with these abnormal sensations and pain, and may need only minimal medication to make them tolerable.

Spasticity may occur as a reflex response to some stimuli or may occur as spontaneous uncontrollable movement of the paralyzed limbs. Spasticity may be so severe that it will impede rehabilitation procedures and interfere with general health. It may interfere with positioning in bed, sitting, exercise regimes and activities of daily living. Relief of spasticity and severe pain through surgical procedures (neurectomy, alcohol block) may be necessary in order to accomplish rehabilitation potentials.

Decalcification of skeletal system and generalized body atrophy occur frequently in spinal cord injury patients, resulting in complications of renal calculi and pathological ossification of muscle. These complications can be minimized by early mobilization, active exercise of non-paralyzed parts, and by the use of the tilt board to get patients in the upright position with their weight on the lower extremities.

Impaired respiratory function occurs in patients with cervical cord lesions. Paralysis of the intercostal and abdominal muscles causes marked protrusion of the abdomen on inspiration as the diaphragm descends. There is little thoracic expansion except for the upper thorax which may be lifted by neck accessory muscles. Without abdominal musculature, forceful expiration is impaired; thus a cough is weak and ineffective, and vital capacity is only about 60 per cent of normal. Since there is little thoracic expansion, the chest cage becomes rigid and the total pulmonary process is lessened. Decreased vital capacity affects energy and tolerance to activity, so patients must be observed closely for signs of fatigue. Positive pressure can force air into the lungs to increase chest expansion and prevent tightness of the rib cage, thus increasing expiratory force for a cough and preventing lung complications such as pneumonia. Glossopharyngeal breathing, a substitute method of breathing which uses muscles of the mouth, tongue, soft palate and throat to force air into the lungs, can also prevent tightness of the rib cage and increase the vital capacity. A study has shown that patients with cervical cord lesions increased their vital capacity to 81 per cent of normal through the use of glossopharyngeal breathing, thus increasing ability to participate in a more active program.[27]

The therapist should be alert for dizziness or "blackouts" which occur when the patient is first brought to the upright position following periods of immobilization in bed. Due to lack of muscle power in the abdominals and lower extremities, blood pools in these areas causing a decrease in blood pressure. If blackouts occur, the therapist should tilt the wheelchair back so that blood flows to the patient's brain. Use of abdominal binders, corsets and Ace bandages on the legs may minimize this problem.

Psychological, Social and Vocational Problems

Immediately post-trauma, the spinal cord injured patient displays anxiety. He develops fears about his health, appearance, sexual functioning, employability, and his separation and loss of status with family and community. He compensates by denying the problem in order to cope with the situation. Upon recognition of the problem facing him, the patient usually becomes depressed, which is the normal reaction of grief and mourning for the loss of function. The family must learn about the patient's needs, probable prognosis and future life problems. They can help prevent further psychological problems if they can visit regularly, become involved in planning for the future, and can assure the patient that he has not lost his role in their lives.

The occupational therapist can assist the patient in making a satisfactory adjustment to his disability by directing the treatment program toward activities that were part of his life before the injury. The activities should be those in which the patient can succeed, so that he will be more highly motivated and regain feelings of self-worth and hope for the future. Opportunity should be provided for social interaction and expression of feelings.

In order to assist the patient in psychological adjustment, the entire rehabilitation staff must encourage the patient to take an active role in his rehabilitation planning, orient him to the reality problems which he will encounter when he takes his place in the family and community, and support him as he is able to set goals and begin solving his own problems.[20] The patient must also be encouraged to set realistic vocational goals if total rehabilitation is to be successful.

If the patient's psychological needs are not met he may react with passivity because of fear of failure or dependency — either overdependency in which he is unable to move without approval, or underdependency in which he is unable to accept appropriate help. He may react with aggression and hostility, in which he strikes out at everyone, or overcompensation in which he becomes a rigid, unbending individual.

Predictors for Recovery and Functional Ability

Prognosis for recovery of function is based on whether the lesion is complete or incomplete. If the lesion in the spinal cord is complete, no motor return is expected, except what can be attributed to nerve root damage. Maximum return from root damage would be expected within 6 months. There is minimal spasticity in the upper extremities of patients having a lesion at the C_6 level or below. Potential function can be determined by the residual muscle power available, especially in the upper extremities.

With an incomplete lesion, there is evidence of sensation or motor function below the level of the cord lesion. This may be manifested by lower extremity sensation or muscle power scattered throughout. There may be an increase in muscle power beginning immediately and progressing over the first several months. When recovery begins to decrease and a plateau is reached and maintained for several months, no new recovery may be expected in the future.[29]

Many authors have equated level of lesion, muscle power and resultant functional ability.[10,11,21,24,25,26,36] It is most important for the occupational therapist to understand the relationship between residual muscle power and potential for function. Key muscles indicate the functional level of the patient and should guide the therapist in anticipating the level of independence that can be attained.

C_4 Functional level. Only the neck muscles and upper trapezius are functional, so the patient will need highly specialized equipment. Equipment comparable to the Rancho Electric Arm, in conjunction with an outside powered hand splint (CO_2 or electric) may be used. This equipment will enable him to perform very limited hand activities such as self-feeding, typing, page turning and manipulating objects on a work surface for recreational activities.[25] This patient will probably be homebound, requiring help for all activities.

C_5 Functional level. When the patient has the use of the biceps, supinator and deltoid, he will need special equipment such as a mobile arm support (ballbearing feeder, balanced forearm orthesis), slings, an outside powered hand splint (CO_2 or electric) or devices for holding equipment. He should be able to perform all the activities described above in addition to some self-care activities of light hygiene (make-up, shaving, brushing teeth, washing the face, combing the hair), writing and using the telephone. The patient is essentially homebound and needs an assistant for preparation or positioning of objects. He may be able to propel the wheelchair for short distances using projections on the hand rims and splints to stabilize the wrists.

C$_6$ Functional level. When the patient has the additional use of the clavicular portion of the pectoralis major and the radial wrist extensors, his functional ability increases markedly. He can now use tenodesis action to grasp objects or use a wrist driven flexor hinge hand splint. He can perform all the activities previously described more efficiently using less equipment. He can roll over and sit up in bed and can assist in transferring to the wheelchair (or may be independent in transfer with use of a sliding board and locking elbows in extension). He can dress (including fastening), can propel his wheelchair with projections on the rims, and can drive a car using hand controls and special steering cuff. He should be able to relieve pressure while sitting and be independent in skin inspection (patients with less function need assistance in these two activities). Patients at this level and below should be able to live independently with minimal help in bowel and catheter care, and should be able to participate in vocational pursuits outside the home, provided no fine hand motion is needed.

C$_7$ Functional level. When the patient has the additional use of triceps, latissimus dorsi and radial wrist flexors, he can perform all the activities previously listed more easily and with less equipment. He can transfer independently and is completely independent in all self-care activities. He should be able to get his wheelchair in and out of his car independently. He may be able to stand in braces, if braced adequately, but ambulation is impractical. Occupations requiring the use of hands are more feasible, but not those requiring fine finger dexterity.

C$_8$ Functional level. The ulnar wrist flexors and extensors and the long finger flexors and extensors are functional at this level. All activities previously described should be performed independently and with ease.

T$_1$ Functional level. Hand intrinsics are functional, permitting the addition of activities requiring fine finger dexterity. The patient lacks trunk stability, but proper bracing makes limited ambulation possible.

T$_6$ Functional level. The thoracic muscles are strong and give the patient respiratory reserve and increased endurance. He can ambulate with braces and crutches using a swing-through gait. He is independent in putting on and taking off braces. He has few vocational limitations in sedentary or semi-sedentary occupations. A wheelchair is usually prescribed for ease in moving around the house.

T$_{12}$ Functional level. The patient has full innervation of the abdominal muscles and can walk with bilateral long leg braces and crutches. A wheelchair may be prescribed for ease in moving around at home.

L$_4$ Functional level. The patient has power in the quadratus lumborum (hip hikers), quadriceps, and hip flexors. He needs short leg braces for ankle stability, can be independent without crutches or canes, but generally uses them because of the deforming effect of an unsupported gait. Some job limitations are present: the patient cannot stand for long periods, and climbing activities should be limited. A wheelchair may still be convenient at home.

ROLE OF THE OCCUPATIONAL THERAPIST

The occupational therapist must carefully assess the patient's function in order to define realistic goals and determine objectives for the treatment program. The patient and his family must participate in the program planning in order to meet the individual needs of the patient.

Objectives of Occupational Therapy

The objectives of occupational therapy are:
1. To prevent or correct deformity, which frequently occurs when spasticity is present.
2. To increase muscle power in the innervated muscles through a graded resistive activities program.
3. To improve functional ability in all self-care activities that are feasible according to the functional level of the patient.
4. To assess the patient for splints, devices and other equipment, and to train him in their use, including use of hand controls in driver education.
5. To improve ability in homemaking tasks utilizing devices and equipment needed to increase independence.
6. To conduct pre-vocational testing and provide job simulation experience in order to assess vocational feasibility.
7. To provide a therapeutic climate, which encourages socialization and develops a feeling of self-worth.

OCCUPATIONAL THERAPY ASSESSMENT PROCEDURES

Careful assessment of physical and functional capabilities must be completed before the therapeutic program is planned, so that all aspects of the problem will be considered.

Physical Assessment

Passive Range of Motion testing determines the limitations in range and potential problem areas that may be caused by spasticity, muscle imbalance or improper positioning. Limitation in joint range may require positioning or splinting to correct contractures.

Assessment of Motor Function

The patient in the spinal shock stage, following initial injury, generally has flaccid paralysis which gradually becomes spastic. The presence or absence as well as the degree of spasticity should be noted. Severe spasticity may be a limiting factor in potential for rehabilitation.

Manual muscle testing reveals which muscles are innervated, indicates muscle weakness, determines where emphasis should be placed in the strengthening program and helps the therapist decide if special orthotic equipment is needed. When applicable, the dynamometer and pinch gauge may be used for measuring strength of gross grasp and pinch.

General tolerance for activity, trunk stability and sitting tolerance must be assessed in order to set goals within feasible limits.

Gross Sensory Testing

Assessment of tactile sensation, proprioception and stereognosis indicate areas of impaired sensation, which guide the therapist in training the patient to be aware of sensory loss and to compensate by use of vision.

Functional Activities or Activities of Daily Living Assessment

Patients should be assessed in the performance of all activities that seem feasible depending on physical capacity. This determines the level of functioning and identifies those areas where training and/or the use of special devices and equipment will increase function.[5]

Assessment for Splints, Devices and Equipment

Manual muscle testing and activities of daily living assessment should indicate whether the patient will require special orthotic equipment such as mobile arm supports, flexor hinge hand splints or self-help devices to increase function. The patient should then be assessed in the use of these devices so that those most functional will be used in training.

The paraplegic and quadriplegic patients must be fitted with adequate wheelchairs in order to increase mobility. The following features are needed for both quadriplegics and paraplegics: 8-in. casters since they are easier to propel; forward locking brakes; non-marking tires; swing-away removable foot rests with heel loops; telescoping foot rests for quick adjustment; seat height so that foot pedal is 3 in. from the floor for clearance; desk-type, padded arm rests, high enough so elbows rest comfortably without drooping of shoulders; seat length adjusted so that one hand can be placed between the seat and knee, and seat width as narrow as possible (just wide enough for hand to fit loosely between skirt guard and hips). The paraplegic will need a heavy-duty chair with pneumatic tires if he will be traveling over uneven surfaces. He should have standard hand rims, a pin lock for arm rests, and a 2- or 3-in. cushion. The quadriplegic patient will need additional height to the seat back (to 1 in. above the inferior angle of the scapula) for trunk support, plasticized or rubber covered hand rims or hand rims with projections, caster locks, and a 3-in. cushion. If endurance is lacking, either an electric wheelchair or a semi-reclining wheelchair may be needed.[12] For some paraplegic and quadriplegic patients the "Stand-Alone"* may provide a means of mobility and opportunity to work in the standing position, thus increasing vocational potential.

Homemaking Assessment and Home Evaluation

If a handicapped person expects to manage his own home or plans to live alone, a homemaking assessment should be done. This includes assessing the patient's ability to get around the kitchen, to reach things in cupboards or in drawers, to make beds, to put up equipment, such as the ironing board, and to lift heavy pots and pans. Sensory impairment is an important safety factor when working around a hot stove. The need for special equipment or devices should be noted. Wheel tables, lapboards and cut-out boards for holding bowls may safely assist the patient in functioning independently.

When it is feasible, the therapist should visit with the patient at home to determine if adjustments are needed and how adaptations can be made to allow more complete independence at home. When a home visit is not feasible, planning may be done with the patient and his family using floor plans and information relative to such things as room sizes, door widths and stair rise.

Prevocational Assessment

When it is feasible for a patient to go back to his former occupation, the job or its component parts may be simulated in the occupational therapy department. This gives the patient the opportunity to perform the job in a protected situation, while helping him to regain self-confidence. When returning to a former job is not feasible, the occupational therapist, working with the vocational counselor, may assess aptitudes and interests to determine areas for potential job placement and training. The patient may be assessed using occupational therapy media, work samples or the "Tower"** tests which have been adapted for the particular needs of the New York area.

OCCUPATIONAL THERAPY – TREATMENT PLANNING AND PROCEDURES

Planning a treatment program on the basis of occupational therapy assessment alone does not give a true picture of the patient's assets and problem areas. Information gained from the medical chart, the physical therapy chart, the members of the rehabilitation team and the patient himself, are necessary for planning a program geared to the individual's

---

* Corporation for Medical Engineering, Whittier, California.
** Institute for Crippled and Disabled, New York, N.Y.

needs. The medical chart can give information relative to premorbid medical patterns, psychological status, and present medical condition. The physical therapist, or the physical therapy chart, can give information relative to lower extremity passive range of motion, residual musculature, sensation and functional ability. Nursing personnel, who are with the patient constantly, can provide information relative to his behavior and his ability to function on the ward. From contacts with families when they visit, nurses may be able to supply impressions relative to family-patient relationships. Social service may supply information relative to the patient's premorbid social and work history as well as feasible discharge planning. The psychologist and/or vocational counselor may provide information relative to the psychological, the cognitive and the vocational potential of the patient which will help in determining long term goals.

With the information gathered from the charts, rehabilitation team members, and assessment procedures, the occupational therapist can plan a program which meets the individual patient's needs. The emphasis of occupational therapy will be in five areas: (1) physical conditioning; (2) training in functional activities, with and without equipment; (3) training in homemaking; (4) exploring vocational and avocational potential; (5) socialization and adjustment to new life patterns.

Physical Conditioning

Physical conditioning includes both strengthening of residual musculature and increasing endurance. Mobile arm supports or slings may be used to provide assistive motion for very weak muscles and to allow strengthening of the available muscles through the use of bilateral activities such as typing (using typing sticks), and bilateral sanding (with hands fastened to sander with gloves or Ace bandages). Progressive resistive activities should be used to strengthen the upper extremity musculature. These may include such activities as woodworking, plastics, weaving and all the activities of daily living that are feasible according to the musculature available. The strength of the wrist extensors is particularly important for dressing and transferring as well as for powering the flexor hinge hand splint. Activities which can develop strength in wrist extensors include grasp and release activities using tenodesis action. Leather stamping may be used as a means of strengthening wrist extensors, resistance being increased by increasing the weight of the hammer.

Triceps and shoulder depressors are important for transferring and can be strengthened through the use of adapted woodworking and weaving activities which require forceful extension. These activities can be used with paraplegics who generally need strengthening of shoulder depressors and triceps for crutch walking. Tools can be

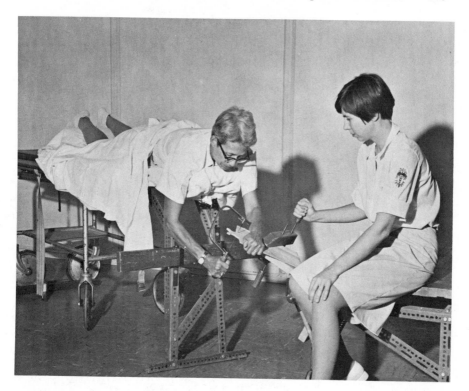

Fig. 10-1   Etter Prone Positioning Litter Extension (EPPLE). Rehabilitation Institute, Detroit.

adapted to provide bilateral motion, and weights can be added to increase resistance. Work can be positioned at optimum height and distance to provide the needed exercise. An inclined plane with weights and pulleys may be used for sanding woodworking projects, thus permitting the use of maximum resistance.

If a patient is unable to sit in a wheelchair because of skin breakdowns or other physical problems, a program of strengthening may be instituted through the use of the EPPLE (Etter Prone Positioning Litter Extension).[1,18] This is an extension for the litter or may be used on the bed. It gives "chest weight support on a narrow surface to allow full range of motion at shoulders and free mobility of the shoulder girdle while maintaining best possible body alignment".[18] For a quadriplegic, a supporting face mask is used.

Using the EPPLE, the patient may be able to begin performing activities such as typing, writing, eating and shaving before he is allowed to sit. He may also be able to perform resistive activities for muscle strengthening in this position, the work being positioned for the desired function. Activities such as woodworking and weaving with an adapted loom are particularly applicable for working in this position. For the paraplegic or quadriplegic patient who must be in the prone position, the EPPLE permits activity which can increase respiratory function, assist urinary function, decrease postural hypotension (blackout when sitting) and increase strength and endurance (see Fig. 10–1).

If desired, assistive exercise and progressive resistive exercises, such as use of overhead pulleys, a skate board and a counter balance sling may be utilized for strengthening of the upper extremities.

Training in Functional Activities (Activities of Daily Living)

Training in activities of daily living may begin while the patient is still in bed. The paraplegic is generally able to do all hand activities without training, but may need some training in dressing, bathing and transfer activities to become proficient in these areas. The quadriplegic patient may begin with light activities such as feeding and brushing the teeth. The C_4 quadriplegic has little residual muscle power available for use; therefore, he will require specialized equipment to allow him to function at a productive level. Many externally powered splints (CO_2 and electricity) and arm devices are being developed to increase the functional ability of these patients.[9,22,23,33,37,38,40] Experiments are also being conducted to utilize functional electrical stimulation devices, or those which stimulate the muscles to perform a function.[13,14] These are still in the experimental stage; however, electronics may provide an answer for increased function for the severely disabled patient in the future.

After the patient has been assessed, he begins training and practice in feeding, selfcare skills and writing, using special devices,[5] adapted equipment or splints as they are needed. The tenodesis, flexor-hinge hand splint may be utilized by those persons who have good power in the radial wrist extensors, reinforcing grasp provided by tendon action.[16,17,28,32,39] The use of these splints greatly increases the functional ability of the quadriplegic patient and requires the use of less adapted equipment. In order for the splints to be of practical value, however, the patient must learn to put them on and take them off in a practical length of time. He must be motivated to use the splints and feel that they increase his function. Tendon tightness may eliminate the need to wear the splints for all activities.

After hand activities are accomplished, training in dressing can begin.[3,31] The patient must have learned bed activities, such as rolling from side to side and coming to the sitting position, and must have developed adequate trunk balance before dressing can be accomplished independently. The first attempts at all of these activities are difficult, frustrating and time consuming, but continued practice increases skill and decreases the time needed to perform them. Many quadriplegics learn tricks of motion which increase their independence.

The patient who can dress himself, shift his weight to relieve ischial pressure, transfer to and from the car, and get his chair in and out of the car is ready for driver training. By using hand controls and a special driving cuff, the quadriplegic as well as the paraplegic can learn to drive a car, and thus attain a higher level of independence.

Homemaker Training

After patients have been assessed relative to function in homemaking tasks, they must be given the opportunity to practice these activities. They must be taught work simplification technics, labor-saving methods including rearrangement of work and storage areas, and energy conservation through careful planning.[6] Weekend visits at home, as soon as medically feasible, will help patients attempt some of the technics and solve some problems but allow them to return for help in difficult areas. Special equipment and devices may be needed to increase independence.

Exploring Vocational and Avocational Potential

The occupational therapist should discuss the patient's future vocational plans with him and concentrate training in the areas related to his vocational goal. For example, if the patient is going to school, extra time may be spent on handwriting to improve note taking. If it is determined that it is feasible for the patient to go back to his former employment, the job tasks may be simulated in occupational therapy so that he will have the skill to perform on his job, when he goes back to work. If new vocational goals are set, such as bookkeeping, or mechanical drawing, the patient may become proficient in performing these tasks using hand splints.

According to studies relative to the vocational potential of spinal cord injured patients, the majority of successful employment opportunities for quadriplegics were in the professional, managerial, sales and clerical areas.[19,34] Few quadriplegics have been successful in manual type occupations. Among the paraplegics it was found that those with the higher educational level were more employable than those who were unskilled or semiskilled. With proper rehabilitation services and manipulation of the environment to maximize abilities, many more spinal cord injured persons can qualify for employment in competitive industry.

Avocational interests should be explored, especially when vocational goals are not feasible, in order to give patients an interest in life. Hobbies such as reading, writing, painting and drawing can be pursued even though physical limitation requires use of a mouth stick to perform many activities.

Socialization and Adjustment to New Life Patterns

The occupational therapist can assist the patient in making satisfactory adjustment to his disability and restore self-confidence by concentrating on accomplishments and capabilities and also by providing opportunities for social interaction. Patients should be encouraged to participate in recreational programs that are provided, and take part in the patient governing bodies which are active in many rehabilitation facilities. To ease the fear of taking part in outside social activities because of "looking different," patients should be encouraged to go on outings, such as bowling, baseball games and movies, while they are in the hospital. These activities make the patient begin to function as a member of a community in preparation for his discharge into his larger home community. Upon discharge, each person should be encouraged to participate in social and community affairs and to attend functions which were part of his life pattern before his injury.

For persons in a wheelchair, there are still architectural barriers which prevent them from participating in many activities. Legislation is being enacted to correct some of these inequities, but it will be many years before all the necessary changes can be made to provide easy access for all handicapped persons.

SUMMARY

The spinal cord injured person must overcome many physical and psychological problems if he is to function in society today. Increased technology is beginning to find answers for some very severe problems, but many are still to be answered. The use of electronic devices may increase the functional ability of the person with a spinal cord injury, and physical complications may be prevented by improvement in medical care, through drugs and equipment. Society must learn to look at capability rather than disability and must learn to accept the individual and provide opportunities for all persons with handicaps. This must be accomplished in order to meet the psychological and social needs of the handicapped.

Some inroads have been made in meeting these problems. Standards have been set which make buildings and facilities accessible to wheelchair patients.[8] Recognizing the need for higher education for the handicapped, many colleges and universities have made provisions for wheelchair students.[15] However, continued effort is needed to meet the needs of spinal cord injured persons, and other handicapped persons, if they are to become integral, contributing members in society.

REFERENCES

Books

1. Etter, M. F.: Exercise for Prone Patient. Detroit, Wayne State University Press, 1968.
2. Friedland, F.: Rehabilitation in spinal cord injuries, IN Licht, S.: Rehabilitation and Medicine. New Haven, Elizabeth Licht, 1968.
3. Frost, A.: Handbook for Paraplegics and Quadriplegics. Chicago, The National Paraplegic Foundation, 1964.
4. Hollinshead, W. H.: Textbook of Anatomy. ed. 2, pp. 204-358. New York, Hoeber Medical Division, Harper and Row, 1967.
5. Lowman, E. W. and Klinger, J. L.: Aids to Independent Living—Self-Help for the Handicapped. New York, Blakiston-McGraw, 1969.
6. May, E. E., Waggoner, N. R., Boettke, E. M.: Homemaking for the Handicapped. New York, Dodd, Mead and Company, 1966.
7. Rusk, H. A.: Rehabilitation Medicine. ed. 2, pp. 498-530. St. Louis, C. V. Mosby Company, 1964.

Journals and Pamphlets

8. American Standards Association: American Standard Specifications for Making Buildings and Facilities Accessible to, and Usable by, the Physically Handicapped. Chicago, National Society for Crippled Children and Adults.
9. Barber, L. M., and Nickel, V. L.: Carbon dioxide powered arm and hand devices. Am. J. Occup. Therapy, 23:215, 1969.
10. Bell, E., Elliott, R. M., and Von Werssowetz, O. F.: Muscle strength and resultant function in cervical cord lesions. Am. J. Occup. Therapy, 15:106, 1961.
11. Bell, E.: Treatment procedures for patients with cervical cord lesions. Study Course III: Dynamic Living for the Long Term Patient, Third International Congress, World Fed. of Occup. Therapists. Dubuque, Iowa, William C. Brown, 1964.
12. Bergstrom, D. A.: Report on a conference for wheelchair manufacturers. Bulletin of Prosthetics Research, 10-3:60, 1965.
13. Dimitrijevic, M. R., Granconin, F., Prevec, T., and Trontelj, J.: Electronic control of paralyzed extremities. Biomed. Engin., January, pp. 8-19, 1968.
14. Doerr, G. M., and Long, C.: Electrical response and electromyograms of upper-extremity muscles in quadriplegia. Orthotics and Prosthetics, 23:20, 1969.
15. Edington, E. S.: Colleges and universities with special provisions for wheelchair students. J. Rehab., 29:14, 1963.
16. Engel, W. H., Kniotek, M. A., Holf, J. P., French, J., Barnerias, M. J., and Siebens, A. A.: Functional splint for grasp driven by wrist extension. Arch. Phys. Med., 48:43, 1967.
17. Engen, T. J., and Ottnat, L. F.: Upper extremity orthotics: a project report. Orthotics and Prosthetics, 21:112, 1967.

18. Etter, M. F.: "EPPLE", Proceedings of the 1961 Annual Conference, American Occupational Therapy Association, pp. 50-54.
19. Felton, J. S., and Litman, M.: Study of employment of 222 men with spinal cord injury. Arch. Phys. Med., 46:809, 1965.
20. Kahn, E.: Social functioning of the patient with spinal cord injury. Phys. Ther., 49:757, 1969.
21. Knapp, M. E.: Practical physical medicine and rehabilitation, spinal cord injury. Postgraduate Medicine, 42:A95 (Part I), 42:A111 (Part II), 1967.
22. Lehneis, H. R.: Application of external power in orthotics. Orthotics and Prosthetics, 22:34, 1968.
23. Long, C., and Masciarelli, V. D.: An electrophysiological splint for the hand. Arch. Phys. Med., 44:499, 1963.
24. Long, C., and Lawton, E. B.: Functional significance of spinal cord lesion level. Arch. Phys. Med., 36:249, 1955.
25. McKenzie, M. W.: The role of occupational therapy in rehabilitating spinal cord injured patients. Am. J. Occup. Therapy, 24:257, 1970.
26. Mead, S.: Spinal cord injuries. Mod. Treatm., 5:949, 1968.
27. Metcalf, V. A.: Vital capacity and glossopharyngeal breathing in traumatic quadriplegia. Phys. Ther., 46:835, 1966.
28. Newsom, M. J., Keenan, G., Maddry, J. and Aguilar, S.: An occupational therapy training program for the C-5-6 quadriplegic. Am. J. Occup. Therapy, 23:126, 1969.
29. Rancho Los Amigos Hospital: Occupational Therapy Treatment Guide for Spinal Cord Patients, Downey, California, Rancho Los Amigos Hospital, 1969.
30. Runge, M.: Follow-up study of self help activities in traumatic spinal cord injury quadriplegics and quadriparetics. Am. J. Occup. Therapy, 20:241, 1966.
31. – – –: Self dressing techniques for patients with spinal cord injury. Am. J. Occup. Therapy, 21:367, 1967.
32. Sabine, C. L., Addison, R. G., and Fischer, H. K.: A plastic tenodesis splint. J. Bone Joint Surg., 47A:533, 1965.
33. Scott, R. N.: Myoelectric control of prosthesis and orthotics. Bulletin of Prosthetics Research, 10-7:93, 1967.
34. Siegel, M. S.: The vocational potential of the quadriplegic. Med. Clin. N. Am., 53:713, 1969.
35. Siller, J.: Psychological situation of the disabled with spinal cord injuries. Rehab. Lit., 30:290, 1969.
36. Symington, D. C., and MacKay, D. E.: A study of functional independence in the quadriplegic patient. Arch. Phys. Med., 47:378, 1966.
37. Trombly, C. A.: Myoelectric control of orthotic devices: for the severely paralyzed. Am. J. Occup. Therapy, 22:385, 1968.
38. Trombly, C. A., Prentke, E. M. and Long, C.: Myo-electrically controlled electric torque motor for the flexor hinge hand splint. Orthopedic and Prosthetic Appliance Journal, 21:39, 1967.
39. Truong, X. T., White, C. F., and Canterbury, R. A.: Modification of flexor tenodesis splint. Arch. Phys. Med., 50:97, 1969.

40. Waring, W., Antonelli, E. E., Fries, D., Runge, M., Stauffer, E. S., and Nickel, V. L.: Myoelectric control for a quadriplegic. Orthotics and Prosthetics, 21:255, 1967.

SUPPLEMENTARY BIBLIOGRAPHY

Books

Kaplan, L., Powell, B. R., Brynbaum, B. B., and Rusk, H. A.: Comprehensive Follow-up Study of Spinal Cord Dysfunction and its Resultant Disabilities. New York, Institute of Rehabilitation Medicine, New York University, 1966.

Journals and Pamphlets

Abramson, A. S.: Modern concepts of management of the patient with spinal cord injury. Arch. Phys. Med., 48:113, 1967.

Bean, L. E.: Car transfer technique of a patient with quadriplegia. Phys. Ther., 49:602, 1969.

Bucy, P. C.: Paraplegia: the neglected problem. Phys. Ther., 49:269, 1969.

Garrett, A. L., Perry, J., and Nickel, V. L.: Traumatic quadriplegia. J.A.M.A., 87:7, 1964.

McDaniel, L. V.: Rehabilitation: then what? Quadriplegia follow up. J. Am. Phys. Therapy Assoc., 45:1042, 1965.

Trombly, C. A.: Principles of operant conditioning: related to orthotic training of quadriplegic patients. Am. J. Occup. Therapy, 20:217, 1966.

ACKNOWLEDGEMENTS

The following registered occupational therapists made suggestions and contributions to this chapter: Carolyn Baum and Trish Collins, Research Hospital, Kansas City, Missouri; Holly Gordon, New England Medical Center, Boston, Massachusetts; Kathleen Lynch, University Hospital, Boston, Massachusetts; and James Sellers, Massachusetts General Hospital, Boston, Massachusetts.

11

Occupational Therapy Management of Cerebrovascular Accident and Hemiplegia

HELEN L. HOPKINS, M.A., O.T.R.

Because of the stress and tension of our society and the increasing number of aged persons in our population, one of the most common disability problems with which the occupational therapist is confronted is that of the cerebrovascular accident (stroke) with a resultant hemiplegia. Hemiplegia is a symptom-complex caused by a lesion in the brain resulting in an upper motor neuron paralysis of the contralateral limbs and lower face.[40] Since the lesion is within the brain substance, many complicating symptoms may be present depending on the location of the lesion. Knowledge about the brain and its function is constantly being expanded through research, but much is still unknown. For example, we cannot determine how much recovery of function is due to spontaneous fading of symptoms and how much is due to the therapeutic regime which has been custom made to meet individual needs. We can, however, keep informed of the research being conducted on brain function and the neurophysiological principles[10, 11] which have evolved regarding overall functioning of the human organism, and apply this information to practice by utilizing technics[5, 6] based on these principles.

IMPACT OF A CEREBROVASCULAR ACCIDENT
ON THE HUMAN ORGANISM

Anatomical Considerations

The lesion in the brain may be caused by an interruption of the blood supply due to a thrombus, an embolus, or a hemorrhage. The resulting symptoms should reflect the location of the lesion. Pathophysiological studies have determined that specific functions are anatomically determined and are disturbed when lesions occur as a result of occlusion or hemorrhage in specific blood vessels.[33,66] If the area of occlusion is known, this information may help the therapist in the assessment and expectation of problem areas.

When the internal carotid artery is occluded, there is an insufficient blood supply to areas of the frontal, parietal and temporal lobes, internal capsule and optic nerve, causing aphasia (dominant hemisphere involvement), contralateral hemiplegia and homonomous hemianopsia. When the anterior cerebral artery is involved, there are disturbances in the anterior part of the internal capsule, the tip of the frontal lobe and the surface of the cerebral hemisphere to the parietal occipital junction, causing contralateral monoplegia (leg), sensory loss, mental confusion, apraxia and aphasia. With involvement of the middle cerebral artery, there are disturbances in the convolutions of the cerebral hemisphere, the lateral orbital frontal region, the internal capsule and anterior thalamus causing contralateral hemiplegia (primarily involving the arm), contralateral facial weakness, aphasia (dominant hemisphere involvement), homonomous hemianopsia and sensory loss. Occlusion of the posterior cerebral artery involves the midbrain, two thirds of the temporal lobe, the middle occipital lobe and the posterior internal capsule causing contralateral hemiplegia, hemianaesthesia, homonomous hemianopsia, ataxia and tremor. When the basilar artery is involved, there are disturbances in the pons, the medulla and the cerebellum causing symptoms from the 3rd to 12th cranial nerves, loss of proprioception and cerebellar dysfunction. Cerebellar artery occlusion creates disturbances in the midbrain, the pons and the cerebellum causing cerebellar ataxia and contralateral loss of pain and temperature.

The anatomy of the circulatory system of the brain is such that blood supply may be re-established through connecting vessels from the opposite side, thus allowing compensation and causing less functional loss than would be expected on a purely anatomical basis.

For this reason, careful assessment is necessary to determine the problems of each individual who has suffered a cerebrovascular accident. The problems are complex and include not only motor loss

CHART 11-1

ARTERY	AREAS OF BRAIN AFFECTED	MANIFESTATION
Internal Carotid	Frontal Lobe Parietal Lobe Temporal Lobe Internal Capsule Optic Nerve	Aphasia (dominant hemisphere) Contralateral Hemiplegia Homonomous Hemianopsia

Anterior Cerebral	Anterior Part of Internal
	  Capsule
	Tip of Frontal Lobe
	Surface of Cerebral Hemi-
	  sphere to Parietal-
	  Occipital Junction
		Contralateral Monoplegia (leg)
		Sensory Loss
		Mental Confusion
		Apraxia
		Aphasia (dominant hemisphere)

Middle Cerebral	Convolutions of Cerebral
	  Hemisphere
	Lateral Orbital-Frontal
	  Region
	Internal Capsule
	Anterior Thalamus
		Contralateral Hemiplegia
		  (primarily arm)
		Contralateral Facial Weakness
		Aphasia (dominant hemisphere)
		Homonomous Hemianopsia
		Sensory Loss

Posterior Cerebral	Midbrain $^2/_3$ Temporal Lobe Middle Occipital Lobe Posterior Internal Capsule	Contralateral Hemiplegia Hemi-anaesthesia Homonomous Hemianopsia Ataxia Tremor
Basilar	Pons Medulla Cerebellum	Symptoms from 3rd to 12th Cranial Nerves Loss of Proprioception Cerebellar Dysfunction
Cerebellar	Midbrain Pons Cerebellum	Cerebellar Ataxia Contralateral Loss of Pain and Temperature

caused by the lesion and the physiological complications which develop secondary to the insult, but also problems having to do with sensorimotor function, intellectual function, communication and psychological, family, social and vocational adjustment.

Physical Problems

The most obvious physical problem occurring with a cerebrovascular accident is the contralateral motor weakness or paralysis of the face, arm and leg. The severity and possibility of return of function are determined by the location and extent of the lesion. There are many complicating physiological factors[7,12,47] which may hinder or limit the extent of rehabilitation, among which are arteriosclerotic or hypertensive heart disease,[42] spasticity, reflex sympathetic dystrophy, vascular complications (such as thrombophlebitis), seizures, decubiti, and bowel and bladder incontinence. A frequently overlooked physiological problem which may limit rehabilitation because of the fatigue factor is the problem of respiratory insufficiency due to paralysis of the respiratory muscles on the hemiplegic side.[38]

Sensorimotor Problems

An area of dysfunction in the hemiplegic which is now being recognized is that of perception and sensorimotor function. Many cerebrovascular lesions cause dysfunction within the parietal lobes of the brain. Since the parietal lobes[1,15] are the major association areas, it is understandable that the hemiplegic patient whose parietal lobe is affected will demonstrate not only motor loss but also perceptual and sensory motor problems.[43] He may have difficulty in integrating and interpreting all the sensory messages from the internal and external environments, and also display a unilateral neglect of space and the body on the contralateral or hemiplegic side.[15] This type of involvement results in:

1. Disturbances in body image and body scheme,[45] causing failure to recognize one's own body or its parts; disturbances in spatial judgment or relative size and distance of objects.
2. Disturbances in speed and time, causing problems of performing too quickly and erratically for safety, or frustration because of poor judgment relative to the passage of time.[31]
3. Impairment of tactile sensation, astereognosis and the coordination of sensory inputs needed to determine spatial relationships.
4. Disturbances in visual perception including judgment of vertical and horizontal.[21]
5. Problems of left-right discrimination.[23,44]
6. Dressing apraxia[25] or inability to dress oneself because of the disorder in the body scheme.
7. Constructional apraxia[15,20,25] or inability to copy two or three dimensional designs, causing problems in carrying out volitional acts using objects in the environment.

The apraxia problems may appear when there is an absence of severe paralysis, sensory loss or cerebellar difficulties, and may be of two types, ideomotor and ideational.[54] Ideomotor apraxia is the inability to imitate gestures or to carry out purposeful movement on command while retaining ability to perform automatic routine activities, such as combing the hair when given a comb. With ideational apraxia there is inability to carry out routine activities such as combing the hair when being presented with a comb and being told to use it in the characteristic fashion. Because of contradictory cues that are received from sight and sensation, there may be problems of strange sensations of unfamiliarity, hallucinations, or illusions of touch.[18,29,37]

According to studies relative to disturbances in the sensorimotor aspect of function, *left* hemiplegics, or persons with lesions in the nondominant hemisphere, have more difficulties in all areas except for the area of left-right discrimination.[20,21,23,34,37,44,45] In the area of left-right discrimination, *right* hemiplegics have more problems possibly due to inability to distinguish the words left and right because of langauge disorders which frequently accompany disorders of the dominant hemisphere. *Right* hemiplegics also demonstrated bilateral apraxic problems.

Communications Problems

Although the right hemiplegic with left dominant hemispheric damage may show fewer sensorimotor disturbances, there is frequently some disability in communication[54,58] which includes both language and social effectiveness. Since it is believed that the left hemisphere is dominant in 97 per cent of people regardless of handedness, and that the dominant hemisphere contains language centers, persons having a lesion in the left hemisphere are most likely to have communications problems.

The use of language and the ability to communicate is a very complicated, highly integrated system in man. It includes speaking, gesturing, body movement, listening, understanding, writing, reading, recognizing, and the ability to abstract and integrate symbols meaningfully. "The patient who has lost his ability to communicate has lost the ability to understand his environment, the ability to structure his thought processes internally in a logical and meaningful order, the ability to formulate language in a logical and meaningful order."[39] Two major speech disorders are the concern of the occupational therapist: namely, aphasia and dysarthria. Aphasia is the loss of language symbols and may be in the expressive area where there is inability to speak, gesture, write or point, and/or the receptive area where there is a problem with understanding spoken language, or what one sees or reads. Dysarthria is the loss of motor function of the speech mechanism.

Intellectual and Cognitive Problems

Intelligence and cognitive ability are dependent on the integrative ability of the brain. Since these integrative processes are impaired by a cerebrovascular accident in the brain, it is not surprising that studies[34,55] demonstrate impairment of specific intellectual functions demonstrated by a drop in performance in the non-verbal intelligence tests regardless of educational level. An overall change in organization and mental abilities is also obvious in the inability to do abstract reasoning. Intellect, communication and sensorimotor ability are frequently involved in a cerebrovascular accident, all of which contribute to learning ability. Therefore, if the individual is unable to perceive and to integrate into thought and action, learning cannot occur, and the rehabilitation potential is limited.

Psychological Problems

If one can look at a cerebrovascular accident from the patient's point of view,[2,4] it is obvious that what has occurred is a catastrophe to the patient. It generally comes on suddenly, not allowing the patient to prepare himself, and, therefore, has a tremendous psychological impact. The patient is confused, stunned, shocked and disoriented. He may first deny his disability in order to keep from being overwhelmed. Then, as denial lessens, he may become depressed. Depression is generally necessary to allow a period of mourning for loss of function. However, if it continues for too long a period it may interfere with participation in rehabilitation and may require psychiatric help. Another emotional factor that may influence rehabilitation potential is emotional lability or disinhibition, which includes loss of self control (inappropriate laughing and crying), reduced tolerance to stress, impulsive behavior, and low self-esteem. Cerebrovascular accident may also cause psychotic-like behavior, regression or egocentricity.[18,52]

Behavioral Manifestations

Because of the impact of the cerebrovascular accident on the psychomotor system there are certain behavioral manifestations which are commonly observed in hemiplegic patients (left hemiplegics more frequently than right). Generally these persons are poor observers of their environment, are highly suggestible and fluctuate in mental ability. They have a limited attention span, show inattention to tasks, are highly distractable and have difficulty in carry-over of learned skills from one situation to another.

Family, Social and Vocational Influences

Success in rehabilitation is dependent on the patient's motivation to participate in treatment programs.[19,59] Both motivation and attitudes toward rehabilitation and recovery are dependent on the premorbid personality and the previous and current life situation. The eventual adjustment of the patient is tied closely to his family and their attitudes toward him and his disability. Therefore, the family must be educated to understand the problems involved in order to establish realistic goals which will fully utilize remaining abilities and maintain adequate levels of social contact for stimulation and attention to life's tasks.[19] When feasible, the rehabilitation goal should include meaningful vocational and/or avocational pursuits in order to increase the sense of worth and self-realization.

Predictors for Recovery

Although the process of recovery may be arrested at any stage and there are no objective criteria to predict which patients will respond to rehabilitation and which will not, there are a few guidelines which may assist prognostically. Studies indicate that motor return occurs chiefly in the first 2 months post insult and appears to be a spontaneous process.[67] Those patients who recovered partial motion recovered more slowly, exhibiting spasticity, with the maximum recovery being reached in the 6th to 7th month. Generally, return of upper extremity function is not as good as that of the lower extremity, and most frequently occurs proximal to distal.

Generally, there is return of sensorimotor function, with most return occurring spontaneously within the first 2 months. When total unilateral neglect of space persists with all the sensorimotor problems (distorted body image, sensory loss, and constructional apraxia), prognosis for complete rehabilitation and independence is guarded.

Complicating factors of bowel and bladder incontinence, severe hypertensive heart disease and excessive brain damage may also be negative predictors for complete rehabilitation.[24] Successful rehabilitation is greatly influenced by the patient's ability to adjust to, comprehend and accept treatment.[3]

ROLE OF THE OCCUPATIONAL THERAPIST

The basic needs of all human beings are self-care, work and play. Thus, the role of the occupational therapist is to help each individual achieve the highest possible level of functioning in these areas. Through a careful evaluation of assets and deficiencies, a therapeutic regime should be devised which meets the individual needs of each person. The occupational therapist must work as an integral member of the rehabilitation team, who share common realistic goals and complement each other in helping the patient achieve his goals. Rehabilitation and planning for discharge should be started upon admission to the program. Total rehabilitation must be carried over into home and community life, where factors must be dealt with which interfere with adjustment and the achievement of basic needs. With changing times and the growing emphasis on community medicine, the entire program of rehabilitation may be carried on in the home environment involving family and community in the progress and adjustment of the hemiplegic. The occupational therapist must first consider the personal goals of the patient and his family, in order to have them participate in program planning and help them feel that they have a measure of control over their destiny.

Objectives of the Occupational Therapy Program

Since spasticity and resultant deformity are common in an upper motor neuron lesion such as hemiplegia, the first objective of occupational therapy is to prevent and correct deformity. Other objectives are (2) to improve sensorimotor function; (3) to improve physical function of the affected side to its maximum while improving skill in the unaffected arm; (4) to improve ability to function in all self-care and daily living activities utilizing devices and equipment where needed for increasing independence; (5) to improve the capacity for organizational and abstract thinking; (6) to improve ability in homemaking tasks utilizing devices and equipment needed to increase independence; (7) to help the patient make vocational adjustments through evaluation and job simulation where indicated and/or develop avocational interests which can be continued at home; (8) to help the patient make plans for home adjustment to meet his present needs and encourage participation in normal activities of the home and community; (9) to provide a therapeutic climate allowing for socialization and a feeling of worth and accomplishment.

OCCUPATIONAL THERAPY ASSESSMENT PROCEDURES

Because the problem of the hemiplegic is a complex one, the occupational therapist is challenged to assess all aspects of function completely and accurately, looking for all factors which can influence function, in order to plan a therapeutic program which will meet his individual needs and help him to achieve his highest functional ability. Assessment must include physical deficits and motor function, sensorimotor function, as well as functional abilities including activities of daily living, cognitive and social factors, homemaking and home assessment and prevocational evaluation. It is important to remember that all areas of function are interrelated and influence each other.

Many factors which influence function can be determined by astute observation on the part of the therapist; however, tests have been devised which assess function in a more standardized fashion. Some of these will be described.

Physical Deficits and Motor Function—Upper Extremity

Passive Range of Motion should be assessed in each joint of the upper extremity, noting any contractures or established deformity as well as joint limitation due to tendon tightness. Tendon tightness may be noted in the finger flexors, manifested clinically by the inability to passively extend and flex the fingers with the wrist in the neutral position. Spasticity should be noted especially in the shoulder adductors, horizontal adductors and internal rotators as well as in all muscle groups of the elbow, wrist and hand. The severity of spasticity should be determined by using a quick stretch to elicit a stretch reflex and to determine the amount of resistance to passive motion. The presence of severe spasticity, edema or pain affects the ability to perform functional tasks.

Gross Motor Patterns [30,51] of the upper extremity should be assessed to determine the base line level of function. Standard manual muscle tests cannot be employed to determine the motor function of the hemiplegic because strength varies with circumstances. Before the patient is able to control individual joint motion he may be able to perform gross motions involving several joints. There are two types: mass flexion and mass extension patterns of "synergies."[27] Motion occurs in more than one joint when a patient is asked to move only one joint. For mass flexion the patient's arm may be positioned straight down at the side and he is asked to bend the elbow as far as he can. Motions occurring at the shoulder, elbow, wrist and hand should be noted.[51] Brunnstrom's[27] variation for eliciting flexion synergies would be to ask the patient to touch his head above his ear with the affected hand. For mass extension pattern the patient's arm is positioned in abduction and external rotation within pain limitation; the elbow is flexed to 90°, and the arm is supported by the therapist if necessary. The patient is then asked to straighten the elbow as far as possible. Motions occurring at the shoulder, forearm, wrist and hand should be noted. Brunnstrom's variation for eliciting extension synergy would be to ask the patient to reach forward and downward to his knees.

Components of the flexion synergy include shoulder abduction, external rotation, elbow flexion and forearm supination. Scapular elevation and retraction may appear. Elbow flexion is the strongest component of the flexion synergy. Components of the extension synergy include shoulder adduction and internal rotation, elbow extension and forearm pronation. Adduction (pectoralis major) is the strongest component of the extension synergy.

The stages of recovery as described by Brunnstrom may be used as a guide in determining level of function.[28]

Stage 1. Unable to perform any motion and there is no resistance to passive movement.

Stage 2. Some components of basic synergy patterns appear as weak associated movements. Spasticity is developing. There is beginning gross grasp.

Stage 3. Basic synergy patterns or some components are performed voluntarily and show definite joint movement. Spasticity is present. Gross grasp and hook grasp are present.

Stage 4. Spasticity is decreasing and movement combinations deviating from basic synergies are developing. Gross grasp is present. Lateral prehension is developing.

Stage 5. There is relative independence from limb synergies and movements can be performed deviating from patterns. Palmar prehension and release are present.

Stage 6. Isolated joint movements are freely performed. Spasticity is disappearing except on rapid movement. Individual finger motion is possible and spherical grasp and release are present.

When determining stages of recovery, it should be noted whether basic synergies can be elicited, reinforced or modified through the use of efferent stimulation such as tonic neck reflexes, labyrinthian reflexes, and cutaneous or proprioceptive stimulation.[27]

Wrist and Hand Recovery[30,51] should be assessed in addition to noting their function within mass motor patterns. With the forearm supported, wrist flexion and extension should be assessed with the elbow first in the flexed, then in the extended position. For hand function, the elbow should be supported on a table top with the elbow flexed to 90° and the forearm in pronation. The patient grasps the dynamometer for gross grasp. The pinch gauge is used to measure lateral and palmar prehension. For mass release the patient is asked to extend his fingers actively. To assess individual finger motion, the patient is asked to touch the tip of each finger with the tip of the thumb. Observations should be made relative to the ease with which these motions are performed.

Movements Deviating from Patterns[30,51] or those that involve the performance of combined motions other than those in mass patterns should be attempted. These include such combined motions as: touching the back of involved shoulder with the hand (shoulder flexion and elbow flexion); touching the examiner's hand, held out to the involved side of the patient (shoulder abduction and elbow extension); picking up an object from the examiner's hand 4 in. above the involved knee (elbow flexion and pronation); and reaching out to receive an object in the palm of the hand (elbow extension and supination). Many other combined motions such as raising the hand to the mouth, tying a bow behind the back or raising the arm over the head may be used to determine motions available for function.[46]

Sensorimotor Function

In studies that have been conducted relative to the relationship between sensorimotor problems and function in the hemiplegic patient, there seem to be some significant correlations, thus indicating the need for more specific testing to determine areas of dysfunction.[56,57,61] No standardized tests of sensorimotor function have been developed for the adult patient. These areas may be assessed in a very gross form through observation of: the patient's posture (verticality), how he dresses himself (apraxia, body image, right-left discrimination, proprioception, gross motor planning), how he writes his name (fine motor planning), recognition of objects placed in his hand (stereognosis), ability to distinguish tactile stimuli (sensation, body image), and ability to copy two and three dimensional designs (visual figure ground, fine motor planning, three dimensional apraxia).

This gross form of assessment cannot evaluate all parameters of sensorimotor function, but may be sufficient to determine the need for further testing in specific areas. If further testing is indicated, the Ayres[16] and Frostig[36] tests which were developed for children may be utilized and/or some of the following tests may be used to identify specific deficiencies in adults.[16,36,51,57]

Upper Extremity Proprioception. With eyes blindfolded, the patient's upper extremity is moved by the therapist to designated positions. The patient is requested to duplicate the position with the unaffected extremity. If pain restricts motion, the examiner adjusts the position to a pain free range. This same procedure may be used for fine proprioceptive sense. The patient's individual fingers are positioned up or down and the patient indicates the position of the finger. Gross error in the proprioceptive area may cause the patient to ignore the arm or fail to use it although functional motion is available.

Sensation. Tactile sensation difficulties may be determined by asking the patient (eyes blindfolded) to locate the finger touched or the place touched on any part of the body. *Two point discrimination* may be assessed by occluding vision of the patient and touching the palmar surface of one or two fingers simultaneously with a divider, the separation of points ranging from 1 to ⅛ in.

Tactile discrimination can be determined by asking the blindfolded patient to discriminate between coarse and fine, smooth and rough, and soft and hard textures. *Object identification* or stereognosis may be assessed by requesting the patient whose eyes are occluded to identify common objects (such as pencil, key, ball) which are placed in either hand.

Body Image. Body parts recognition and finger recognition may be determined by asking the patient to point to or move a body part as it is named. For body visualization, the patient may be presented with statements concerning the relative location of body parts such as "the head is higher than the arm" and patient indicates yes or no. The Man Puzzle, consisting of a simple six piece puzzle, may be presented to the patient as another means of determining body visualization. Draw-a-Person test may also be used for determining body image. The patient is told to draw a person, explaining that artistic ability is not important. The examiner should note whether body parts are distinguishable and/or are inappropriately placed and/or are missing. For right-left discrimination the patient is asked questions regarding his right or left side and the right and left side of the examiner.

Spatial Judgment. Graphic skill which requires making free-hand reproductions of geometric designs as seen on stimulus cards, tests two-dimensional apraxia. Drawing of common objects such as a box, a house, a clock or a flower, indicates the patient's orientation to space.[37] Absence of parts, misplacement or indistinguishable parts may indicate unilateral neglect of space. Form constancy or the ability to recognize the same shape, though varied in size and placement, may be tested by having the patient trace around all of the geometric designs that are the same (i.e., all the circles) on a sheet containing many varied designs. Ayres Space Test assesses the patient's ability to discriminate visually shape and position of objects, while geometric puzzles assess the ability to visualize parts that make up the whole, when using 2 or 4 blocks to fill in a cut-out on a form board.

3 *Dimensional Constructional Praxis* is tested by using a series of 6, 8 and 15 block structures.[20] The blocks necessary to reproduce each series are presented in separate boxes. Progressing from the least to the most difficult, a block structure is placed in front of the patient who is instructed to build an identical model from the blocks in the box.

Vertical and horizontal perception are assessed by having a patient indicate when he judges a rod to be straight up and down (vertical) or exactly straight across (horizontal).[21] Testing is first conducted in the light, then in the dark, to determine if the patient compensates using visual cues.

Figure Ground. Visual figure ground is assessed by asking the patient to identify single objects as presented on cards. The examiner then presents one card at a time with two or three of the previously identified objects superimposed or embedded in a configuration. The patient names the objects as soon as he recognizes them. For auditory figure ground the patient, with eyes occluded, is asked to identify auditory stimuli such as a bell, a gong or a cymbal and then to identify two sounds made simultaneously. Patients may also be asked to locate the direction from which the sounds come.

Motor Planning. For Fine Motor Planning the patient is given a device with a free moving grommet on an irregularly curved wire attached to a handle. He is asked to manipulate the handle so that the grommet slides along the full course of the wire.

Intellectual Functioning

The occupational therapist can get some basic idea of the patient's cognitive ability by probing his awareness of himself and those around him, asking a few questions relative to his orientation to time (What day is this?), place (Where are you?), and person (What is your name?). Questions about recent events (i.e., What did you have for breakfast this morning?) will give cues regarding recent memory. Asking a patient to solve simple mathematical problems with or without paper or to solve simple riddles or puzzles gives cues relative to abstract reasoning. The patient's ability to stick to and complete a task, recognize errors, follow instructions and use good judgment in working out a task gives the therapist cues relative to other parameters of intellectual functioning. These observations will help the occupational therapist to determine how minutely each task must be broken down into its component parts and how simple and concrete the instructions must be for the successful completion of tasks. Problems in communication skills may make it difficult to assess intellectual functioning.

Functional Testing

Self-Care Ability – Activities of Daily Living. All areas of self-care should be assessed including self-feeding, grooming, personal hygiene, dressing, written communications, use of household fixtures (faucets, light switches, etc.), and other pertinent hand activities such as striking a match, handling money and winding a watch. The type and amount of assistance needed, inconsistency of performance, impractical amount of time needed, unusual positions of the patient during testing and where testing is being done (bedside, bathroom, in bed, in wheelchair) should be recorded.

Spontaneous Use of Hand and Functional Activities Use Testing.[17,30,51] Patients are asked to perform activities that normally require two hands, not being told to use the affected hand so that it may be used in a spontaneous fashion. Activities include such things as holding down paper while writing, opening a bottle with an opener and peeling a fruit or vegetable. These simple functions require only limited control. The test items increase in complexity requiring higher levels of sensory and motor control up to the ability to use individual finger motion in bilateral touch typing. Speed and precision of reciprocal movements and coordination of the arm and hand during activities should be noted.

Evaluation of Devices and Equipment. The initial assessment for self-care ability should give the therapist an indication of the need for and value of special one-handed devices and equipment to improve functional ability. Some of these devices may be used as a temporary measure for increasing independence and can be discarded when patient's skill has increased. However, some may need to be used permanently (see Chapter 8 on ADL). When walking is impractical because of lack of muscle power, undue fatigue, or other complicating factors, the patient should be evaluated for the proper wheelchair. Generally a wheelchair for a hemiplegic should have padded fixed arm rests which are high enough to support the affected arm, removable foot rests with a heel loop on the involved side, the seat low enough to allow the patient to propel the chair with his unaffected leg, and a 2-in. foam cushion for comfort. If edema or thrombophlebitis of the leg is present, an elevating leg rest may be indicated.

Homemaking Evaluation and Home Assessment[9]

Homemaking goals should be established according to the needs as well as the physical capacities of the patient. If the patient has been assuming all the duties in maintaining a household and hopes to reassume them, she should be assessed in all the duties required to maintain a household including cleaning, cooking (diet control), bed making, laundry and shopping; as well as taking responsibility for planning and supervising family or paid help. If, however, the physical capacity or needs of the patient indicate a lower level of functioning, she should be assessed only in areas of capability and need. A man may need to be assessed in limited homemaking functions, or as a home manager, if his physical capacity will not allow him to go back to work and his wife must become the wage earner for the family.

Special devices, especially those which allow activities to be done with one hand, may be needed in order to increase independence (see Chapter 8 on ADL). When possible, a home visit should be made with the patient while he is still in the hospital in order to assess the feasibility of modifications and/or changes that will allow for optimum functioning at home. If weekend visits are part of the rehabilitation plan, the patient should try as many activities as practical while on visits, so that problem areas may be worked out in the treatment program. If a home visit is impossible, the patient, the family and the therapist may plan for modifications or changes using floor plans as guides.

Need for socialization and opportunities for socialization within the individual's community should be equated and the patient should be encouraged to participate in community activities whenever possible.

Prevocational, Vocational and Work Tolerance Evaluation

An occupation often serves as an index of an individual's worth in society, both economically and socially, and defines his role in the community. Thus, it is frequently a high priority need of the individual to return to some type of remunerative occupation if physically and psychologically feasible. The individual may need to be assessed in his ability to perform tasks required on his job in order to determine if he can return to the previous occupation. This may be accomplished by simulating the job itself or through the use of tasks that require similar skills. If, because of inability to perform the needed skills it is determined that a new occupation is in order the occupational therapist, working with the vocational counselor, may plan a prevocational testing program which will take into account the interest and needs of the patient and the practical aspect of the community's occupational opportunities. Occupational therapy media or tests such as the "Tower System,"* may be adapted to meet the occupational needs of the community and be utilized to test potential ability. Training then should be done in vocational rehabilitation training centers, qualified trade schools or other specialized training programs.

The area of work tolerance for the hemiplegic must not be overlooked because fatigue and decreased tolerance are common problems. Thus, a patient's sitting and standing tolerance must be checked constantly from his first day of treatment by checking blood pressure, pulse and respiration as well as closely observing for signs of fatigue such as tremor, diffuse perspiration, weakness, lethargy and pallor. As tolerance increases, time and energy expenditures may be increased until the patient reaches a level of optimum functioning within his physical limitations. Limited work tolerance may be the factor which prevents a person from returning to remunerative occupation. When age or physical limitations prevent a person from returning to work, his interests should be explored to find an avocation which may add meaning to his life and increase his feelings of self-worth.

OCCUPATIONAL THERAPY – TREATMENT PLANNING AND PROCEDURES

Before beginning an occupational therapy program on the basis of an assessment, information which will help to guide in treatment planning and treatment precautions should be obtained from the medical

*Institute for Crippled and Disabled, New York.

chart and from members of the rehabilitation team. The medical chart can supply information relative to premorbid and current medical problems, social and psychological status. The physical therapist can provide information relative to lower extremity sensory and motor status, as well as transfer and ambulation ability. It is of value to correlate the treatment program in occupational therapy and physical therapy. Members of the nursing staff are with the patient constantly and can provide valid information relative to patient's behavior and ability to function consistently. Close collaboration with the nursing staff is especially important in the self-care area. Social service provides information relative to the patient's premorbid social and work history, his home situation and a feasible discharge plan. Vocational or rehabilitation counselors and/or the psychologist and/or the speech pathologist can provide information relative to emotional, cognitive and communications factors which suggest the most effective means of relating to and communicating with the patient.

Once the patient has been assessed and the information from the charts and from the other rehabilitation personnel has been collected, the specific goals and objectives can be determined for each individual patient and treatment can be planned to meet these objectives.

Among the goals that will have to be considered for each patient are maintaining passive range of motion, upper extremity strength and functional use, activities of daily living and homemaking. Treatment technics will then have to be devised to accomplish these goals.

Increasing Pain-Free Passive Range of Motion

Use of Splints or Slings for Positioning. When the patient has no voluntary control over the musculature of the shoulder and the shoulder girdle, the scapula is allowed to rotate downward, eliminating the natural shelf which retains the integrity of the joint, thus permitting the shoulder to subluxate. By using an overhead suspension sling attached to the wheelchair, some degree of arm support is given to the wheelchair patient. The hand and arm may be elevated if edema is present. The spring may assist weak shoulder musculature and improve the function of the arm. If a sling is not desired, an arm trough or a mobile arm support (balanced forearm orthosis) may be fastened to the wheelchair arm to support the involved shoulder. Precautions must be taken so that circulation is not cut off by the retaining straps, and so that the arm does not fall out because of spasticity and get caught in the spokes of the wheelchair. If the patient becomes ambulatory before he has control over the shoulder musculature, a cloth or webbing sling may be used for support during ambulation and when transferring.

There has been much controversy over the use of slings for the hemiplegic patient because they reinforce flexion synergy patterns and may contribute to deformity patterns in the arm unless full range of motion for all joints is retained.[53] Special attention should be given to the position of the scapula during range of motion exercises in order to help prevent subluxation.

When spasticity begins to develop, static hand splints are frequently used to prevent flexion deformity of the wrist and fingers. Differing opinions have arisen from studies regarding the relative value of dorsal versus ventral splinting for the hemiplegic hand, but all agree that splinting does reduce flexor spasticity.[32, 62, 63] However, it was found that the use of a static splint at night and a dynamic rubberband finger extension assist splint for 4 hours a day while doing grasp and release activities caused diminishing of the stretch reflex and a decrease in release time.[62]

Experimental splints are being devised which use electrotherapy,[64, 65] whereby stimulation causes muscle contraction that has a functional purpose such as producing wrist extension or finger prehension. These splints have many limitations but may soon be perfected and be of functional value to hemiplegic patients.

Passive Range of Motion Exercises. Patients can be taught to move the affected extremities through full range of motion passively. When self ranging is utilized precautions must be taken if the patient has weak or no motion. Full range is contraindicated because of the tendency for supporting joint structures to become loosened. Instability can lead to pain and subluxation, especially in the shoulder joint. The range should be limited to 90° of flexion or abduction of the shoulder with external rotation limited to 30 to 35°. Elbow range should be from 20° extension to 120° flexion, pronation to 90° supination to neutral, wrist 20 to 30° of extension.

Activities. Using the suspension sling, activities such as bilateral sanding, weaving on a floor loom with long shuttles, or other gross activity with the placement of the projects on an elevated surface, will help increase pain-free passive range of motion.

Exercise Technics. If the therapist thinks that it is within his jurisdiction, exercise technics such as the ball-bearing exercise skate (49) and wand exercises may be utilized for increasing range of motion.*

Increasing Dexterity in Uninvolved Upper Extremity

While the programs for strengthening and use of the involved upper extremity are being carried out, the uninvolved extremity must become more skilled in order to perform one-handed activities.

*In the opinion of the editors it is not within the occupational therapist's jurisdiction.

Upper Extremity Strengthening

Muscle Re-education. The nervous system works on a facilitory-inhibitory principle requiring stimulation, integration response and feedback in order to have a balanced system which responds purposefully to the environment. When a cerebrovascular accident causes a brain lesion, one or more of these functions is disturbed, resulting in faulty sensory input, poor integration, inadequate motor response and faulty feedback. Through the use of increased stimulation to the exteroceptors in the skin, eyes, etc., and the proprioceptors in the muscles and tendons, an attempt can be made to "rebalance the nervous system by conditioning remaining circuits, training new pathways, connectors and reflexes."[11] This is done by strengthening or facilitating the weak muscles and weakening or inhibiting the antagonistic strong muscles, through the use of tapping, brushing, icing, patterning and positioning, thus initiating motion or assisting a part through the available range of motion.

The specific sensorimotor technics of Fay, Doman-Delacato, Kabott-Knott, Bobath, Brunnstrom and Rood are described in another chapter.[6,22,27,28,35,48] Several of the following principles are important to remember when treating the hemiplegic patient:[5]

1. Gross motor patterns should be established before fine skills are attempted.
2. Resistance properly applied and graded in total movement patterns enhances motor output.
3. Various sensory and proprioceptive stimuli influence the motor system and can inhibit or facilitate it depending on the method and area of application.
4. The motor system learns through repetition on a subconscious level.

Activities for Strengthening. Once motor patterns have been established through sensorimotor technics, they should be followed by activities that are geared to the patient's functioning level. The patient should enjoy the activities and should be motivated to perform them so that the actual exercise is on a subconscious level. Motor function must be subcortical until it becomes integrated, then it may be used on the cortical level. In other words, the patient must learn to move by "how it feels" before he can learn to move by "thinking about it." Activities must be adapted to give correct exteroceptive and proprioceptive stimulation to enhance motor output. A hemiplegic can get postural support if he does gardening or scrubs floors on all fours. Weaving and woodworking are good to use for extension of the upper extremity—with resistance to extension. Bilateral activities such as raking, sawing, planing, mopping and pushing a vacuum cleaner incorporate spiral diagonal patterns.[5] Recreational activities such as playing ball, and other games that require bilateral motion may cause spontaneous movement at the subcortical level which later can be motor planned at the cortical level.

Tools or equipment may need specially shaped, built-up or adapted handles. The tonic neck reflex may be utilized to produce easier elbow extension, and motion may be reinforced by incorporating sensory and proprioceptive stimuli (therapist produced) into the activity program.

Exercise Technics for Strengthening. If the therapist thinks that additional exercise technics are indicated both for assistance and for progressive resistance, counterbalance pulley exercises, ball-bearing skate exercises,[49] track exercises[41] and theraplast exercises[51] may be used, along with the sensorimotor technics and activities.*

Trunk and Lower Extremity Strengthening

Sitting and standing balance are very important in the rehabilitation of the hemiplegic patient. By gradually increasing sitting time and utilizing bilateral activities or activities stimulating balance reactions, trunk balance can be improved and sitting tolerance increased. Standing tolerance can be increased in like fashion; standing initially in the standing table, gradually decreasing support while increasing time. Stimulating balance reactions, while standing, can also be accomplished through the use of activities requiring both hands and by recreational activities such as ball playing.

When reciprocal motion is needed in the lower extremities, the bicyle jig saw can give the needed motion while simultaneously increasing muscle power by adding resistance. Resistance can be added through a brake or spring system in the mechanism itself and by cutting or sanding increasingly thicker and harder materials. The treadle sander provides reciprocal ankle motion and strengthening. By cutting or sanding a project, the patient is able to coordinate motion in all four extremities.

Increasing Functional Use

The patient should be trained to use his affected extremity as much as possible for performing functional activities. The therapist should demonstrate how the arm may be used for a specific activity and may need to place the patient's hand or arm in the desired position. The patient should practice using the arm daily in activities that require a particular arm function, such as stabilization, so that he may learn to use it for all activities that require stabilization. As strength and con-

*In the opinion of the editors it is not within the occupational therapist's jurisdiction.

trol increase he should go on to activities which require the use of this improved function.

The person who has minimal voluntary control may only be able to use the arm to stabilize or weight objects. As a mass flexion pattern develops with gross grasp, he may be able to hold objects while using the other hand to perform the activity. As the mass flexion pattern becomes stronger and some elbow extension and lateral prehension appear he may assist in two-handed activities, such as pulling on and taking off shoes and socks. As more shoulder control, coordinated motion and pinch and release develop, the affected hand can be used to assist in finer coordinated activities.[51]

Activities of Daily Living

Assessment in activities of daily living should determine areas of dysfunction. Once problem areas are determined, the patient should be trained in those areas through daily practice, using the affected hand as a helping hand when possible, or one-handed devices when necessary. Activities should be broken down into minute detail and instructions should be very concrete to decrease the chance of failure. The right hemiplegic who may be suffering from language problems generally profits more from non-verbal instruction (demonstration and gestures) than from verbal instruction. The left hemiplegic generally profits more from verbal instruction than from non-verbal. The right hemiplegic may have a tendency to perform too slowly but will be error free while the left hemiplegic may perform too quickly, impulsively and erratically. Suggestions to the left hemiplegic to slow down and take things step-by-step may improve performance.[34] Because of the factors of fatigue and frustration, sufficient time must be allowed for patients to accomplish self-help tasks. It may be necessary to give frequent rest periods, to give assistance or to stop an activity if the frustration level gets too high. Specific step-by-step dressing technics for the hemiplegic patient have been worked out at Highland View Hospital and may be used as a guide.[26] It is important to have the patient try to use the affected hand in every possible way as a helping hand. However, where little functional return has occurred in the affected arm and hand, patients may be able to become independent through the use of selected one-hand devices.[8,13,14,60] (See chapter 8 on ADL.) The therapist should be sure that the patient is well trained in the use of these devices.

Reinforcement is a necessary part of learning self-care activities. These activities should be carried out daily at the normal time, with patients dressing in the morning and remaining in street clothing the entire day. If this is impossible, as in a general hospital, the patient's family should bring in street clothes so the patient can be assessed and trained in dressing in occupational therapy. There must be good communication and a close working relationship with the nursing personnel in order to assure consistent function. Before the patient's discharge, the family should be instructed regarding self-care technics and equipment used by the patient, so that they can be carried over into his normal living pattern at home.

Communications and Speech

Loss of communications skills causes much frustration for the hemiplegic patient. The occupational therapist can assist the speech pathologist by encouraging functional speech and providing stimulation and support which encourage participation in verbal communication. The occupational therapist may stimulate functional speech by increased auditory and visual stimuli, but the therapist must learn to give the patient sufficient time to express himself. He should speak in short simple sentences and give only one direction at a time.[50] In both spoken and written communication, the occupational therapist works on the motor aspect, getting the cues for content from the speech department.[58]

Homemaking Training and Home Planning

When a woman has been evaluated relative to needs and ability in homemaking, she should begin a training program which includes not only practice in performance of homemaking activities but also methods of work simplification, and energy conservation. To do this she will have to learn how to rearrange work and storage areas and plan work more efficiently. Whenever possible, the affected arm should be used in homemaking activities. However, some one-handed methods may have to be learned and one-handed devices may be needed to increase independence.[8,9,13,14] The patient's judgment and the ability to solve problems must be considered, as these factors may be the ones which determine independence.

   If the patient is to be discharged to her home where she will be responsible for homemaking tasks, it is important that family members be made aware of her capabilities and limitations, so that needed adjustments in living patterns may be made. They should also be made aware of the patient's need for constant reassurance and support. Adaptations in the home require cooperative planning for maximum function plus an understanding on the part of the patient's family. A home visit should be made, if possible, both pre- and post-discharge to help both patient and family make changes necessary for satisfactory adjustment.

Socialization

There is some opportunity for socialization of patients in the occupational therapy program but the major opportunity for socialization usually occurs when the treatment program is over. Patients should be encouraged to participate in the recreational programs that are provided, and also take some part in the patient government bodies which are active in many rehabilitation facilities. These activities make the patient begin to function as a member of a community in preparation for his discharge into his larger home community.

When the individual is discharged from the hospital, it is important that he be able to take his place in the community again. He should be encouraged to attend social affairs, join Golden Age Clubs, or attend those types of functions which were part of his life pattern before his cerebrovascular accident.

For patients in a wheelchair there are still architectural barriers which prevent them from participating in many activities. Legislation is being enacted to correct some of these inequities, but it will be many years before all the necessary changes can be made to provide easy access for all handicapped persons.

SUMMARY

A cerebrovascular accident has a catastrophic impact on the human organism causing problems which are very complex and interdependent. An attempt has been made to delineate the component parts of the problem, to define occupational therapy measures for assessing function and to outline treatment technics which can be used to help the patient reach his highest potential. The procedures described here are not complete and will need to be changed as more information relative to neurophysiological function and treatment technics are obtained through research. Methods for assessment and treatment in occupational therapy will have to be modified constantly to incorporate new principles as they develop.

REFERENCES

Books

1. Critchley, M.: The Parietal Lobes. New York, Hafner Publishing Co., 1966.
2. DeForest, R. E. (ed.): Proceedings of the National Stroke Congress. Springfield, Charles C Thomas, 1966.
3. Fields, W. S., and Spencer, W. A.: Stroke Rehabilitation — Basic Concepts and Research Trends. St. Louis, W. H. Green, 1967.
4. Hodgins, E.: Episode — Report on the Accident Inside My Skull. New York, Atheneum, 1968.

5. Huss, J.: Controversy and confusion in physical dysfunction treatment techniques—clinical aspects, in Zamir, L. J.: Expanding Dimensions in Rehabilitation. Springfield, Charles C Thomas, 1969.

6. ———: Clinical applications of sensorimotor treatment techniques in physical dysfunction, in Zamir, L. J.: Expanding Dimensions in Rehabilitation. Springfield, Charles C Thomas, 1969.

7. Licht, S. (ed.): Rehabilitation and Medicine. New Haven, Elizabeth Licht, 1968.

8. Lowman, E. W., and Klinger, J. L.: Aids to Independent Living—Self Help for the Handicapped. New York, Blakiston-McGraw, 1969.

9. May, E. E., Waggoner, N. R., and Boettke, E. M.: Homemaking for the Handicapped. New York, Dodd, Mead and Co., 1966.

10. Moore, J. C.: The developing nervous system in relationship to techniques in treating physical dysfunction, in Zamir, L. J.: Expanding Dimensions in Rehabilitation. Springfield, Charles C Thomas, 1969.

11. ———: Structure and function of the nervous system in relation to treatment techniques, in Zamir, L. J.: Expanding Dimensions in Rehabilitation. Springfield, Charles C Thomas, 1969.

12. Rusk, H. A.: Rehabilitation Medicine. ed. 2, p. 590. St. Louis, C. V. Mosby, 1964.

Journals and Pamphlets

13. American Heart Association: Do it yourself again—Self help devices for the stroke patient. New York, American Heart Association, 1965.

14. American Rehabilitation Foundation: Rehabilitation Nursing Techniques Booklets. Minneapolis, American Rehabilitation Foundation, 1964.

15. Anderson, E. K., and Choy, E.: Parietal lobe syndromes in hemiplegia. Am. J. Occup. Therapy, 24:13, 1970.

16. Ayres, A. J.: Ayres Perceptual Motor Tests. Los Angeles, Western Psychological Services, 1968.

17. Bard, G., Hirschberg, G. G., and Tolleson, G.: Functional testing of the hemiplegic arm. J. Am. Phys. Therapy Assoc., 44:1081, 1964.

18. Bardach, J. L : Psychological factors in hemiplegia. J. Am. Phys. Therapy Assoc., 43:792, 1963.

19. Belmont, I., Benjamin, H., Ambrose, J., and Restuccia, R. D.: Effect of cerebral damage on motivation in rehabilitation. Arch. Phys. Med., 50:507, 1969.

20. Benton, A. J., and Fogel, M. L.: Three dimensional constructional praxis. Arch. Neurol., 7:347, 1962.

21. Birch, H. G., Proctor, F., Bortner, M., and Lowenthal, M.: Perception in hemiplegia: judgment of vertical and horizontal by hemiplegic patients. Arch. Phys. Med., 41:19, 1960.

22. Bobath, B. and Cotton, E.: A patient with residual hemiplegia and his response to treatment. Phys. Ther., 45:849, 1965.

23. Boone, D. R. and Landes, B. A.: Left-right discrimination in hemiplegic patients. Arch. Phys. Med., 49:533, 1968.

24. Bourestom, N. C.: Predictors of long-term recovery in cerebrovascular disease. Arch. Phys. Med., 48:415, 1967.

25. Brain, W. R.: Visual disorientation with special reference to lesions of the right cerebral hemisphere. Brain, 64:244, 1944.
26. Brett, G.: Dressing techniques for the severely involved hemiplegic patient. Am. J. Occup. Therapy, 16:262, 1960.
27. Brunnstrom, S.: Motor behavior of adult hemiplegic patients. Am. J. Occup. Therapy, 15:6, 1961.
28. ⸻: Motor testing procedures in hemiplegia. Phys. Ther., 46:357, 1966.
29. Burt, M. M.: Perceptual deficits in hemiplegia. Am. J. Nurs., 70:1026, 1970.
30. Caldwell, C. B., Wilson, D. J., and Braun, R. M.: Evaluation and treatment of the upper extremity in the hemiplegic stroke patient. Clin. Orthop. 63:69, 1969.
31. Casella, C.: Perception of time by hemiplegic patients. Arch. Phys. Med., 48:369, 1967.
32. Charait, S. E.: A comparison of volar and dorsal splinting of the hemiplegic hand. Am. J. Occup. Therapy, 22:319, 1968.
33. Dacso, M. M.: Rehabilitation of the stroke patient. Mod. Treatm., 5:971, 1968.
34. Diller, L.: Perceptual and intellectual problems in hemiplegia: implications for rehabilitation. Med. Clin. N. Am., 53:575, 1969.
35. Fox, J.: Cutaneous stimulation—effects on selected tests of perception. Am. J. Occup. Therapy, 18:53, 1964.
36. Frostig, M.: The developmental program in visual perception. Chicago, Follett, 1966.
37. Gordon, V., Young, J. S., Cobb, C., and DeTurk, J.: Functional significance of disturbances in cortical integration in the nondominant hemiplegic patient. Proceedings of the 1960 Annual Conference, Am. Occup. Therapy Assoc., p. 28, 1960.
38. Haas, A., Rusk, H. A., Pelosof, H., and Adam, J. R.: Respiratory function in hemiplegic patients. Arch. Phys. Med., 48:174, 1967.
39. Hagen, A. C.: Communication disorders of the stroke patient. Clin. Orthop. 63:112, 1969.
40. Hastings, A. E.: Patterns of motor function in adult hemiplegia. Arch. Phys. Med., 46:255, 1965.
41. Herring, M., Fairbanks, P., and Gralewicz, A.: A manual for occupational therapists—program for re-establishing motion. Cleveland, Mrs. Marjorie Herring, 1967.
42. Iseri, L. T., Smith, R. V., and Evans, M. J.: Cardiovascular problems and functional evaluation in rehabilitation of hemiplegic patients. J. of Chronic Diseases, 21:423. 1968.
43. Kent, B. E.: Sensory-motor testing: the upper limb of adult patients with hemiplegia. Phys. Ther., 45:550, 1965.
44. Lucas, M. E.: Perceptual disorders of adults with hemiplegia. Phys. Ther., 49:1078, 1969.
45. MacDonald, J. C.: Body scheme disturbances in hemiplegia. Study Course III. Dynamic Living for Long Term Patient, Third Int. Congress, World Fed. Occ. Therapists, Dubuque, Iowa, Wm. C. Brown, p. 47, 1964.

46. Michels, E.: Evaluation of motor function in hemiplegia. Phys. Therapy Rev., 39:589, 1959.
47. Moskowitz, E.: Complications in the rehabilitation of hemiplegic patients. Med. Clin. N. Am., 53:541, 1969.
48. Northwestern University—special therapeutic exercise project. Proceedings: an exploratory and analytical survey of therapeutic exercise. Am. J. Phys. Med., 46:732, 1967.
49. Newall, B.: Ball bearing platform for increased arm mobility in treating quadriplegic and hemiplegic patients. Am. J. Occup. Therapy, 24:290, 1970.
50. Norton, C., and Towne, C. C.: Occupational therapy for aphasic patients. Am. J. Occup. Therapy, 22:506, 1968.
51. Rancho Los Amigos Hospital: Occupational therapy treatment guide— adult hemiplegia. Downey, California, Rancho Los Amigos Hospital, 1968.
52. Rigoni, H. C.: Psychologic consideration in evaluating and treating the stroke patient. Clin. Orthop., 63:94, 1969.
53. Robins, V.: Should patients with hemiplegia wear a sling? Phys. Ther. 49:1029, 1969.
54. Sarno, J. F., and Sarno, M. T.: The diagnosis of speech disorders in brain damaged adults. Med. Clin. N. Am., 53:561, 1969.
55. Shanan, J., Cohen, M., and Adler, E.: Intellectual functioning in hemiplegic patients after cerebrovascular accidents. J. Nerv. Men. Dis., 143:181, 1966.
56. Taylor, M. M.: Analysis of dysfunction in left hemiplegia following stroke. Am. J. Occup. Therapy, 22:512, 1968.
57. Taylor, M. M., Schaeffer, J. N., Blumenthal, F. S., and Grisell, J. L.: Controlled Evaluation of Percept-Concept-Motor Training Therapy after Stroke Resulting in Left Hemiplegia. Detroit, Rehabilitation Institute Inc., 1969.
58. Taylor, M. L.: Aphasia. Study Course III, Dynamic Living for the Long Term Patient, Third Int. Congress, World Fed. Occ. Therapists. Dubuque, Iowa, William C. Brown, p. 42, 1964.
59. Ullman, M.: Behavioral changes in patients following strokes. Springfield, Charles C Thomas, 1962.
60. U.S. Public Health Service, Division of Chronic Diseases, U.S. Dept. of Health, Education and Welfare: Up and Around. Distributed by: American Heart Association, New York, 1965.
61. Williams, N.: Correlation between copying ability and dressing activities in hemiplegia. Am. J. Phys. Med., 46:1332, 1967.
62. Wolcott, L. E.: Orthotic management of the spastic hand. Southern Med. J., 59:971, 1966.
63. Zislis, J. M.: Splinting of hand in a spastic hemiplegic patient. Arch. Phys. Med., 45:41, 1964.
64. Dimitrijevic, M. R., Brancanin, F., Prevec, T., and Trontelj, J.: Electronic control of paralyzed extremities. Biomed. Engin., January, 1968, p. 8.
65. Liberson, W. T., Holmquest, H. J., Scot, D., and Dow, M.: Functional electrotherapy: stimulation of the peroneal nerve synchronized with the swing of the gait in hemiplegic patients. Arch. Phys. Med., 42:101, 1961.

66. McHenry, L. C., and Valsamis, M. P.: Pathophysiology of cerebrovascular insufficiency. G. P., 33:78. 1966.
67. Bard, G. and Hirschberg, G. G.: Recovery of voluntary motion in upper extremity following hemiplegia. Arch. Phys. Med., 46:567, 1965.

SUPPLEMENTARY BIBLIOGRAPHY

Books

Ayers, G. E.: Vocational rehabilitation counseling. In Zamir, L. J.: Expanding Dimensions in Rehabilitation. Springfield, Charles C Thomas, 1969.

Journals and Pamphlets

American Heart Association: Aphasia and the Family. New York, Am. Heart Assoc., 1965.

American Heart Association: Strokes (A Guide for the Family). New York, Am. Heart Assoc., 1964.

Berstrom, D. A.: Report on a conference for wheelchair manufacturers. Bulletin on Prosthetics Research, 10-3:60, 1965.

Covalt, D. A.: Rehabilitation of the patient with hemiplegia. Mod. Treatm., 2:84, 1965.

DiAngeles, L.: Evaluation of the hemiplegic patient. Study Course III, Dynamic Living for the Long Term Patient. Third Int. Congress, World Fed. Occ. Therapists. Dubuque, William C. Brown, 1964.

Goble, R. E.: The role of the occupational therapist in disabled living research. Am. J. Occup. Therapy, 23:145, 1969.

Haese, J. B., Trotter, A. B., and Flynn, R. T.: Attitudes of stroke patients toward rehabilitation and recovery. Am. J. Occup. Therapy, 24:285, 1970.

Johannsen, W. J., Jones, D. and Thill, M. K.: Effectiveness of homemaker's training for hemiplegic patients. Arch. Phys. Med., 48:244, 1967.

Michels, E.: Motor behavior in hemiplegia. Phys. Ther. Assoc., 45:759, 1965.

Olsen, J. Z., and May, B. J.: Family education: necessary adjunct to total stroke rehabilitation. Am. J. Occup. Therapy, 20:88, 1966.

Perry, J.: Orthopedic management of the lower extremity in the hemiplegic patient. Phys. Ther., 46:345, 1966.

Peterson, J. C., and Olsen, A. P.: Language problems after a stroke. Minneapolis, American Rehabilitation Foundation, 1964.

Smith, C. R.: Home planning for the severely disabled. Med. Clin. N. Am., 53:703, 1969.

Trombly, C. A.: Effects of selected activities on finger extension of adult hemiplegic patients. Am. J. Occup. Therapy, 18:233, 1964.

Troyer, B. L.: Sensorimotor integration—a basis for planning occupational therapy. Am. J. Occup. Therapy, 15:51, 1961.

Twitchell, T. E.: The restoration of motor function following hemiplegia in man. Brain, 74:433, 1951.

U.S. Public Health Service, Chronic Disease Program, U.S. Dept. of Health, Education & Welfare: Strike Back at Stroke. Distributed by American Heart Association, New York, 1960.

Acknowledgements

The following Registered Occupational Therapists made suggestions and contributions to this chapter: Carolyn Baum and Trish Collins, Research Hospital, Kansas City, Missouri; Ann Gill, St. Francis Hospital, Pittsburgh, Pennsylvania; Holly Gordon, New England Medical Center, Boston, Massachusetts; and Katherine LaQue, Cardinal Cushing Rehabilitation Center, Holy Ghost Hospital, Boston, Massachusetts.

12

Occupational Therapy For Cerebral Palsy

ANITA SLOMINSKI, B.A., O.T.R. and
CELESTINE HAMANT, B.A., O.T.R.

INTRODUCTION

The purpose of this chapter is to provide the student of occupational therapy with an overview of cerebral palsy and the methods used by occupational therapists to treat patients with this disability. It presents an overview and does not attempt to cover all aspects of medical theory or treatment modalities. For the student who needs more detailed information, supplementary sources are listed in the bibliography and reference section at the end of this chapter.

According to Denhoff and Robinault,[5] relief carvings simulating spastic diplegia were found in Egyptian monuments. Ancient Greek and Hebrew scriptures refer to cripples, and the New Testament refers to the beggar, "lame from his mother's womb" (Acts 3:2). Both Raphael and Poussin, Renaissance artists, painted people with deformities representing cerebral palsy. Pediatric textbooks carried medical descriptions of this condition as early as 1497 (by Metlinger) and 1656 (by Felix-Wurl). The clinical description of the spastic diplegic was first reported by W. J. Little in 1843.[16] However, almost an entire century passed before the confused concepts and pessimistic attitudes toward treatment were clarified and overcome.

Freud described childhood cerebral palsy in 1843,[13] and Osler wrote about it in 1889. Much confusion existed, however, between the results of childhood poliomyelitis and early brain damage. In 1861, Little recognized the abnormal mental and physical conditions, especially the spastic-rigidity which he related to obstetric difficulties. Today this is documented by detailed records and research.

Prior to World War II, Phelps and Crothers pioneered in the treatment of children passed over by others as hopeless cripples. Phelps coined the term "cerebral palsy" to separate those children with combinations of motor and sensory abnormalities from those who were primarily mentally deficient with mild motor impairment.[20]

DEFINITION

In 1952 Perlstein defined the condition, stating: "cerebral palsy is a disorder characterized by paralysis, weakness, incoordination, or any other aberration of motor function due to pathology of the motor control centers of the brain, resulting from maldevelopment, injury, or disease caused by a variety of factors that operate prenatally, natally, or postnatally."[19]

In 1949 Denhoff described cerebral palsy; not as a definitive entity, but as merely "one component of a broader brain-damage syndrome comprised of neuromotor dysfunction, psychologic dysfunction, convulsions, and behavioral disorders of organic origin. Mental retardation or deficiency, visual, aural, or perceptual problems, as well as speech, behavioral, and emotional disturbances, are included as associated handicaps reflecting a damaged brain."[5] Therefore cerebral palsy is recognized as neuromotor dysfunction with numerous associated handicaps usually present.

Representing the Nomenclature and Classification Committee of the American Academy for Cerebral Palsy, Minear, in 1956, combined the experts' opinions when he said: "Cerebral Palsy comprises those motor and other symptom complexes caused by nonprogressive brain lesion (or lesions). The characteristic thing about cerebral palsy is that it is a well-defined entity with a variety of etiologies and pathologies."[18]

The following chart (12-1) is a combination and simplification of several classification tables which the authors believe will aid the student of occupational therapy in understanding cerebral palsy, its etiology, pathology, distribution and complex symptomatology.

ACCOMPANYING DISORDERS

Because cerebral palsy is caused by damage to the brain, the likelihood of that same damage causing other problems is quite high. The problems accompanying cerebral palsy can be, and often are, more handicapping to the patient than the neuromuscular disorder itself. They can add immeasurably to the complexity of treatment of the cerebral palsied patient.

CHART 12-1

CLASSIFICATION OF CEREBRAL PALSY
(Condensed from classification tables according to Ingram, and Denhoff and Robinault)

I. Etiology — causative factors
  A. Prenatal
    1. Hereditary
      a. Static
      b. Progressive
    2. Acquired in utero
      a. Infection
      b. Anoxia
      c. Cerebral hemorrhage
      d. Blood incompatibility (RH factor, etc.)
      e. Maternal metabolic disturbances
  B. Paranatal
    1. Anoxia
    2. Trauma and hemorrhage
      a. Malposition
      b. Sudden pressure change
      c. Prolonged labor
  C. Postnatal
    1. Trauma
    2. Infection (high temperature)
    3. Vascular accidents
    4. Toxic causes (lead poisoning)
    5. Anoxia (carbon monoxide poisoning, drowning)
    6. Neoplasm

II. Distribution — topographical involvement of extremities
  A. Monoplegia: one extremity
  B. Paraplegia: lower extremities (both legs)
  C. Hemiplegia: one half of the body vertically;
                        arm and leg on the same side of the body
  D. Triplegia: three extremities involved; fourth normal
  E. Quadriplegia or
     tetraplegia: all four extremities equally involved
  F. Diplegia: bilateral symmetrical involvement, but lower
                        extremities more severe than upper extrem-
                        ities (definition used by Cerebral Palsy Academy)
  G. Double hemiplegia: bilateral symmetrical involvement, but
                        upper extremities more involved than lower
                        extremities (definition used by Cerebral
                        Palsy Academy)

III. Pathology Related to Motor Symptoms
  A. Pyramidal tracts   Spasticity — hyperactivity of the
                                 pathologic stretch
                                 reflex which shows
                                 abnormal on a muscle
                                 myographic record.

CHART 12-1 (continued)
CLASSIFICATION OF CEREBRAL PALSY
(Condensed from classification tables according to Ingram, and Denhoff and Robinault)

III. Pathology Related to Motor Symptoms (continued)		
B. Extra-pyramidal tracts and/or their connections	Athetosis—	bizzarre purposeless movements—involuntary throughout waking hours (non-tension, tension, tremor, dystonic)
C. Cerebellum	Ataxia—	disturbance of kinesthetic or balance sense characterized by loss of equilibrium, dyssynergies, and often astereognosis, with lack of depth perception.
D. Diffuse damage	Rigidity—	disturbance of agonist-antagonist relations in slow passive motion of both muscle groups
	Mixed—	having any combination of motor impairment

Mental Retardation

Nearly three fourths of all cerebral palsied children are mentally retarded to some extent, ranging from near normal intelligence to profound retardation. The most commonly accepted scale of intelligence is as follows:[21]

Normal	85 – 110
Borderline Retardation	69 – 84
Mildly Mentally Retarded (educable)	51 – 68
Moderately Mentally Retarded (trainable)	36 – 50
Severely Mentally Retarded (trainable)	21 – 35
Profoundly Mentally Retarded	0 – 20

Perceptual-Motor Dysfunction

A problem found in about half of all cerebral palsied patients is perceptual-motor dysfunction. It is so common that it is often referred to as the "hidden problem" in cerebral palsy. It challenges the therapist to find new approaches to attain treatment goals when learning ability is decreased because of perceptual-motor dysfunction. (see Chapter 14 by Gilfoyle and Grady.)

Seizures

Some children with brain damage exhibit epileptic seizures. These can be any of the various types (e.g., grand mal, petit mal, Jacksonian) but petit mal (characterized by a brief lapse in consciousness) seems to be the most common. Anti-convulsant medication can very often bring this problem under control.

Sensory Disorders

Vision

Many common visual disorders are found in the normal population; cerebral palsied persons tend, in a somewhat higher incidence, to have strabismus (deviation of the eye which the patient cannot overcome) and/or nystagmus (continuous rolling movement of the eyeball). These problems can seriously hinder or distort visual reception.

Hearing

Hearing loss or deafness is a less frequent disorder accompanying cerebral palsy, but one of which the therapist needs to be aware. It is often associated with such etiologic factors as blood incompatibility and maternal rubella.

Sensation

Loss or decrease in sensations of pain, position, temperature, touch, location, or stereognosis frequently accompany cerebral palsy. Such problems are often found in hemiplegic extremities but may be noted in any affected limb. They can seriously impede functional use of the extremity.

Speech and Language

Speech and language disorders are not uncommon in the normal population, but the incidence is increased in the cerebral palsied population. Incoordination of the speech musculature, aphasic disorders, and even the deprivation brought about by lack of normal life experiences can cause serious delay in the development of speech and language.

EVALUATION

One of the most important activities of the occupational therapist is the evaluation of the patient. This not only precedes treatment but accompanies it and proceeds throughout treatment. Only by continually evaluating the patient can the therapist decide when to begin treatment, when to change it, and when to terminate it.

One must evaluate the patient's abilities as well as his disabilities; for in order to treat the areas of dysfunction, one must capitalize on abilities already present. Nor is it sufficient simply to note and to proceed to concentrate treatment on disability areas. It is important first to consider *why* the patient is unable to perform certain tasks. Is it because of physical disability, abnormal reflex patterns, mental retardation, perceptual dysfunction, or some other factor? Or is it a combination of all of these? The evaluation guide (see Chart 12–2) is meant only to provide the occupational therapist with guidelines for evaluating the cerebral palsied patient. It is not a form to be filled out.

Treatment goals must be realistic for cerebral palsied patients in order to prevent discouragement on the part of the patient, his family, and the therapist. These patients are often treated on an out-patient basis, so the therapist must depend on the family to carry out the treatment program in the home. Therefore, it is necessary to evaluate thoroughly the home situation as well as the patient. This can be done through parent interviews, but home visiting is an even more effective method.

With a thorough background in child development one can determine by evaluating the child and interviewing the family, the general stage at which the patient is performing and why. There are many forms and test batteries that can be used for this purpose:

The Gesell Developmental Evaluation
Denver Developmental Evaluation
Milani-Comparetti Developmental Examination
Reflex Testing Methods for Evaluation of Central Nervous System
    Development
Southern California Perception Test Battery
The Purdue Perceptual-Motor Survey
Developmental Test of Visual Perception

Information is also often needed from other sources before an adequate treatment program can be set up. The occupational therapist must request this information from other medical services such as ophthalmology, audiology and speech, psychology, physical therapy, social service, and education.

TREATMENT

Today's treatment usually follows one or a combination of the sensorimotor approaches (e.g., Rood, Bobath, Kabot-Knott, Phelps, Deaver, Brunnstrom, and Doman-Delacato). For detailed descriptions of these refer to Chapter 13 by Huss.

Positioning

Correct positioning is basic to the treatment of any patient. Whether he is lying down, standing or sitting in a chair, correct body alignment

CHART 12–2

EVALUATION GUIDE – CEREBRAL PALSY

I. General
   A. Attitude
      1. Child
      2. Parents
   B. Co-operation
   C. Attention span
   D. Discipline
   E. Cleanliness
   F. Follows directions
      1. Verbal
      2. Demonstrated

   G. Vision
      1. Nystagmus
      2. Strabismus
   H. Speech
   I. Hearing
   J. Intelligence
   K. Seizures
   L. Condition of teeth and mouth

II. Motor
   A. Head control
   B. Trunk control (Scoliosis)
   C. Crawling
   D. Sitting
   E. Creeping
   F. Standing
   G. Cruising

   H. Walking
   I. Walks with aids
      1. Braces
      2. Crutches
      3. Walker
   J. Wheelchair (Chair-fast)

III. Activities of Daily Living
   A. Feeding
      1. Dependent
         a. Lip closure
         b. Tongue thrust
         c. Tongue lateralization
         d. Swallowing
         e. Straw drinking
         f. Texture of food eaten
      2. Feeds self with assistance
      3. Independent
         a. Finger feeds
         b. Spoon
         c. Cup or glass
         d. Straw
         e. Fork
         f. Knife (cutting, spreading)
         g. Serves, passes food
         h. Pours liquid
         i. Eats most foods
   B. Dressing
      1. Does not cooperate
      2. Cooperates, but dependent
      3. Needs some assistance
      4. Independent
         a. Coat, sweater, cardigan
            blouse

         b. Pants, trousers
         c. Shoes, slippers, boots
         d. Socks
         e. Pullover shirt
         f. Bra
         g. Braces
         h. Fastenings (zipper,
            shoelaces, buttons)
         i. Gloves, mittens
      5. In what position does patient
         dress (is patient dressed)

   C. Toilet Activities
      1. Toileting
         a. Not toilet trained
         b. Toilet trained, but depend-
            ent
         c. Needs assistance with cloth-
            ing, transfers or braces
         d. Independent
      2. Bathing
         a. Dependent
         b. Can bathe self with assist-
            ance
         c. Independent
         d. Can wash hands and face at
            wash basin

CHART 12–2 (continued)

III. Activities of Daily Living (continued)
    3. Hygiene
      a. Wash hair
      b. Set hair
      c. Comb and brush hair
      d. Brush teeth
      e. Cut, clean and file nails
      f. Shave face
      g. Menstrual care
      h. Apply make-up, deodorant. etc.
      i. Shave legs and underarms

IV. Upper Extremities
    A. Bilateral discrepancy in strength or ROM
    B. Dominance
      1. Preferred
      2. Established
    C. Use of pencil or crayon
    D. Sensation
    E. Stereognosis
    F. Grasp-release pattern
    G. Fine finger dexterity
    H. If chair-fast, can patient propel self, transfer independently

V. Socialization
    A. Does patient get along well with others
      1. At home
      2. At school (work)
      3. In the neighborhood
    B. If a child, does he play
      1. Constructively with toys
      2. By himself
      3. With siblings
      4. With normal peers
    C. If an adolescent or adult, does patient have opportunity for socialization
      1. In the home
      2. Outside the home

VI. Academic
    A. School
      1. Name of school
      2. Grade level
      3. Kind of school (for mentally retarded, etc.)
      4. Does patient perform at grade level in
        a. Reading
        b. Spelling
        c. Writing
        d. Mathematics
      5. If in high school, has patient seen vocational counselor
    B. Pre-School
      1. Concept of color
      2. Concept of size
      3. Concept of shape
      4. Ability to match and discriminate
      5. Number concepts
      6. Form imitation (Gesell)
      7. Form copy (Gesell)
      8. Draw a man (Gesell)
      9. Is perceptual testing indicated

VII. Equipment
    A. Transportation
      1. Stroller
      2. Wheelchair
      3. Car seat
    B. ADL
      1. Feeding aids
      2. Bathing aids
        a. Lift
        b. Tub seat
      3. Toileting aids
        a. Commode chair
      4. Dressing aids
        a. Adapted clothing
        b. Floor seat

VIII. Future Plans
    A. Live and work independently
    B. Self care (supervised)
    C. Cared for at home
    D. Residential placement

for comfort and function must be considered. The sitting position is most important since eating, eliminating, and most school work and employment tasks are accomplished from the seated position.

The average person sits at a standard height table top 30 in. from the floor, resting his elbows on the table, his feet flat on the floor, his trunk leaning forward over the table. His head is centered over his trunk, and his thighs are slightly abducted. If a patient cannot achieve or maintain this "position of function," he must then be helped to do so by adapting the equipment in which he is sitting. This may be accomplished by a simple adjustment such as a foot rest, a seat belt or by raising or lowering a table. For a patient who is wheelchair-fast yet unable to sit in the "position of function," adaptations are necessary. Correct positioning is even more critical. It should precede any activity session and be a part of any treatment program.

The position of the patient often determines not only his own attitude, but also the kind of care and attention he will receive from others. The bedfast cerebral palsied patient receives limited stimulation from his surroundings and often looks hopeless to those who care for him. By placing him in a "position of function," he himself may be able to accomplish some things by himself, and activities can much more easily be done for and with him. It is often necessary to build or modify each individual's chair to meet his needs.[2]

The procedure for positioning a moderately to severely handicapped cerebral palsied patient in a wheelchair is as follows:

1. Evaluate the patient. Head balance, trunk balance, abnormal reflex patterns causing extensor thrust or postural deformities, scoliosis, dislocated hips, adduction deformities, involuntary movement.

2. Measure the patient. Seat the child on a firm surface, a flat board placed under the buttocks will do or a chair with a flat hard seat. Hold the child upright so that accurate measurements can be taken. (The measurements as described by the Everest & Jennings Company are helpful).

Seat width. When seated on a flat firm surface, the thighs automatically abduct; measure from the outside of the knees; check and see if the buttocks are wider than the knee spread. If the person lacks lateral balance, then chair sides (close to the hips) attached to the seat will help him to stabilize himself or to be stabilized in the middle of the chair (See Fig. 12–3).

Seat depth: Measure femoral length by placing the measuring tape at the curve of the buttocks and taking the measurement at the flexed knee. If a dislocated hip makes one leg shorter than the other, use the shorter dimension. To avoid pressure on the hamstring tendons, subtract 1 in. from this dimension (or two fingers behind the knee). Because of adductor spasm, it has been found helpful to raise the seat

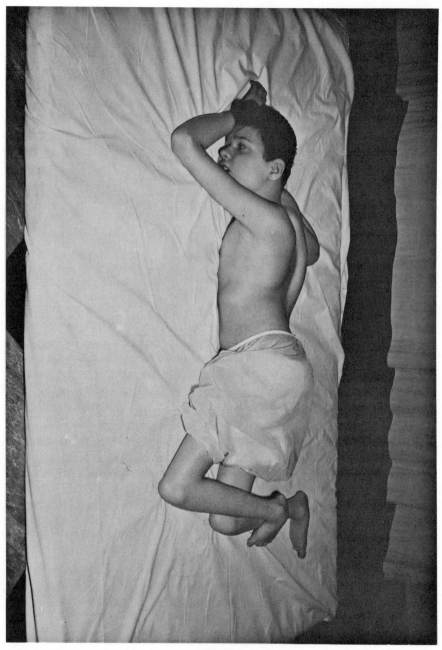

Fig. 12–1.

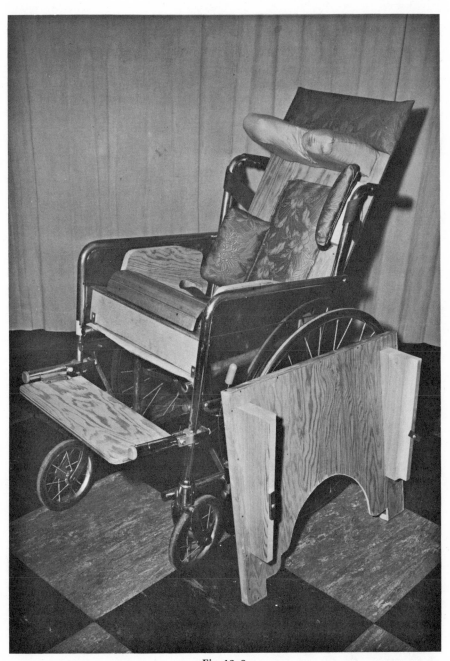

Fig. 12–2.

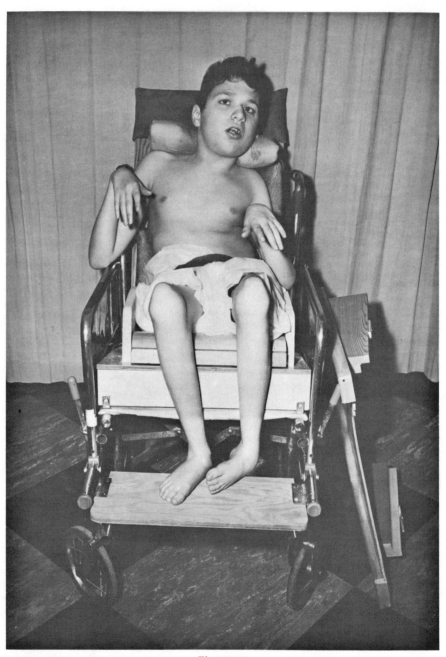

Fig. 12–3.

under the knees, increasing the angle of hip-flexion approximating 7°
to 10°. This flexion can be achieved in either of two ways:

1. Adding a plastic sponge wedge cushion of 1½ in. at the front
   graduated to ½ in. at the rear.
2. Preferred at the Cerebral Palsy Clinic, Indiana University Medical
   Center, is the rolled wooden seat (Fig. 12–2) inducing hip flexion.
   The latter is preferred because it conforms more naturally to the
   curve of the thigh. The uncovered wood is cooler, the wooden
   slats allow air to circulate and prevent skin breakdown, and the
   four coats of varnish on the wood prevent it from absorbing the
   odors that stay with plastics or upholstered materials. When one
   or both hips are dislocated or subluxed, it is sometimes necessary
   to use the sponge wedge because the leg lengths are unequal. For
   the patient with severe adductor tightness, thigh cuffs are sometimes used (Fig. 12–6).

Seat back height: Measure from the flat surface of the seat to the
scapulae of the seated patient. If a head support is needed, continue
measuring to the top of the head. The back is fixed at 90° to the seat unless the person needs to be forward flexed (cases of extensor thrust). A
less than 90° seated position can be achieved by reducing the right angle of seat and back: 5° forward and 5° by raising the front of the seat ½
to 1 in. or more if necessary. For the patient who must be reclined,
maintain the 90° or less angle by raising the seat as the back is reclined (See Fig. 12–2).

Foot-rest height: The foot-rest depth must equal the whole shoe,
heel to toe, in order to give firm support to the foot. For the patient
with extensor thrust, a single foot-rest for both feet is preferred to
the flip-up pedals because the pedals are more apt to slip when unequal pressure is applied by abnormal postural thrusting (See Fig. 12–3).
The height is taken from the sole of the shoe to the flexed knee to assure
that the femurs rest comfortably on the seat and that the legs are not
hanging down unsupported. This prevents decrease in circulation,
edema and nerve pressure. It may be necessary to use ankle straps, heel
back boards, or slight flexion of the toes (5° to 10°) to prevent extensor
thrusting and to inhibit clonus (See Figs. 12–6,7).

Lap-board (wheelchair tray): To stabilize and encourage vertical
trunk balance, each chair-fast person must have a lap-board. The fore-
arms should rest comfortably at the normal elbow flexion position with
the humerus perpendicular to the floor and close to the trunk. If the
person can wheel his own chair, the lap-board should be inside the
chair arm to encourage the mobility of the patient (See Fig. 12–7). A
large second table top can be added for a work surface if necessary. If
the person will be cared for by someone else and self-propulsion is im-

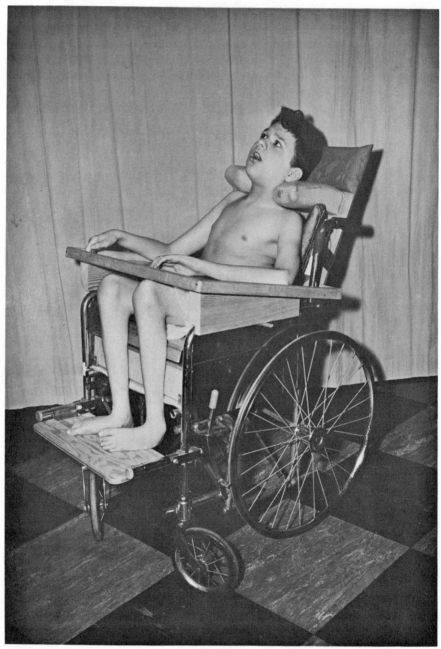

Fig. 12–4.

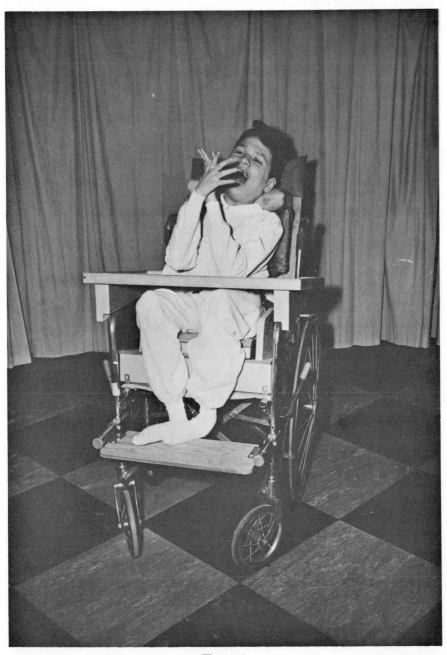

Fig. 12–5.

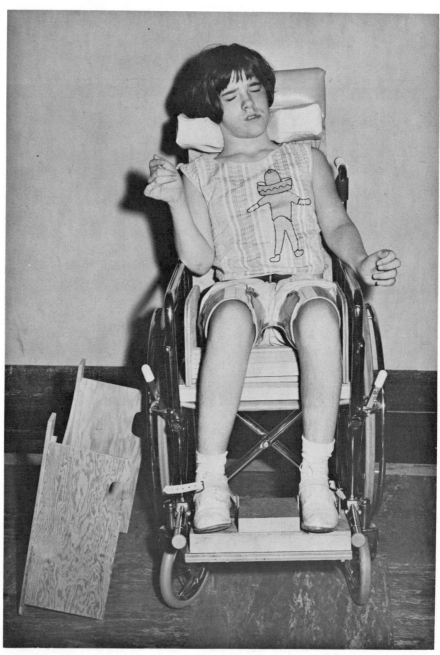

Fig. 12–6.

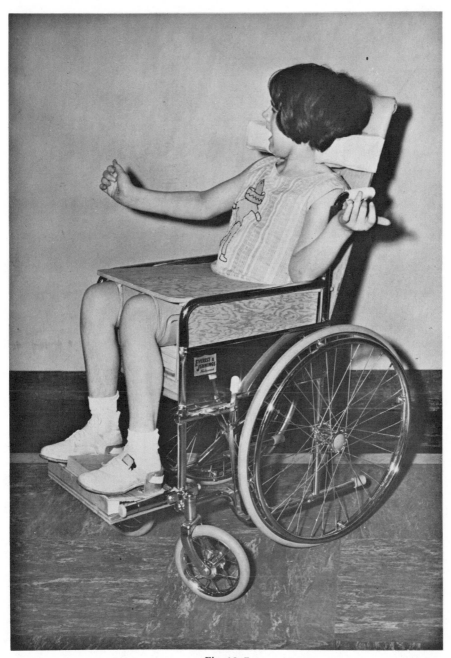

Fig. 12–7.

possible, a larger than arm-frame lap-board may be considered to encourage forearm support and upper extremity use (e.g., assistive self-feeding, or playing with toys (See Figs. 12–4,5). The waist cut-out of the lap-board is measured to allow the therapist's fingers to fit easily between the lap-board and the patient. This will allow for additional cold weather clothing. Measure the waist from left to right for width; then place the measuring tape at the back of the chair and come forward to the waist belt line. This will give the lap-board cut-out depth.

If scoliosis or rib-cage deformities interfere, allow for these. Only rarely is padding of the lap-board cut-out necessary. The use of the lap-board will encourage voluntary trunk balance if this is possible. The fit of the tray does not permit the patient to get his arm caught between the tray and his waist. The tray fits like a loose belt.

Seat-belts: These are used in all chairs and are placed just like those in an airplane or automobile so that the pull is across the hips over the thighs and to the rear of the buttocks with no pressure over the groin, stomach, or genital area. Seat belts of cotton twill do not cut into the skin as much as nylon seat belts. Two inch cotton twill trunk straps are fine for junior or adult sized chairs; 1½ inch straps work well for a Tiny Tot wheelchair. The chest is never restricted by strapping, as this can impede breathing. If additional upper trunk support is needed, a vest is used or the chair back is reclined.

Head-neck supports: These are made to fit between the ears and shoulders, touching the base of the occiput without irritating cervical nerves I, II, and III, which stimulate extension of the head and neck as well as the entire body (Figs. 12–4,6). These are used as training devices as well as head supports. Often the patient learns to support his own head as a result of being carefully positioned to inhibit abnormal reflexes over long periods of time.

3. Care of Equipment. Persons responsible for the care of equipment should keep it clean and dry. Frequent cleaning is necessary only if the patient is incontinent. A wheelchair, like an automobile, should be serviced regularly if it is in constant use. Servicing prolongs the life of any mechanical equipment.

4. Gains from Correct Positioning. Getting severely handicapped or bed-fast cerebral palsied patients up in wheelchairs extends their horizons because they are mobile. They are able to be moved outside and into groups for learning and socialization. Furthermore, the prolonged use of fitted equipment with improved and maintained posture inhibits abnormal reflexes (tonic neck reflexes, extensor thrust). Peer and group contacts often encourage the desire to do more for oneself, so that increased function is a frequent by-product of positioning. Other positive results include an increase in visual and auditory stimulation, a lengthening of the attention span, and better general health (e.g., less pneumonia and constipation).

Activity

Once the initial evaluation has been done and the patient has been properly positioned, activity can begin.

In all aspects of treatment of cerebral palsied patients, it is well to keep in mind their high rate of perceptual-motor dysfunction. Use of a multisensory approach is recommended, thus stressing the gradation of tasks from internal (centered on patient himself) to external (centered on patient's relation to his environment), from gross to fine activities, and variation in activity, so as to avoid the development of splinter skills (specific skills learned in the absence of the general concept). See Chapter 14 by Gilfoyle and Grady.

As in the treatment of any other patient, it is important to remember to treat the "whole person." It is easy, but disastrous, to concentrate on the patient's upper extremities and to forget his emotional and psychological needs, his place in his family, his school, and his community.

The treatment program depends on the age, potential, and problems of the particular patient for whom it is planned, but certain activities are commensurate with the various stages of development.

For the infant, feeding may be the area of primary concern, and careful positioning coupled with facilitation technics for mouth closure and swallowing may be in order. Stimulation toward response to people and toys, visual tracking, the use of hands, head control, and movement of all body parts are other important treatment considerations for infants.

Gross motor activities, verbalization, increased use and control of the upper extremities, and finger feeding are areas of consideration in working with the cerebral palsied toddler. By this stage, seating equipment is in order if the child is not able to sit alone. Hand splinting may be recommended by the physician at any stage of the patient's development.

At pre-school age, more complex ADL skills take priority. If it is within the child's ability, stress is placed on independence in eating (adapted feeding equipment is sometimes necessary), toilet training, and at least basic dressing skills, with undressing always preceding dressing. Upper extremity strength, range of motion and coordination must be maintained and increased, and the child's interest in pre-school activities (coloring, painting, pasting, drawing, cutting, and matching and differentiating objects) can be capitalized on to achieve these goals. It is not too early to begin work habit training at this stage, looking forward to eventual vocational goals. The importance of attending to directions, taking turns, sharing, cleaning up, finishing

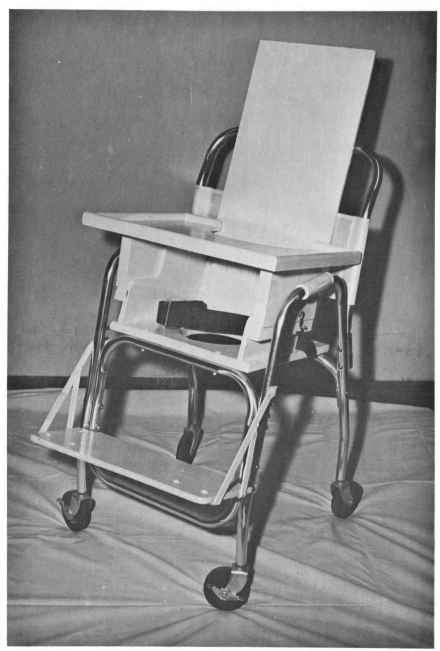

Fig. 12–8.

tasks, putting things away, and using good manners, should be inculcated into all aspects of treatment.

During the school-age years, independence in dressing, toileting and bathing should be emphasized. Adapted equipment may be necessary and clothing may need to be altered. Care of the hair and nails should not be overlooked. Girls must learn to handle their own menstrual care, and boys must master shaving.

Special writing and typing patterns and devices may be needed during this time. Household responsibility is essential to the latency-aged child's feeling of importance and should be part of any home program for this age group.

For the pre-adolescent and adolescent, prevocational exploration and vocational evaluation and training become critical areas of concern. In addition, recreation and activities outside the home are extremely important.

The adult cerebral palsied patient who is not able to work will need recreational programs and peer contacts as well as maintenance of mobility and equipment.

For the patient, severely involved both mentally and physically, for whom total care will always be necessary, it is important that the occupational therapist make that care as easy as possible. Priority treatment goals for these patients are feeding and toilet training as well as increased use of the upper extremities. Adapted equipment for wheelchairs, lifts, commode chairs (Fig. 12–8), bathtub seats, car seats, and other special devices are often needed.

Operant conditioning technics have been used successfully with trainable and profoundly retarded patients to modify their behavior and make them easier to care for.

The severely physically disabled patient with normal or near normal intelligence is often seriously frustrated by his lack of ability to do things. This type of patient is a challenge to the creativity of the occupational therapist in terms of activity planning. Special considerations include mouth-stick typing (Fig. 12–10), painting, and the use of a word or spelling board if speech is not understandable.

Group treatment has been tried with all age levels of cerebral palsied patients. It has been as effective or more effective in nearly all cases than individual treatment, primarily from a motivational viewpoint (Figs. 12–12,13). Many patients will try harder and persevere longer if they see that others are working hard too.

In many centers, therapy is referred to as "work," and the children come to "work" in occupational therapy. The rationale behind this is that many of the activities required of the children are not necessarily fun, although every effort is made to prevent their being unpleasant

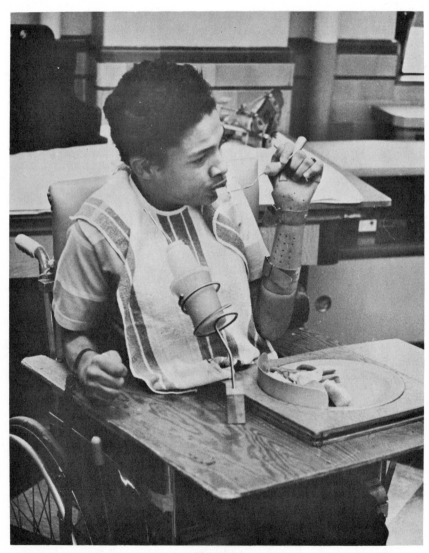

Fig. 12–9.

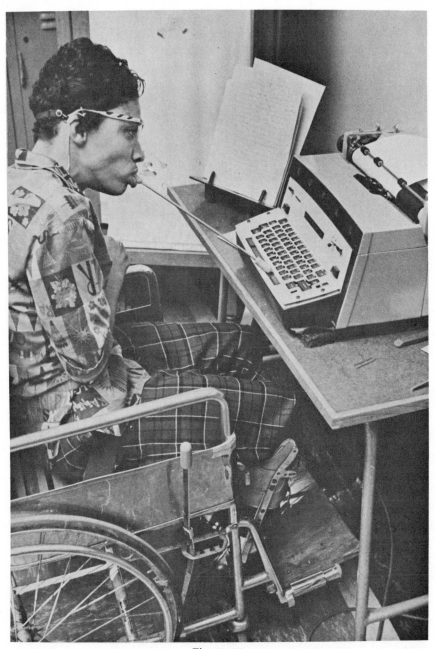

Fig. 12–10.

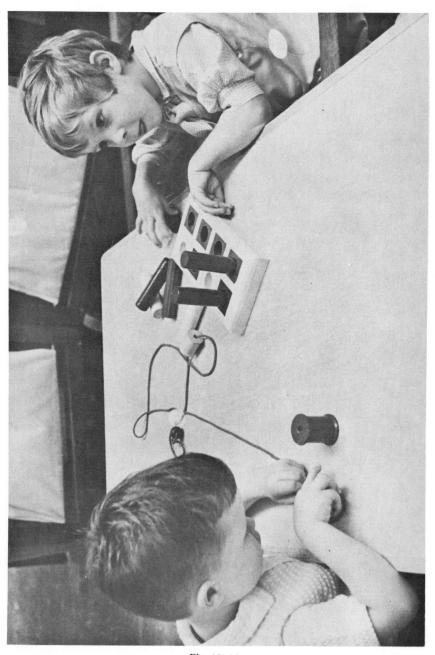

Fig. 12–11.

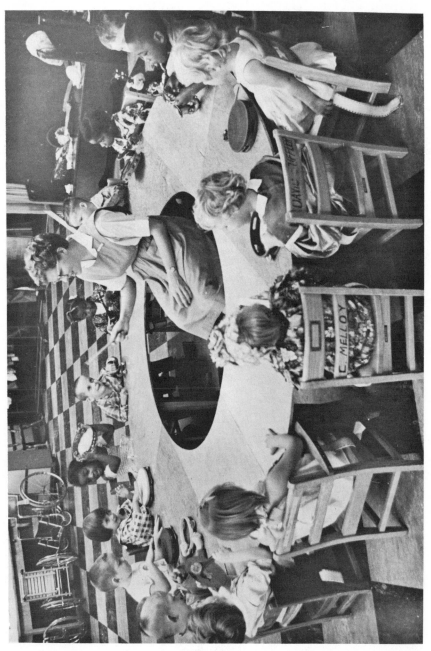

Fig. 12–12.

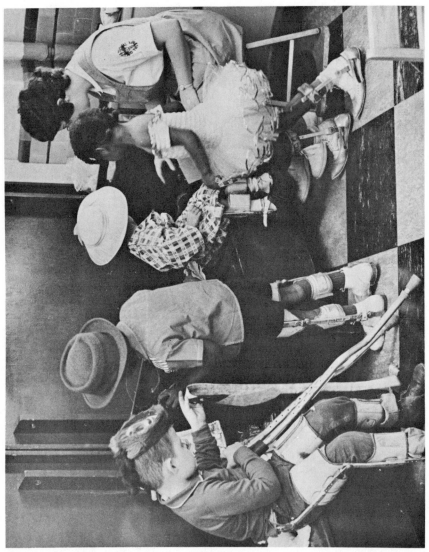

Fig. 12–13.

(Fig. 12–11). Therefore, just as father and mother do "work" that is not fun, so does the child.

As with all other children, it is important that success be rewarded with praise. However, praising a child for success, when he has actually failed, fools no one, least of all the child. With cerebral palsied patients (children or adults) it is often necessary to break goals down so that success can be realistically achieved.

Perhaps one of the most important decisions an occupational therapist has to make besides determining if a patient needs treatment, is deciding when treatment should be terminated. Only by keeping a careful record of progress will this be feasible. When a patient no longer needs or no longer benefits from treatment, it should be stopped. This is not to say that it should not be begun again if conditions warrant.

TEAM APPROACH

Cerebral palsy is one of the conditions which most clearly points out the need for a team approach to treatment. It is essential that occupational therapists work with parents, physicians, other allied health personnel, and volunteers to best meet the needs of the patients.

Parents

The parents or persons responsible for the care of the cerebral palsied patient, as well as the patient himself, when possible, must participate in planning and carrying out the treatment program. They must understand both the rationale behind what they are asked to do and the anticipated results.

It is extremely important to be realistic with parents in relation to their child's potential for improvement. Treatment goals must be kept small and should be possible to achieve within a reasonable period of time. Expecting too much or too little of the patient can have equally disastrous results in terms of frustration and discouragement for the patient, the parents, and the therapist.

Many parents fear that if the patient does not improve, the medical personnel working with him will give up, leaving them with nowhere to turn for support and help. On the one hand, it is wrong to continue to treat a patient intensively when he is no longer able to benefit from treatment; on the other hand, it is equally wrong to completely withdraw support from the parent or person responsible for the patient, leaving them to attempt home treatment and care programs without guidance.

Some centers have solved this problem by having patients seen routinely by the treatment team once a month, or once every two or three months. On this basis, both progress and problems can be noted and the home treatment program can be reviewed and renewed. As the patient reaches stages where more intensive therapy is indicated, he is seen several times a week for a period of weeks or months to work on such areas as feeding training, dressing skills, mouthstick typing, or perceptual-motor training. Parents are given the added option of calling in for appointments when they feel the need.

Patients who are placed in residential institutions should be seen periodically by the "treatment team," even if they are in a situation where therapy is available. Close communication between the team and the residential staff will help to maintain the patient's level of function and prevent regression. The patient's adapted wheelchair equipment will have to be checked periodically and adjusted for growth.

Physicians

The occupational therapist is responsible for maintaining communication regarding the patient's progress with his physician. This can be either a family doctor or a specialist.

Allied Health Personnel

Considering the complexities of cerebral palsy, it is not difficult to realize that concomitant problems are frequent. Parental guilt and overprotection, sibling rivalry and jealousy, financial problems, anxiety over the care of the patient, educational placement—all of these difficulties and many more require the skills of many disciplines of allied health personnel.

The occupational therapist must work effectively and efficiently with the physical therapist, the speech therapist, the social worker, the nurse (Public Health Nurse, Visiting Nurse Association), the special education teacher, psychologist, psychometrist, orthotist, and dietician to insure the best in medical care for the patient.

Volunteers

When properly trained, volunteers can be of great assistance to the occupational therapist in treating cerebral palsied patients by assisting with and carrying out routine or repetitious aspects of therapy. They can be extremely helpful to parents as baby-sitters or workers in day care centers. Volunteers at home can prepare materials to be used in the therapy program or by individual patients (i.e., papers and toys for perceptual training, adapted clothing or equipment for individuals or departments).

CASE I (see Fig. 12–13, Boy with fur hat at age 7 years.)

Name:	LT (male)
Diagnosis:	Spastic Quadriplegia (moderately involved)
Age:	12 years
Accompanying Disorders:	Perceptual dysfunction

Patient was born 2 months prematurely, had difficulty breathing at birth, was hospitalized for 1 month and had problems with feeding. He was diagnosed at age 2½ years when his family realized that he was not going to outgrow his slowness. He was referred to occupational therapy where a program of neuromuscular facilitation was used for 4 years. He learned to feed himself, worked on dressing skills and showed an increase in attention span. Pelvic band long-leg control braces and crutches were used for one year. After he learned to walk, the bracing was gradually discontinued. Psychological testing indicated normal intelligence. At age 7, he was accepted in a public school for the physically handicapped. The occupational therapist continued to work on dressing, teaching him to recognize clues in clothing for right and left, back and front. Writing skills and fine coordination were stressed. Now, at age 12 years, LT is being referred to a regular public school and will enter at seventh grade. He is ADL independent, using no special devices or walking aids.

CASE II (see Figs. 12–1 through 5)

Name:	PW (male)
Diagnosis:	Mixed Quadriplegia (athetoid and spastic) (severely involved)
Age:	20 years
Accompanying Disorders:	Blindness, seizures, microcephaly, profound mental retardation

Condition was the result of a full-term, extremely difficult forceps delivery. Patient had blade marks on his face and head. He had his first convulsion at age 1 month and was hospitalized in opisthotonic posture and with breathing difficulties. He was referred to occupational therapy at age 10 for aid in care. He was bedfast and had fixed contractures of all extremities. A wheelchair was constructed to position him to improve circulation, elimination and respiration. Mrs. W., his mother, found that feeding him was much easier in the wheelchair and that, with his head supported there was less spillage. Her washing of bedding and clothing was reduced considerably. Mrs. W. was instructed in the use of a lift for transfer from bed to wheelchair and from wheelchair to bathtub, etc.

At age 20, PW is still cared for at home by his mother. With the adapted wheelchair and the lift, she can manage him without undue fatigue. He eats all meals in his wheelchair, weighs 120 pounds and is in good health; his seizures are controlled with medication. In the summer, Mrs. W. enjoys taking PW outside on the porch and neighbors come over to visit with her.

CASE III

Name:	MS (male)
Diagnosis:	Spastic Quadriplegia (moderate – severely involved)
Age:	26 years
Accompanying Disorders:	Visual problems, perceptual dysfunction, moderate mental retardation (educable)

Patient was born at 7 months gestation weighing 4 pounds, had diarrhea at 2 weeks of age and returned to the hospital, remaining there for 6 weeks. He sat poorly, stood at 18 months. Occupational therapy was initiated at 3½ years for self-help skills. Hand use was adequate except for fine movements (e.g., coloring and bead stringing). He always moved very slowly (as in a slow motion film). Five different surgical procedures were completed on his lower extremities during a period of 8 years. Psychological testing showed perceptual deficits primarily in eye-hand coordination and spatial relations. Activities were devised by the occupational therapist and school teacher to be carried out at home. MS has problems with visual acuity which glasses relieve to some extent. He completed high school at 18 years of age. Today at age 26, MS is independent in ADL but very slow (1 hour to dress). He walks laboriously with short leg braces and axillary crutches. His writing is legible but slow and tedious. He works at home, making rubber stamps with a punch machine; he does not make enough money to pay taxes. His physical ability seems to be diminishing with age and years of sitting. He is not motivated to do the prescribed exercises, so it is anticipated that he will become wheelchair-fast within the next ten years.

CASE IV

Name: PG (female)

Diagnosis: Athetoid Quadriplegia
          (moderately involved)

Age: 15 years

Accompanying Disorders: Dull normal intelligence;
          speech disorder

Patient was the product of a full term difficult delivery. After 12 hours of labor the patient was born with the cord wrapped around her neck. She had severe respiratory distress and a subdural hematoma.

PG was referred for therapy at age 2. Since she is from a rural area, she has been hospitalized on six occasions for intensive training. Over the years, she has gained in head, trunk, and extremity control. She feeds herself with adapted feeding equipment and drinks through a straw. She is able to dress herself except for fastenings and transfer in and out of her wheelchair with the use of rails at the toilet. She can bathe herself with some assistance and care for a very simple attractive hair style. She manages her menstrual needs with sanitary pants.

With an adapted device in her hand and a key guard, she does her homework on an electric typewriter. PG has a tutor, since there are no schools for the handicapped in her area. She is at her grade level and expects to finish high school.

She moves about the house well in her wheelchair, and helps her mother with cleaning and cooking chores. Her speech is difficult but understandable, even to strangers.

PG has a pleasant, outgoing personality and is corresponding with several other teenage shut-ins in the state.

This patient is scheduled for re-admission for therapy in the summer. Occupational therapy goals include total independence in bathing and dressing. Physical therapy will begin ambulation with a walker, and vocational evaluation and counseling will be started.

CASE V (Figs. 12–9,10)

Name: VC (female)

Diagnosis: Tension Athetoid Quadriplegia
          (severely involved)

Age: 43 years

Accompanying Disorders: Moderate mental retardation
          (educable); unintelligible speech

This patient was referred for therapy at age 34 years. She was untreated prior to that time.

Her birth history was normal except for difficulty in breathing. Parents were told that the child was "hopeless" when she was 6 years old. She has had no education. At referral, her condition was one of knee flexion contractures of 75°, she was unable to sit upright, her arms were held in elbow and wrist flexion, symmetrical and asymmetrical tonic neck reflexes were dominant. She had unintelligible speech, blinking eyes for "yes" and frowning for "no" responses. Occupational therapy adapted a wheelchair and used a hand splint in conjunction with her tonic neck reflexes to initiate self feeding. The opposite wrist was restrained in neutral position. Facilitation of mouth and lips for better closure and speech were used. The patient was seen in occupational therapy twice weekly and the family was instructed in a home program. Within 3 months, the patient could feed herself independently with adapted equipment. Another patient tutored VC so that by the end of 1 year she could read and eventually progressed to the third grade level. The occupational therapist worked with a dentist to introduce mouth-stick typing, so that the patient could type letters and address mailing labels for family members. Various medications were tried with some success to relieve tension. This is maintained today. At age 43 years, VC resides in a county home for the aged. Her typing is a useful pastime and keeps her in touch with family members. Her ability to self-feed relieves the nursing personnel in her 6 bed ward. Her adapted wheelchair enables her to be out of bed the entire day (Figs. 12–9,10).

CASE VI

Name: BL (male)

Diagnosis: Spastic Right Hemiplegia
                    (mildly involved)

Age: 5 years

Condition was the result of an uneventful pregnancy and normal delivery. Nothing unusual was noticed until about age 6 to 9 months when he did not use his right hand to reach out or play with toys. He was referred for treatment at age 1 year, at which time he cruised around furniture, holding onto objects with his left hand for support. His right hand was kept fisted. He walked on his right toes with a circumducted gait.

Neuromuscular facilitation was used for the right arm and leg. Normal and bilateral activities were encouraged. BL was seen weekly, then bi-monthly until he was three years old. Progress was good. He began to use his right hand as a helper. Biweekly therapy in a nursery-school age group began. General but steady improvement was recorded at a normal rate for his age. At age 3½ he was independent in ADL except for over the head clothing and buttoning. At age 4, a hand splint was devised to prevent thumb subluxation. This was discontinued at age 5. He can now actively supinate his forearm, extend his wrist and abduct his thumb. A hand night splint will be used for maintenance purposes. He uses his right hand well as an assist. BL will enroll in public school kindergarten in September of this year.

REFERENCES

1. Barsch, R. H.: The Parent of the Handicapped Child. Springfield, Illinois, Charles C Thomas, 1968.
2. Bensberg, G. J. (ed): Teaching the Mentally Retarded. pp. 51–97. Atlanta, Georgia, Southern Regional Education Board. 1965.
3. Courville, C. B.: Cerebral Palsy. Los Angeles, San Lucas Press, 1954.
4. Denhoff, E.: Cerebral Palsy – The Preschool Years. Springfield, Illinois, Charles C. Thomas, 1968.
5. Denhoff, E. and I. Robinault: Cerebral Palsy and Related Disorders, A Developmental Approach to Dysfunction. New York, McGraw-Hill, 1960.
6. Ibid. pp. 10, 11.
7. Finnie, N. R.: Handling the Young Cerebral Palsied Child at Home. New York, Dutton & Co., 1970.
8. Gesell, A. and C. S. Amatruda: Developmental Diagnosis, Normal and Abnormal Child Development. New York, Paul B. Hoeber, 1941.
9. Gesell, A., et al.: The First Five Years of Life. New York, Harper & Row, 1940.
10. Gutman, E.: Wheelchair to Independence; Architectural Barriers Eliminated. Springfield, Illinois, Charles C Thomas, 1968.
11. Hatton, D. A.: Understanding Cerebral Palsy for the Parents of the Cerebral Palsied Child. Erie, Pa., Erie County Crippled Children's Society, 1969.
12. Holt, K. S.: Assessment of Cerebral Palsy. London, Lloyd-Luke (Medical Books) Ltd., 1965.
13. Ingram, T. T. S.: Pediatric Aspects of Cerebral Palsy. Edinburgh and London, E. & S. Livington Ltd., 1964.
14. Ibid. pp. 3, 7–12.
15. Kamenetz, H.: Wheelchair Book-Mobility for the Disabled. Springfield, Illinois, Charles C Thomas, 1969.
16. Little, W. J.: On the Influence of Abnormal Parturition, Difficult Labours, Premature Birth, and Asphyxia Neonatorum on the Mental and Physical Condition of the Child, Especially in Relation to Deformities (Trans. Obster. Soc. London). 1861. London, Longmans, Green, Longmans and Roberts, 1862.
17. Lowman, E. W., and Klinger, J. L.: Aids to Independent Living. McGraw-Hill, 1969.

18. Minear, W. L.: A classification of cerebral palsy. Pediatrics, 18:841–852, 1956.
19. Perlstein, M. A.: Infantile cerebral palsy, classification and clinical correlations. J.A.M.A., 149:30–34, 1952.
20. Phelps, W. M.: Cerebral Palsy, in Allen O. Whipple (ed.): Nelson New Loose-Leaf Surgery, pp. 180–0–180–S. New York, Thomas Nelson & Sons, 1947.
21. Robinson, H. B., and Robinson, N. M.: The Mentally Retarded Child; A Psychological Approach. p. 463. New York, McGraw-Hill, 1965.

For Bibliography or additional information write:
United Cerebral Palsy Association, Inc.
66 East 34th Street
New York, New York 10016
   or
National Society for Crippled Children and Adults
2023 W. Ogden Avenue
Chicago, Illinois

13

Sensorimotor Treatment Approaches

A. JOY HUSS, M.S., O.T.R., R.P.T.

INTRODUCTION

This chapter will attempt to provide the reader with an historical overview of the various sensorimotor treatment approaches, their current status, a simplified approach to the neurophysiological rationale, a brief statement regarding the application of these principles to occupational therapy and an extensive bibliography for greater depth by those interested. It is not intended to be an exposition in depth for those already thoroughly familiar with one or more of these approaches, but rather to open the door for the beginner or the uninitiated, to intrigue and perhaps to challenge. They are not hailed as a cure-all that will help everyone, but do provide the occupational therapist with one more tool which when used appropriately may assist in hastening the patient's rehabilitation.

OVERVIEW

Fay—Doman—Delacato

Neuromuscular Reflex Therapy

Temple Fay, M.D., neurosurgeon, was the forerunner of these approaches beginning in the early 1940's. For nearly two decades he observed, discussed, demonstrated and wrote about "neuromuscular reflex therapy" which he defined as the "utilization of reflex levels of response to the highest level possible."[3] Much of his work was done prior to the present knowledge and understanding regarding the central nervous system and was based on the work of Sherrington. His basic premise was that ontogeny recapitulates phylogeny. Therefore an individual's neurological development parallels the evolution from fish to amphibian, to reptile, to anthropoid. Since human movement is based on patterns of muscle activity, not on individual muscle response, he believed that if reflex patterns were elicited and utilized properly functional movement could be established.

As a result, his treatment program involved the following six concepts:

1. After careful observation of the patient's level of functioning, including existing reflexes and automatic responses, treatment began with simple patterns of movement utilizing these reflexes.
2. Since in normal development each stage lays the foundation for the next stage so in treatment it is essential that lower levels of mobility be developed before expecting higher levels.
3. Reflexes in and of themselves are not abnormal, but may indicate pathology if they interfere with refined coordinated movement. Therefore reflexes can be utilized to develop muscle tone, inhibit antagonists and lead to higher levels of coordinate movement.
4. Passive exercise patterns which involve the total extremity, not isolated joints, can enhance the sensory feedback mechanisms important for movement.
5. Patterns done repeatedly actively or passively will in time lead to the spontaneous development of higher level patterns.
6. The patterns utilized are prone patterns of forward propulsion that can be observed in normal human infants as well as in amphibian and reptilian life forms.[3]

The three basic patterns used are homologous (bunny hop), homolateral (camel walk) and crossed-diagonal (reciprocal).

Homologous is a bilateral-symmetrical pattern. With the head in midline with some flexion and extension of the neck, the upper extremities are flexed at the shoulder while the lower extremities are extended at the hip. The extremities are then reversed rhythmically. In prone this is not too effective for propulsion, but in the all-fours position it is commonly called the bunny hop.

Homolateral is an ipsilateral pattern with the head, thorax and pelvis turned toward the flexing upper and lower extremities with extension of the contralateral extremities. The pattern is then reversed leading with the head. In the all-fours this provides a gait similar to that of a camel.

Crossed-diagonal is a more highly integrated pattern with flexion of the upper extremities and extension of the lower extremities on the face side with extension of the upper limbs with flexion of the lower limbs on the opposite side. In the all-fours this provides the typical reciprocal gait pattern seen in higher mammals and human infants.

Following the prone position are the all-fours (hands and knees), planti-grade (hands and feet) and the erect postures. All three patterns are utilized in the first three positions. Homolateral and crossed-diagonal are utilized in the erect position. Depending on the level of development, patterns are done passively, active-assistively, or actively. The key elements in determining the program planned for a patient are intellectual and functional motor development levels. Chronological age is less important.

Dr. Fay's work has provided the basic foundation for the approach now advocated by Carl Delacato, Ed.D., Robert Doman, M.D., and Glenn Doman, physical therapist. The same patterns of movement are utilized. In addition the program includes selective use of sensory stimulation such as heat, cold, brushing and pinching, procedures to establish hand dominance and a breathing exercise routine to increase the vital capacity.

The program for any given patient is administered at least 4 times per day, for 5 minutes, 7 days a week. Each treatment requires at least three adults because each extremity must be manipulated smoothly and rhythmically in the proper pattern.

Kabat—Knott—Voss

Proprioceptive Neuromuscular Facilitation

Around 1946, Herman Kabat, M.D., physiatrist and neurophysiologist, began the development of a therapy system based on neurophysiological principles outlined by Sherrington, Coghill, McGraw, Gesell, Hellebrandt and Pavlov. The major emphasis is stimulation of the proprioceptors with active participation by the patient. These principles were expanded and utilized in treatment by Margaret Knott and Dorothy Voss, both physical therapists. "Proprioceptive neuromuscular facilitation enlists the less involved parts, to promote a balanced antagonism of reflex activity, of muscle groups and of components of motion."[76]*

As stated by Knott and Voss in the second edition of *Proprioceptive Neuromuscular Facilitation* the philosophy of treatment is

> . . . based upon the ideas that all human beings respond in accordance with demand; that existing potentials may be developed more fully; that movements must be specific and directed toward a goal; that activity is necessary to the best development of coordination, strength, and endurance; and that the stronger body parts strengthening weaker parts through cooperation lead toward a goal of optimum function.[76]**

*p. xiv.
**p. 3.

The technic is therefore defined as "methods of promoting or hastening the response of the neuromuscular mechanism through stimulation of the proprioceptors."[76]*

There has been a gradual evolution of the present day technic since the 1940's. Initially greatest emphasis was placed on the use of maximal resistance throughout the range of motion. Patterns of movement were utilized which allowed action at two or more joints and required two component actions of a given muscle. Other factors considered important were *stretch* for proprioceptive stimulation, *positioning* to enhance contraction, *motion* beginning in the strongest part of the range progressing to the weaker part, incorporation of *reflexes* and reinforcement through *resistance.*

In 1949, based on Sherrington's law of successive induction, *rhythmic stabilization* and *slow reversal* procedures were added to enhance facilitation of the weaker muscles. In 1951, the patterns of movement were analyzed more thoroughly. In order to apply stretch to maximally elongated muscles it was found that patterns that were spiral and diagonal were most effective and that they also corresponded more nearly to normal, functional patterns of movement.

Since that time the above principles have been incorporated into mat, gait and self-care activities to assist in motor learning and the development of strength and balance.

Current technics being used are: maximal, but not overpowering resistance; quick stretch; postural and righting reflexes; mass movement patterns with spiral and diagonal components; reversal of antagonists—rhythmic stabilization and slow reversal; ice is used generally for inhibition and occasionally for facilitation.

The patient is evaluated developmentally and treatment begun appropriately. In all cases, beginning treatment utilizes the strongest groups of muscles and the most coordinated movements the patient has for reciprocal innervation, irradiation and summation. Movement patterns are reinforced through simple verbal commands which utilize the patient's voluntary control.

Bobath

A Neurodevelopmental Approach

The Bobath approach has been developed in England by Karl Bobath, M.D., neuropsychiatrist, and Mrs. Berta Bobath, F.C.S.P., physical therapist. Work was begun in the 1940's with cerebral palsy patients and also with adult acquired hemiplegic patients. The treatment, however, is suitable for other disorders of central nervous system function.

*p. 4.

Principles are based on the work of Magnus, Sherrington, deKleijn, Schaltenbrand and Walshe.

The basic principle upon which treatment is based is the inhibition of primitive, phasic and tonic reflex activity, followed by immediate facilitation of righting and equilibrium reactions in proper sequential development leading to skilled activities. The patient is so handled that the abnormal patterns are blocked and higher level reactions elicited. As this handling is repeated the patient's nervous system learns the feel of more normal tone and movement patterns and more normal spontaneous movement begins to take place. *Reflex inhibiting patterns are not static nor are the muscles relaxed. The patterns of movement are changed so that postural set can be adjusted to fit the activity.*

> In changing the abnormal patterns, it is seldom desirable to fix the entire body of the patient in a new pattern, or to hold him securely, making movement either unavailable or unlikely. Only those parts of the body are held from which it has been found possible to control the state of tone in other parts, and only sufficient control is used to prevent return to abnormal patterns and to stimulate or facilitate the desired activity.[3]*

The key points which are most effective for this control are the proximal regions such as head, neck, shoulder girdle, trunk and pelvis. From these key points the therapist can facilitate righting and equilibrium reactions which bring one to the upright position, turn one around and maintain balance when the center of gravity is changed.

Evaluation of the patient is a systematic determination of the distribution of muscle tone, its interference with movement, and the effect which hypertonus in one area has on another area of the body. Thus, one is looking at postural set and the movement patterns which are superimposed. Those readers not familiar with the basic reflexology of development are referred to Bobath[18] and Fiorentino[41] for this information.

Bracing is incompatible with this approach because it shifts the hypertonus to other non-stabilized joints creating problems elsewhere. Also bracing does not allow the system to make the necessary postural adjustments.

In addition to the reflex inhibiting patterns and the stimulation of righting and equilibrium reactions a technic called *tapping* is employed. Tapping is used to increase or set postural tone and provides both exteroceptive and proprioceptive input. The most effective input appears to be that which stimulates joint receptors. The procedures are described by Semans.

*p. 739.

The purpose of tapping is to bring about an increase in postural tone sufficient to support functional movements as well as body posture *versus* gravity. There is danger, however, in overstimulating in these procedures, and there is a need for carefully grading the stimuli so that the nervous system can handle the input and effectively organize it.[3*]

As the tone shifts and more normal functional movement takes place activities appropriate to the level of development are initiated.

Brunnstrom

Around 1951, Miss Signe Brunnstrom, physical therapist, became concerned with the lack of rehabilitation of the upper extremity in acquired hemiplegia. She studied the research on reflex responses in decerebrate cats and hemiplegia in man. From the research efforts of Riddoch and Buzzard, Magnus and deKleijn and Simons she selected the effects of associated reactions initiated either by voluntary effort on the non-involved side or by reflex stimulation; *postural reactions* resulting from tonic neck and tonic labyrinthine reflexes; and the *flexion* and *extension synergies*. After careful observation of over one hundred hemiplegic patients she delineated the stages of recovery, and technics to facilitate the patient's progression from one stage to the next. Thus treatment consists of developing the potential for "co-ordinate movement with reflex-like mechanisms, sensory cues, volitional effort and gradation of demand through the stages of recovery."[3*]

The stages of recovery follow a definite sequence and the patient never skips a stage. However, he may plateau at any one of the six stages which are:

1. Immediately following the vascular insult there appears to be flaccidity with no voluntary movement in the affected extremities.
2. Spasticity begins to develop. The flexion and extension synergies can be stimulated reflexively. They first appear with co-contraction but gradually become more distinct with the flexion synergy dominating the upper extremity, and the extension synergy dominating the lower extremity.
3. Spasticity becomes quite severe. However, the synergies can now be voluntarily initiated with some range of motion. Any attempt to use the extremity voluntarily results in a synergy pattern.
4. Spasticity begins to decrease. Simple, uncoordinated movements which differ from the basic synergies can be performed slowly and deliberately. Also beginning to develop are reciprocal movements within the synergies.

*p. 758.
*p. 794.

5. Spasticity continues to decrease to the point that the patient can perform some functional activities although still slowly and deliberately without eliciting synergies. Some independence of the synergy patterns is achieved, and isolated individual joint movement is possible.
6. Spasticity has almost disappeared. Individual joint motion is freer and has controlled speed and direction. With rapid, reciprocal movement some incoordination may still be present.

Because of the degree of cortical control necessary for hand control recovery of function in the hand is more difficult and less predictable. Mass grasp does precede mass extension and thumb motion precedes finger motion.

After evaluation of the patient's stage of recovery and sensory status, treatment aimed at reflex training follows.

1. Motion synergies are *elicited* on a reflex level. Reflexes used include:
   a. tonic neck reflex
   b. tonic labyrinthine reflex
   c. tonic lumbar reflex
   d. resistance to voluntary contraction of non-involved limb.

It is important to note that in the upper extremities resistance to flexion of the non-involved extremity facilitates flexion in the involved extremity and vice versa. In the lower extremities resistance to flexion in the non-involved extremity facilitates extension of the involved extremity and vice versa.

   e. Sensory stimulation includes quick stretch, passive movement, tapping over a muscle belly, surface stroking, positioning and pressure on muscle belly or tendon.
2. Motion synergies are *captured*, that is, an effort is made to establish voluntary control of the synergies. This is accomplished by utilization of the following stages:
   a. repetition using facilitation
   b. repetition without using facilitation
   c. working from proximal to distal, concentrating on various components of the synergy with and without the use of facilitation. Reciprocal motion between the two synergies is started with a goal of diminishing the time lag between contraction and relaxation of antagonistic muscles.
3. The motion synergies are next *conditioned* by combining elements of antagonistic synergies starting with the stronger components. At this point time is also spent on muscles which do not partici-

pate in the synergies such as the serratus anterior and the pero-
neals.[3] As progress occurs, more complex motions with rapid
reciprocation are initiated.
4. And finally the last and most difficult step, the *elicitation* of voluntary hand and finger function. Maneuvers such as "Souque's
phenomenon" and "imitation synkinesis" are helpful.[3*]

Postures and positions used during treatment include supine, sitting
and standing. Visual and verbal cues are used throughout. Volitional
effort and functional activities are initiated early and are considered
necessary if there is to be carryover by the patient.

Rood

A Neurophysiological Approach

Miss Margaret S. Rood, occupational therapist and physical therapist,
frustrated by the slow improvement of patients with cerebral palsy
began to delve into the neurophysiological and developmental literature in the late 1930's. Based on the works of Sherrington, Gesell,
Denny-Brown, Eldred, Hooker, Magoun, Cooper, Boyd, and others a
method of treatment has evolved since the 1940's.

The basic principles utilized are as follows:

1. Motor output is dependent upon sensory input. Thus sensory
stimuli are utilized to activate and/or inhibit motor responses.
2. Activation of motor responses follows a normal developmental
sequence. All muscles progress through the following stages of
development.
   a. Full range of shortening and lengthening with the antagonist.
   Phasic movement—reciprocal innervation.
   b. A pattern of co-contraction in which antagonistic muscles of
   one or more joints work together for a holding action. Stability-
   tonic postural set.
   c. A pattern of heavy work movement superimposed on the co-
   contraction. Movement in weight-bearing position.
   d. Skill or coordinate movement. Movement in nonweight-bear-
   ing position with stabilization at the proximal joints.
3. Since there is interaction within the nervous system between
somatic, psychic and autonomic functions stimuli can be used to
influence one or more directly or indirectly.[3]

This treatment approach can thus be defined as "The activation,
facilitation and inhibition of muscle action, voluntary and involuntary,
through the reflex arc."[102]

*p. 791, 794.

CHART 13-1
SKELETAL DEVELOPMENTAL SEQUENCES

(1) Reciprocal Innervation	(2) Co-innervation	(3) Heavy Work Movement	(4) Skill
1. Withdrawal— Total flexion in supine	4. Co-contraction of neck with vertebral extension		
2. Roll over; flexion top side, extension bottom side.	5. Prone on elbows static holding with co-contraction neck and shoulder	6. Push back 7. Pull forward	8. Belly crawling
3. Pivot prone— total extension except for elbows.	9. All fours— static holding.	10. Shifting weight backward-forward side to side alternate arm-leg	11. Creeping
	12. Standing— static	13. Shifting weight backward-forward side to side.	14. Walking—must analyze stance, push off, pick up and heel strike.

S. Randolph, J. Huss, 1966

This treatment approach assumes that an exercise *per se* is not treatment unless the pattern of response is correct and results in feedback which enhances learning of that response. Treatment or therapy is not in the form of a motor act alone, but rather is the application of stimuli to activate a response, followed by sensory input from a correct response with additional stimuli given to facilitate or inhibit elements in the pattern. The use of stimuli is an integral part of treatment, since sensory factors are essential for the achievement and maintenance of normal motor functions.[3*]

Developmental sequences are as outlined in Charts 13–1 and 2. These patterns are used to evaluate the patient's level of development which determines the level of treatment.

Sensory stimulation is provided for the exteroceptors by brushing and icing. Brushing is done with a soft brush attached to a battery powered mixer. The dermatonal representation for those muscles to be

*p. 903.

CHART 13-2
VITAL FUNCTION DEVELOPMENTAL SEQUENCES

(1) Reciprocal Innervation	(2) Co-innervation	(3) Heavy Work Movement	(4) Skill
1. Inspiration 2. Expiration	3. Sucking	4. Swallowing fluids 6. Chewing 7. Swallowing solids	5. Phonation 8. Speech

J. Huss, 1966

activated is brushed for approximately 5 seconds. Ice is applied to the same area with pressure for approximately 5 seconds. Ice is never applied to the posterior trunk, neck and head because it will increase reactions of the sympathetic portion of the autonomic nervous system.

Proprioceptors are stimulated with a rubbing pressure into the muscle belly, pounding with finger tips into a muscle belly, quick stretch (sudden elongation) of a muscle and/or alternating resistance to muscle contraction and vibration. Muscles without dermatonal representation such as the gluteus medius must be stimulated through the proprioceptors and not exteroceptors. Joint compression is used either to inhibit tight musculature around a joint or to facilitate co-contraction in a pattern of extension. Light compression will cause the first response. Strong compression will elicit the second response. Joint traction induces a flexion response. Vestibular stimulation through fast movement such as rolling or swinging is important in establishing overall muscle tone in a hypotonic patient.

Inhibitory procedures used by Miss Rood include slow stroking, neutral warmth and slow rolling for overall relaxation and pressure to the muscle insertion for specific relaxation.

Slow stroking is an alternate stroking of the posterior primary rami with a firm but light pressure. One hand starts at the occiput and progresses to the coccyx. As the first hand finishes, the second hand starts. Thus there is always contact with the patient. This is done for 3 minutes. If the hair growth pattern is irregular this may be irritating to the patient.

Neutral warmth is the wrapping of part or all of the patient in a cotton towel or blanket for 10 to 20 minutes. Slow rolling from supine to side and return is also generally inhibitory. The rolling continues until relaxation is seen.

Depending on the type of muscle tone and developmental level of the patient a treatment program may be all inhibitory, inhibitory and facilitory, or all facilitory.

Cortical demand for voluntary effort on the part of the patient is directed through activities which utilize the patterns which have been stimulated. The patient's attention is thus directed to the activity, not to specific movement or stabilizing patterns.

Fuchs
Orthokinetics

Julius Fuchs, M.D., orthopedic surgeon, dissatisfied with the static approach of braces, casts and splints, created devices which provided immediate mobilization as well as support. His work was done in the 1920's and was published in German in 1927. A description was not published in English until 1951. The principles were applied originally to fractures, scoliosis and other orthopedic problems. The application to neurological and arthritic dyskinesias was done by Manfred Blashy, M.D., physiatrist, Elsbeth Harrison and Ernest Fuchs, both occupational therapists, in the 1950's.

The basic idea is the use of a segment or cuff composed of elastic and inelastic parts. Several of these put together form the orthokinetic tube. The inelastic or *inactive fields* cover those parts where support and muscle inactivity are desired. The elastic or *active fields* cover those parts where muscle activity is desired. The inactive field thus becomes the inhibitory field, and the active field the facilitory field.

Originally these cuffs were made of leather and molded directly to the patient. Currently they are made of Ace bandages or sewing elastic 1 to 6 in. wide, depending on the size of the area of application. The device is usually 2 or 3 layers thick for the active field and 3 to 4 layers thick in the inactive field. The layers are stitched firmly together to provide the inactive field and left free for the active field. The cuff can be fastened with velcro.

Among the results claimed by Fuchs and others are:
1. Rapid relief of pain
2. Increase of muscle strength
3. Increase of range of motion
4. Muscle re-education
5. Improvement of coordination

This author has also noted an increase in girth as muscle bulk fills in.

The cuffs are worn repeatedly to increase the effects. They can be worn all day while the individual is active. This provides continuous sensory input. The greater the imbalance initially between agonist and antagonist muscle groups the quicker the effects will be noticed.

This is an effective, inexpensive procedure which supplies continuous input when the patient is not "in therapy." It should be further investigated by occupational and physical therapists as to its value as an adjunct to treatment.

SUMMARY

In looking at all of the sensorimotor treatment approaches it is helpful to place them in a continuum of control needed by the patient.

The Fay—Doman—Delacato approach is initially one of passive movement superimposed upon the patient. Only later does this call for active participation on the part of the patient.

Rood uses a strong mixture of exteroceptive and proprioceptive input in developmental patterns followed by activity utilizing the stability and mobility of the patterns. The individual's attention is directed to the activity, not to the patterns per se.

Orthokinetics provides a continuous exteroceptive input followed by proprioceptive feedback as muscles are facilitated and inhibited. The individual is able to use the resultant muscle function in activities of daily living.

Bobath inhibits primitive patterns and then facilitates righting and equilibrium reactions controlling at key points so that the nervous system receives feedback only from more normal movement. Whenever possible cortical control of movement is demanded.

Brunnstrom uses the initial synergy patterns seen in recovery from cerebral vascular insult on both a reflexive level and with conscious control by the patient. Using exteroceptive and proprioceptive input as well as the cortical control these patterns are then broken up leading to functional movement.

Kabat—Knott—Voss place primary emphasis on proprioceptive input reinforced by visual and verbal cues which demand cortical control by the patient. Exteroceptive stimulation is considered primarily in the placement of the therapist's hands.

Thus when the patient is at a level in which cortical control hinders movement, approaches such as Rood, Fuchs, Bobath and Fay can be utilized. Once cortical control begins to develop and strengthening is needed Brunnstrom and Kabat—Knott—Voss approaches become appropriate.

Many of the technics of the various approaches are quite similar. It is very often feasible to employ technics from various approaches at any given time with any individual. The therapist must know and understand normal human development, neurophysiology and technics of evaluation in order to use effectively these treatment approaches.

NEUROANATOMICAL AND NEUROPHYSIOLOGICAL FACTORS

The nervous system is the mediator of all that occurs within an organism, be it a one-celled creature or a human. It is an extremely complex system in man. To date our knowledge of how it functions is only partial.

To facilitiate understanding man has arbitrarily divided the nervous system into two parts: the central nervous system (CNS) and the peripheral nervous system (PNS). Any nervous system structure that is located inside of bony structure is CNS, and conversely that outside of bone is PNS. A functional distinction is that the CNS is the headquarters for organization and consists of the brain and spinal cord. The PNS is responsible for carrying sensory information to and motor information from the CNS. That functional part of the total system which regulates smooth muscle, cardiac muscle and glands is called the autonomic

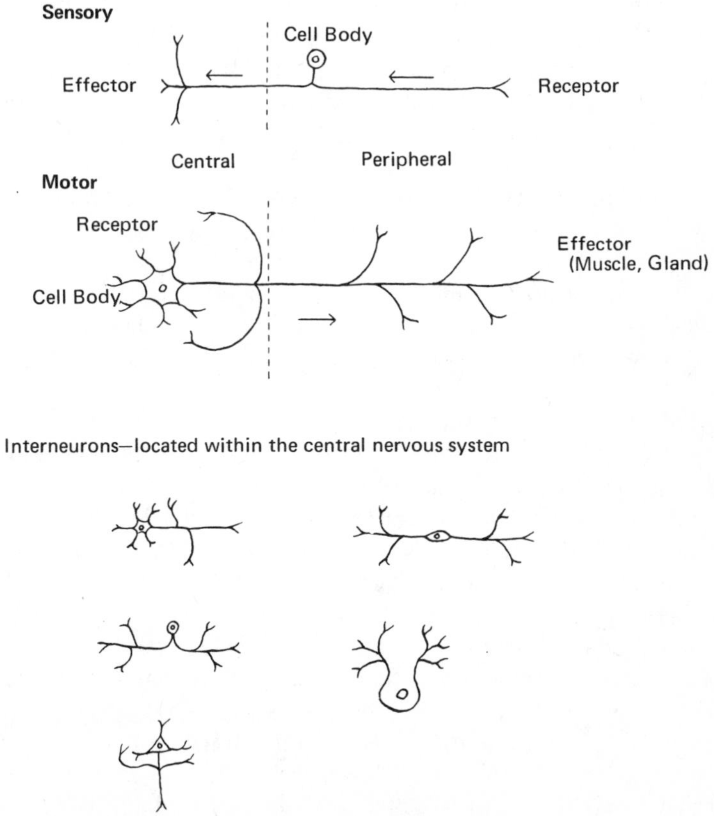

Fig. 13–1 Types of neurons.

nervous system (ANS). The ANS consists of the sympathetic division (SNS) and the parasympathetic division (PSNS). The SNS is often referred to as the thoracolumbar division as its neurons come from the thoracic and lumbar regions of the spinal cord ($T_1 - L_2$ or $_3$). The PSNS is also called the craniosacral division as its neurons are found in cranial nerves III, VII, IX, X and XI and sacral nerves 2, 3, 4.

The *structural* and *functional* unit of the nervous system is the neuron. There are over 20 billion neurons within man's system. In addition the CNS contains glial cells (glue) which have to do with phagocytosis, myelination of the neurons and possibly memory storage.

There are three basic types of neurons. *Sensory* neurons receive information concerning the environment and the state of the organism and pass it on to the CNS. Motoneurons take information out of the CNS and cause a response. This response will be mediated by either skeletal muscle, smooth muscle such as that found in blood vessels, spleen, liver, etc., cardiac muscle or glands. *Interneurons* or *internuncials* are those neurons interposed between the sensory and motoneurons and make up the bulk of the nervous system. They are extremely important in the check and balance system. See Figure 13–1 for a diagrammatic representation of each type of neuron.

Collaterals or branches off most neurons may synapse (or connect) with the receptor for the same neuron or on the receptor area of other neurons. There may be synapses on as many as 100 to 1,000 other neurons (neuron pool), many glands or few. Thus the avenue is present for much interaction between neurons and the organs supplied for either inhibition or facilitation.

Figure 13–2a depicts diagrammatically a reflex arc integrating the sensory neuron, interneurons and motoneuron. Figure 13–2b depicts the servomechanism [feedback] concept of the function of the nervous system.

At birth the nervous system has a full complement of structure, but it is not fully developed functionally until 18 to 20 years of age. Initially it is a gross, facilitory system with no ability to fractionate movement. There are few inhibitions or controls of movement. Reactions are subcortically controlled. Volitional or voluntary movement is not possible. Reactions are controlled at spinal cord and brain stem levels. As higher centers develop and begin to function a cortical, inhibitory overlay begins to take over control of movement. As the facilitory and inhibitory centers begin to work together fractionation of movement becomes possible, and the organism moves from gross to fine coordination. In the fully developed, normal nervous system facilitation and inhibition work together for control. If this balance is destroyed or never develops the organism will function either with too much facilitation (hyperkinetic and/or hypertonic) or with too much inhibition (hypotonic).

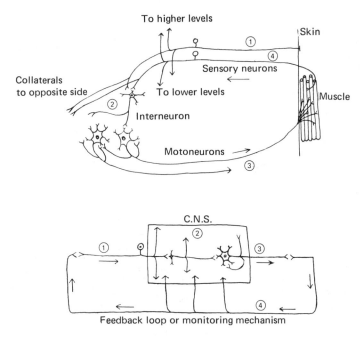

Fig. 13–2 (Top) Reflex arc.
(Bottom) Servomechanism.

Each neuron has a threshold, which is the amount of electrical energy required to cause a propagation of the impulse. If the resting threshold is too high or the stimulus raises the threshold, then the neuron is said to be inhibited. If the threshold lowers so that it is more easily fired off or fires automatically, then it is said to be facilitated. One of the purposes of the technics discussed in the first section is to influence the threshold levels for either inhibition or facilitation.

Built into the nervous system is a mechanism called *homeostasis* or balance within the system (or maintenance of the status quo). Thus the nervous system will react only to a change in stimuli in an effort to bring the system back into balance.

It is also a *redundant* system. There are different areas responsible for the same function with differing degrees of control. Therefore, if damage occurs it is possible that some other area may be able to take over and learn to control those functions lost, although possibly not to the same level of control.

The exact mechanisms of the learning process are not as yet known. However, it is known that the nervous system is dependent upon sensory input for learning to occur. Also learning takes place at least at three different levels. *Cortical* or conscious learning, is the slowest and

Chart 13-3 RECEPTORS

EXTEROCEPTIVE	PROPRIOCEPTIVE	INTEROCEPTIVE
GENERAL	**UNCONSCIOUS**	Pain (Diffuse or Non-Specific)
Now have two kinds: OLD-via spinotectal and retic. Deep pain, diffuse-throbbing longer lasting. Xed-unxed NEW-sharp pain, well localized via sp-thal. trs. Xed.	Neuromuscular Spindle A. Nuclear bag fiber B. Nuclear chain fiber	Stretch or Contraction to an Abnormal Degree
Temperature	Neurotendinous Spindle	Olfaction*1
Light Touch, Light Pressure, and Crude Tactile Sense	Vestibular (Labyrinth)	Gustatory*1
SPECIAL	**CONSCIOUS**	
Vision	Pressure Superficial and Deep*2	
Hearing	Vestibular (Labyrinth)*2	
	Joint, Ligament, Fascia, Periosteum*2	
Olfaction*1	Vibratory	
Gustatory*1	Tactile Discrimination*3	
	a. deep pressure	
	b. spatial localization	
	c. perception of size, shape, texture	
	d. skin drawing and 2-point tactile	

*1 can be considered as either an exteroceptive or interoceptive type of receptor, according to different authors.
*2 Kinesthetic Sense: receptors which let one know where their body is in space. Also called position sense. Consists of those receptors starred and probably others.
*3 Also called sterognosis.

J. C. Moore

most poorly retained. *Subcortical* learning by the *reticular formation* is the fastest and easiest and is retained the longest. The *basal ganglia* level is semiautomatic and produces stereotyped responses. It is the second fastest area. The *alpha-gamma linkage system* (or fusimotor system) at the *spinal cord* level is probably necessary for motor learning. The more senses and levels that can be used, the faster learning takes place.

Sensory input which is necessary for function to occur is received from the external world through *exteroceptors*, from the muscles, joints, tendons, fascia and ligaments through *proprioceptors*, and from the internal organs through *interoceptors*. These receptor classifications are outlined in Chart 13–3.

The *exteroceptive* input is both specific and non-specific or conscious and subconscious in its effects. The *specific* inputs provide a conscious awareness of the external environment which includes vision, hearing, light touch, temperature and pain. These are mediated over direct pathways via the thalamus to the cortex. The non-specific inputs are handled basically by the reticular formation for correlation with all other sensory input and motor output. These are brought to the conscious level only when there is a sudden change in stimuli (i.e., clothing which is generally ignored as a stimulus until it is either too loose or too tight), or the temperature of a room which "suddenly" becomes too hot or too cold or too stuffy.

Two of the major proprioceptive mechanisms used in all of the approaches mentioned in section one of this chapter are the receptors responding to muscle stretch and muscle contraction: the *neuromuscular spindle* and the *neurotendinous organ*.

The neuromuscular spindles lie imbedded within the muscles and are in parallel with the muscle fibers. They are attached at their polar ends to muscle or fascia. The spindles are both a sensory (afferent) and a motor (efferent) mechanism. A spindle is composed of long nuclear bag fibers which extend beyond the capsule wall, and shorter nuclear chain fibers which are within the capsule wall. Both of these fiber types contain contractile muscle tissue called *intrafusal fibers* as compared with the muscle which is called *extrafusal*. These intrafusal fibers are supplied by gamma motor neurons. The extrafusal are supplied by alpha motor neurons. There are two sensory endings located within the spindle. The *primary ending*, formerely called annulospiral, is wrapped around the equatorial region of the bag and the chain fibers. It has the lowest threshold and responds to being stretched. The input via Group Ia sensory fibers is to both the alpha and the gamma motor neurons for a contraction of the extrafusal muscle followed by contraction of the intrafusal muscle in which the

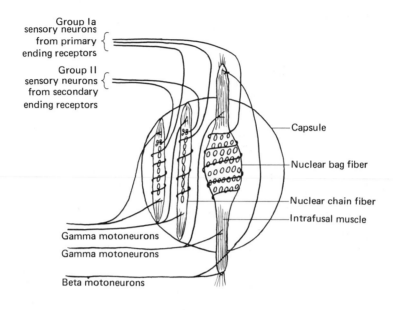

Group Ia
sensory neurons
from primary
ending receptors

Group II
sensory neurons
from secondary
ending receptors

Capsule

Nuclear bag fiber

Nuclear chain fiber

Intrafusal muscle

Gamma motoneurons

Gamma motoneurons

Beta motoneurons

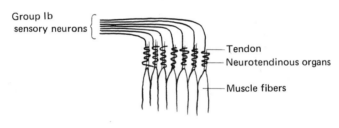

Group Ib
sensory neurons

Tendon
Neurotendinous organs

Muscle fibers

Neurotendinous organs

Fig. 13-3 (Top)   Neuromuscular spindle.
(Bottom)   Neurotendinous organs.

endings lie. If the extrafusal and intrafusal fibers remain in ratio, with both contracting, then the spindle is said to be *biased* and can be re-fired. If only the extrafusal fibers contract, then the spindle is placed on slack, and the primary ending cannot refire (Fig. 13-3). In the normal individual this mechanism is responsible for maintaining muscle tone and increasing the ability to maintain a contraction. The primary ending is facilitory to the same muscle in which it lies.

The *secondary ending*, formerly called myotube or flowerspray, in man is probably located on the nuclear chain fibers (Fig. 13-3). It has a higher threshold and responds only to stretch. The input via Group II sensory neurons is to the alpha motoneuron pool. This ending is always facilitory to either flexors, adductors or internal rotators.

Thus if it is fired off in an extensor it will facilitate the antagonistic flexor. If it is fired in a flexor it will facilitate that same muscle. In therapy, therefore, it can be used to inhibit extreme extensor tone, but it should not be used if there is too much flexor tone. The same applies to external rotators versus internal rotators and abductors versus adductors respectively.

The neurotendinous organs are located at the junction of muscle fibers and tendon. These were formerly called Golgi Tendon Organs. These are squiggly organs and arranged in series, which enables them to respond to either a stretch or a contraction of the muscle in which they lie (Fig. 13–3). The threshold is generally higher than in the primary and secondary endings. However, the threshold within the organ itself apparently is lower for contraction than for stretch. Since it probably is a protective mechanism to prevent muscle tearing, it is inhibitory to the muscle in which it lies. In the range of stretch there is pain associated with this, such as when one twists an ankle and finds the muscles around the joint inhibited and severe pain occurs. When fired with a maximal contraction against maximal resistance there is no pain, and the range of free movement is increased. Input is mediated over Group Ib fibers to the alpha motoneuron pool.

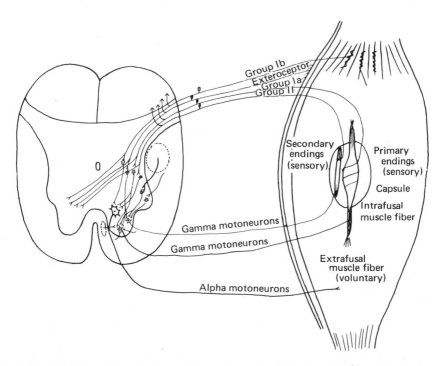

Fig. 13–4 Composite of exteroceptive and proprioceptive input with motor output.

Figure 13–4 is a composite showing the mechanisms of exteroceptive input, the neuromuscular spindles, neurotendinous organs, alpha and gamma motoneurons and supraspinal influences on the alpha and gamma motoneurons. It will be noted that this is a highly complex system and that the gamma motoneurons play an exceedingly important role via the alpha-gamma linkage system in motor control.

The *reticular formation* is a loose network of cells located in the central core of the brain stem extending from the medulla to the thalamus. It consists of both ascending and descending portions. The ascending is usually referred to as the *Reticular Activating System* (RAS). It is responsible for keeping the organism awake and alert. It functions at all times thus making waking and sleeping active processes. It receives either directly (nonspecific sensory input) or indirectly via collaterals (specific sensory input) all sensory input from outside of and within the organism. It monitors this sensory information and then alerts the cortex as to which inputs should be consciously handled. Thus, new and strange sounds, for instance, are heard by the organism and handled appropriately. If this sound continues repetitively it drops from the conscious level and is ignored. If it suddenly changes pitch or position the conscious levels are realerted. Or if the sound suddenly ceases the cortex is alerted. Thus the individual living near a railroad track no longer responds to every train that goes by while the visitor is acutely aware of each one regardless of the hour, day or night.

The descending portion of the reticular formation receives all outgoing motor information from higher and lower centers as well as information from the RAS. It has both facilitory and inhibitory centers and assists in maintaining a balance between these effects. Its major influence is on the gamma motoneurons. It appears that the descending reticular formation may be one of the controlling agents of proximal, postural muscle tone and righting reactions as well as deglutition.

There is a definite neurological tie-up between non-specific sensory stimuli, the reticular formation and the gamma loop system. Thus sensory stimuli applied appropriately are going to have not only a direct effect on the gamma and alpha motor neuron pools, but also will enhance feedback and reverberating circuits for continued input to these neurons by way of the reticular system.

The functions of the autonomic nervous system are extremely pertinent to the discussion at hand. It is basically a system of checks and balances. The PSNS functions to conserve and restore homeostasis. The SNS alerts and prepares the organism for fright, fight, or flight. In an SNS state the organism is less able to think clearly and react appropriately to the situation at hand. Thus if a therapist or anyone else is trying to teach something to someone an effort should be made to keep it on a PSNS basis.

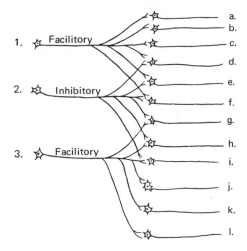

Fig. 13–5   Release phenomenon. Neurons c through i are receiving both facilitory and inhibitory stimuli. If neuron #2 was destroyed, then neurons c through i would be released from the inhibitory influence and receive only facilitory input.

When there has been injury or trauma to the nervous system the clinical picture one sees is that for which the nervous system cannot compensate. This is called a *release phenomenon*. Each neuron is receiving both facilitory and inhibitory input. If the inhibitory overlay is lost or diminished the clinical picture will be one of too much facilitation with athetosis, spasticity or similar muscle tone (Fig. 13–5). While conversely with too much inhibition the thresholds will be too high and the picture will be flaccid, floppy or paralyzed type of muscle tone.

To reiterate, the nervous system is a highly complex mechanism in man with redundancy, reverberating circuits, and repetitive sensory input necessary for motor output. Thus, the therapist is provided with possibilities for improving the functional usage by the individual. The next question is how does this apply to occupational therapy?

It is the opinion of this author that the approaches discussed above are *preliminary to and not a replacement for* the gamut of standard occupational therapy principles and activities. The reader is referred to other chapters in this text for these principles. The procedure for treatment should be evaluation, preliminary sensory input and finally utilization of the motor output through meaningful activity done in the proper position and developmental sequence. Thus one cannot merely stop with evaluation, nor with sensory input. Neither can one start with motor output on a cortical conscious level if there is damage to the nervous system. For many years the emphasis has been on the motor output. But since motor output is dependent upon sensory input there must be correlation of the two followed by appropriate functional use. This material should be integrated into a total evaluation-treatment approach. Frustration of patient and therapist will result if the emphasis is on only sensory input or motor output.

The sensorimotor treatment approaches are not an end in themselves. They only comprise one tool in the total armamentarium of the occupational therapist.

BIBLIOGRAPHY

1. Adams, S. L.: The Sequential Development of the Nervous System As a Guide to Therapy (Master's Thesis, U.S.C.), 1959.
2. Adrian, E. D.: Sensory Integration, Liverpool, University Press, 1949.
3. American Journal of Physical Medicine (Nu-Step), 46, 1967.
4. Andersen, P., and Sears, T. A.: The role of inhibition in the phasing of spontaneous thalamo-cortical discharge, J. Physiol. Lond., 1964.
5. Andrew, B. L. (ed.): Control and Innervation of Skeletal Muscle. Dundee, Scotland, D. C. Thomson & Co., 1966.
6. Ashworth, B., Grimby, L., and Kugelberg, E.: Comparison of voluntary and reflex activation of motor units. J. Neurol. Neurosurg. Psychiat., 1967.
7. Ayres, A. J.: Occupational therapy for motor disorders resulting from impairment of the central nervous system. Rehab. Lit., 21:10, 1960.
8. ———: Perceptual-Motor Dysfunction in Children, Monograph from Greater Cincinnati District, Ohio Occ. Ther. Assoc. Conf., 1964.
9. Barker, D.: Symposium on Muscle Receptors. Hong Kong, Hong Kong Univ. Press, 1962.
10. Basmajian, J. V.: Control and training of individual motor units. Science, 1963.
11. Basmajian, J. V.: Primary Anatomy. ed. 6, Baltimore, Williams & Wilkins, 1970.
12. Bekesy, G. von.: Sensory Inhibition. Princeton, N.J., Princeton Univ. Press, 1967.
13. Bell, C., Buendia, N., Sirra, G., and Segundo, J. P.: Mesencephalic reticular responses to natural and to repeated sensory stimuli. Experientia, 1963.
14. Biancomi, R. and Van der Meulen, J. P.: The response to vibration of the end organs of mammalian muscle spindles. J. Neurophysiol., 1963.
15. Blashy, M.: Manipulation of the neuromuscular unit in the periphery of the central nervous system. J. So. Med. Assoc., 1961.
16. Blashy, M., and Fuchs, R.: Orthokinetics: A new receptor facilitation method. Am. J. Occup. Therapy, 1959.
17. Blashy, M., Harrison, H. E., and Fuchs, E. M.: Orthokinetics — a preliminary report on recent experiences with a little known rehabilitation therapy. V. A. Bulletin, 1955.
18. Bobath, B.: Abnormal Postural Reflex Activity Caused by Brain Lesions, London, Wm. Heinemann Med. Bks. Ltd., 1965.

19. Bosma, J. F. (ed.): Symposium On Oral Sensation And Perception. Springfield, Ill., Charles C Thomas, 1967.
20. Bouman, H. D.: Some considerations of the physiology of sensation. J. Am. Phys. Therapy Assoc., 1965.
21. Boyd, I. A.: The Structure and Innervation of The Nuclear Bag Muscle Fibre System and The Nuclear Chain Muscle Fibre System in Mammalian Muscle Spindles. Phil. Trans. Roy. Soc. Lond., Ser. B, 1962.
22. Boyd, I. A., Eyzaguire, C., Matthews, P. B. C., and Rushworth, G.: The Role of The Gamma System In Movement And Posture. ed. 2, N.Y., Assoc. For Aid of Crippled Children, 1968.
23. Calne, D. B., and Pallis, C. A.: Vibratory sense: A critical review. Brain, 1966.
24. Carpenter, D. O., and Henneman, E. A.: A relation between the threshold of stretch receptors in skeletal muscle and the diameter of their axons. J. Neurophysiol., 1966.
25. The Child With Central Nervous System Deficit—Report of Two Symposiums. U.S. Dept. of Health, Educ. & Welfare, 1965.
26. Crosby, E. C., Humphrey, T., and Lauer, E. W.: Correlative Anatomy of The Nervous System. N.Y., Macmillan, 1962.
27. Crosby, E. C., Schneider, R. C., DeJonge, B. R., and Szonui, P.: The alterations of tonus and movements through the interplay between the cerebral hemispheres and the cerebellum. J. Comp. Neurol., 1966.
28. Crowe, A., and Matthews, P.C.B.: The effects of stimulation of static and dynamic fusimotor fibers on the response to stretching of the primary endings of muscle spindles. J. Physiol. Lond., 1964.
29. Decker, R. (ed).: Motor Integration. Springfield, Charles C Thomas, 1962.
30. deGail, P., Lance, J. W., and Neilson, P. D.: Differential effects on tonic and phasic reflex mechanisms produced by vibration of muscles in man. J. Neurol. Neurosurg. Psychiat., 1966.
31. Denny-Brown, D.: The Cerebral Control of Movement. Liverpool, Liverpool Univ. Press, 1966.
32. Doman, G., and Delacato, C.: Children With Severe Brain Injuries. J.A.M.A., 74, 1960.
33. Eklund, G., and Hagbarth, K. E.: Motor effects of vibratory muscle stimuli in man. Electroenceph. Clin. Neurophysiol., 1965.
34. Eklund, G., and Hagbarth, K. E.: Normal variability of tonic vibration reflexes in man. Exp. Neurol., 1966.
35. Eldred, E., and Fujimori, B.: Relations of The Reticular Formation To Muscle Spindle Activation in Jasper, H. H. (ed.): Reticular Formation of Brain, Boston, Little, Brown, 1958.
36. Elliott, H. C.: Textbook of Neuroanatomy, Philadelphia, J. B. Lippincott, 1963.
37. Engberg, I., Lundberg, A., and Ryall, R. W.: Reticulospinal inhibition of transmission in reflex pathways. J. Physiol. Lond., 1968.
38. ———: Reticulospinal inhibition of interneurones. J. Physiol. Lond., 1968.
39. Fay, T.: Basic considerations regarding neuromuscular and reflex therapy. Spastics Quarterly, 3, 1954.

40. Fay, Temple, Neuromuscular Reflex Therapy For Spastic Disorders, J. Florida Med. Assoc., 44, 1958.
41. Fiorentino, M.: Reflex Testing Methods For Evaluating C.N.S. Development. Springfield, Charles C Thomas, 1963.
42 Gatz, A. J., and Manter, J. T.: Essentials of clinical neuroanatomy and neurophysiology, ed. 4, Philadelphia, F. A. Davis, 1970.
43. Gillette, H. E.: Systems of Therapy in Cerebral Palsy, Springfield, Charles C Thomas, 1969.
44. Gilman, S. and McDonald, W. I.: Cerebellar facilitation of muscle spindle activity. J. Neurophysiol., 30, 1967.
45. Gilman, S., and McDonald, W. I.: Relation of afferent fiber conduction velocity to reactivity of muscle spindle receptors after cerebellectomy. J. Neurophysiol., 1967.
46. Granit, R. (ed.): Nobel Symposium I—Muscular Afferents And Motor Control. N.Y., John Wiley & Sons, 1966.
47. Granit, R.: Receptors And Sensory Perception, New Haven, Conn., Yale Univ. Press, 1955.
48. ——: The gamma loop in the mediation of muscle tone. Clin. Pharmacol. Ther., 1964.
49. Granit, R., and Henatsch, H. D.: Gamma control of dynamic properties of muscle spindles. J. Neurophysiol., 1956.
50. Grimby, L. and Hannerz, J.: Recruitment order of motor units in voluntary contraction: changes induced by proprioceptive afferent activity. J. Neurol. Neurosurg. Psychiat., 1968.
51. Guyton, A. C.: Textbook of Medical Physiology. ed. 3. Philadelphia, W. B. Saunders Co., 1966.
52 Hagbarth, K. E., and Eklund, G.: Motor Effects of Vibratory Muscle Stimuli In Man in Granit, R. (ed.): Proceedings of The First Nobel Symposium, Muscular Afferents And Motor Control. Stockholm, Almquist & Wiksell, 1966.
53. Hagbarth, K. E., and Eklund, G.: Tonic vibration reflexes (TVR) in spasticity. Brain Research, 1966.
54. ——: The effects of muscle vibration in spasticity, rigidity and cerebellar disorders. J. Neurol. Neurosurg. Psychiat., 1968.
55. Hall, V. E. (ed.): Annual Review of Physiology, Palo Alto, Annual Reviews, Inc. published yearly.
56. Hellmuth, J. (ed.): Exceptional Infant, 1, The Normal Infant, N.Y., Brunner/Mazel, 1967.
57. Hernandez-Peon, R.: Reticular Mechanisms of Sensory Control. Sensory Communication, N.Y., John Wiley & Sons, 1961.
58. Hollingshead, W. H.: Functional Anatomy of The Limbs And Back, ed. 3, Philadelphia, W. B. Saunders, 1969.
59. Houk, J., and Simon, W.: Responses of golgi tendon organs to forces applied to muscle tendon. J. Neurophysiol. 30, 6, 1967.
60. Howard, I. P., and Templeton, W. B.: Human Spatial Orientation. N.Y., John Wiley & Sons, 1966.

61. Huss, A. J.: Application of Rood technique to treatment of the physical handicapped child. O. T. for The Multiply Handicapped, 1965.
62. Huss, A. J.: An Introduction To Treatment Techniques Developed By Margaret Rood, 1967.
63. Huss, A. J.: An Overview of Sensorimotor Treatment Techniques — Present and Future. Unpublished lecture, 1967.
64. Huss, A. J.: The Role of the Descending Reticular Formation in Motor Activity. Unpublished, 1968.
65. Huss, A. J.: Clinical Application of Sensorimotor Treatment Techniques in Physical Dysfunction, Controversy and Confusion in Physical Dysfunction Treatment Techniques — Clinical Aspects, Expanding Dimensions in Rehabilitation, Springfield, Ill., Charles C Thomas, 1969.
66. Jansen, J. K. S.: Spasticity — Functional Aspects. Acta. Neurol. Scand., 1962.
67. Jansen, J. K. S., and Matthews, P. B. C.: The central control of the dynamic response of muscle spindle receptors. J. Physiol. Lond. 1962.
68. Jasper, H. (ed.): Reticular Formation of the Brain. Boston, Little, Brown, 1958.
69. Johnston, R. M., Bishop, B., and Coffey, G. H.: Mechanical vibration of skeletal muscles. J. Amer. Phys. Therapy Assoc., 50, 1970.
70. On The Treatment of Spastic Pareses, Journal of Swedish Association of Registered Physical Therapists, 27, 1969.
71. Kabat, H.: Central facilitation: the basis of treatment for paralysis. Permanente Fnd. Med. Bull, 10, August 1962.
72. Kenshalo, D. R. (ed.): The Skin Senses. Springfield, Charles C Thomas, 1968.
73. Kimble, D. P. (ed.): The Anatomy of Memory, Learning, Remembering and Forgetting, Palo Alto, Calif., Science & Behavior Books, Inc., 1965.
74. Knighton, R. S., and Dumke, P. R. (eds.): Pain, Henry Ford Hospital International Symposium, Boston, Little, Brown, 1966.
75. Knott, M.: Bulbar involvement with good recovery, J. Amer. Phys. Therapy Assoc., 1961.
76. Knott, M., and Voss, D. E.: Proprioceptive Neuromuscular Facilitation: Patterns and Techniques. ed. 2, N.Y., Harper & Row, 1968.
77. Lang, A. H., and Vallbo, A. B.: Motoneurone activation by low intensity tetanic stimulation of muscle afferents in man. Exp. Neurol., 1967.
78. Lindblom, U.: On the treatment of spastic paresis. J. Swedish Assoc. Reg. P. T., 27, Reprint, 1969.
79. Llinas, R., and Terzuolo, C. A.: Mechanisms of supraspinal actions upon spinal cord activities: reticular inhibitory mechanisms upon flexor motoneurons., J. Neurophysiol. 1965.
80. Luria, A. R.: Human Brain and Psychological Process. N.Y. Harper & Row, translated 1966.
81. MacConaill, M. A., and Basmajian, J. V.: Muscles and Movements: A Basis for Human Kinesiology. Baltimore, Williams & Wilkins, 1969.
82. Magni, F., and Willis, W. D.: Cortical control of brain stem reticular neurons. Arch. Ital. Biol., 1964.

83. ——: Subcortical and peripheral control of brainstem reticular neurons. Arch. Ital. Biol., 1964.

84. ——: Afferent connections to reticulo-spinal neurons. Prog. Brain Res., Elsevier, 12, 1964.

85. Magoun, H. W.: The Waking Brain. ed. 2, Springfield, Ill., Charles C Thomas, 1963.

86. Matthews, P. B. C.: Muscle spindles and their motor control. Physiol. Rev., 1964.

87. ——: The reflex excitation of the soleus muscle on the decerebrate cat caused by vibration to its tendon. J. Physiol., 1966.

88. Moore, J. C.: Neuroanatomical and Neurophysiological Factors Basic to Use of Neuromuscular Facilitation Techniques in West, W. (ed.): Occupational Therapy for Multiply Handicapped Child, 1965.

89. ——: Neuroanatomy Simplified. Dubuque, Iowa, Kendall-Hunt, 1969.

90. ——: Unpublished class notes course on Neuromuscular Facil. Neurophysiological Concepts and Application in O.T., Dept. of Post-graduate Medicine, Univ. of Michigan, 1969.

91. Morgan, C. T.: Physiological Psychology. ed. 3, New York, McGraw-Hill, 1965.

92. Mountcastle, V. B. (ed.): Medical Physiology. ed. 12, St. Louis, C. V. Mosby, 1968.

93. Neff, W. D. (ed.): Contributions to Sensory Physiology ed. 2, N.Y., Academic Press, 1967.

94. Netter, F.: Nervous System, Ciba.

95. Noback, C. R.: The Human Nervous System. New York, McGraw-Hill, 1967.

96. Pederson, E. (ed.): Spasticity and neurological bladder disturbances. Acta. Neurologica. Scand., Supplementum 3, 38, 1962.

97. Peele, T. L.: The Neuroanatomic Basis for Clinical Neurology. ed. 2, New York, McGraw-Hill.

98. Quiring, D. P.: The Head, Neck and Trunk. Philadelphia, Lea & Febiger, 1958.

99. Ranson, S. W., and Clark, S. L.: The Anatomy of the Nervous System—Its Development And Function. ed. 10, 622 pp. Philadelphia, W. B. Saunders, 1965.

100. Rasmussen, A. T.: The Principal Nervous Pathways. New York, Macmillan Co., 1957.

101. Reuck, A. V. S., and de Knight, J. (ed.): Myotatic, Kinesthetic and Vestibular Mechanisms, London, Churchill, 1967.

102. Rood, M. S.: Unpublished class notes 1958, 1959, 1965, 1970, taken by J. Huss.

103. Rood, M. S.: Use of Reflexes As An Aid In O.T., delivered at World Fed. of O.T., Copenhagen, Denmark, Aug. 1958.

104. Ruch, T. C., et. al.: Neurophysiology ed. 2, Philadelphia, W. B. Saunders, 1966.

105. Rushworth, G.: Some aspects of the pathophysiology of spasticity and rigidity. Clin. Pharmacol. Ther., 1964.

106. Rushworth, G., and Young, R. R.: The effect of vibration on tonic and phasic reflexes in man. J. Physiol. (Lond.), 1966.
107. Sattely, C. (ed.): Approaches to The Treatment of Patients With Neuromuscular Dysfunction. Dubuque, Iowa, William C. Brown, 1962.
108. Scheibel, M. E., and Scheibel, A. B.: The response of reticular units to repetitive stimuli," Arch. Ital. Biol., 1965.
109. Schultz, D. P.: Sensory Restriction—Effects on Behavior. New York, Academic Press, 1965.
110. Schwartzman, R. J., and Bogdonoff, M. D.: Behavioral and anatomical analysis of vibration sensibility. Exp. Neurol., 1968.
111. Segundo, J. P., Takenaka, T., and Encabo, H.: Electrophysiology of bulbar reticular neurons. J. Neurophysiol., 30, 1967.
112. ———: Somatic sensory properties of bulbar reticular neurons. J. Neurophysiol. 30, 1967.
113. Semans, S.: Physical therapy for motor disorders resulting from brain damage. Rehab. Lit., April, 1959.
114. Sherrington, C.: The Integrative Action of The Nervous System. New Haven, Yale Univ. Press, 1961.
115. Shimazu, H., Hongo, T. and Kubota, K.: Two types of central influence on gamma motor system. J. Neurophysiol, 1962.
116. Smith, K. U.: Delayed Sensory Feedback and Behavior. Philadelphia, W. B. Saunders, 1962.
117. Smith, K. U., and Smith, W. M.: Perception and Motion. Philadelphia, W. B. Saunders, 1962.
118. Suda, I., Koizumi, K., and Brooks, C.: Reticular formation influences on neurons of spinal reflex pathway. J. Neurophysiol., 1958.
119. Takano, K., and Homma, S.: Muscle spindle responses to vibratory stimuli at certain frequencies. Jap. J. Physio., 1968.
120. Timo-Iaria, C., and Antunes-Rodriques, J.: Reticular influences on a spinal reflex arc. Acta Physiol. Lat. Am., 1963.
121. Tokizane, T., and Shimaza, H.: Functional Differentiation of Human Skeletal Muscle. Tokyo, Univ., Tokyo Press, 1964.
122. Troyer, B.: Sensorimotor integration: a basis for planning occupational therapy. Am. J. Occup. Therapy. 15, No. 2, 1961.
123. Wagman, I. H., Pierce, D. S., and Burger, R. E.: Proprioceptive influence in volitional control of individual motor units. Nature (Lond), 1965.
124. West, W. (ed.): Occupational Therapy for the Multiply Handicapped Child. Chicago, Univ. of Illinois Press, 1965.
125. Widen, L. (ed.): Recent Advances in Clinical Neurophysiology, Pro. 6th Intern. Congr. Electroencepholog. Clin. Neurophysiol 1965, Elsevier, Amsterdam, 1967.
126. Wolstencroft, J. H.: Effects of afferent stimuli on reticulospinal neurons. J. Physiol, 1961.
127. Woodburne, L. S.: The Neural Basis of Behavior. Columbus, Ohio, C. E. Merrill, 1967.
128. Yamanaka, T.: Effects of High Frequency Vibration on Muscle Spindles In The Human Body. Zhiba Igakkai Zasshi 40, 1964.

129. Zamir, L. J. (ed.): Expanding Dimensions in Rehabilitation, Springfield, Ill., Charles C Thomas, 1969.
130. Zimmerman, M.: Dorsal root potentials after c-fiber stimulation. Science, 1968.

ACKNOWLEDGEMENT

The author wishes to express her appreciation to Josephine C. Moore, Ph.D., O.T.R., for her tireless efforts over the years to simplify and integrate the author's understanding of the neuroanatomical and neurophysiological bases for these approaches.

14

Cognitive-Perceptual-Motor Behavior

ELNORA M. GILFOYLE, B.S., O.T.R. and
ANN P. GRADY, B.S., O.T.R.

INTRODUCTION

Knowledge of human development is of paramount importance in occupational therapy. Cognitive-Perceptual-Motor functioning is a crucial factor in this developmental process.[2,29,37] Development is dependent upon the maturation of the nervous system. There is a correlation between the nervous system's maturation, purposeful environmental stimuli, and the motor response.[20,40] When the nervous system is deprived of meaningful stimuli; when the nervous system cannot make a meaningful response to this process, effective maturation cannot take place.[47] The resulting central nervous system maturation may lead to dysfunction in Cognitive-Perceptual-Motor developmental behavior.[2,3,40]

One therapeutic role of the occupational therapist is the evaluation and treatment of Cognitive-Perceptual-Motor (CPM) dysfunction.[37] Proficiency in this role depends upon the therapist's basic knowledge of the developmental process of normal CPM behavior and the effect of the integration of the sensory motor process.

This chapter discusses a developmental concept of CPM behavior, the theoretical principles of dysfunction, and general background information regarding the evaluation and treatment procedures for the occupational therapist.

Factual knowledge regarding CPM development and dysfunction is in the descriptive stage. When evaluation-treatment procedures are recommended, the occupational therapist must be aware that the categorization of CPM behaviors and the theories of treatment go far beyond what has been derived from scientific facts. Similarly, the material presented in this chapter must be considered provisional.

DEFINITION OF COGNITIVE-PERCEPTUAL-
MOTOR BEHAVIOR

Perception is here defined as a process of sensory judgment: the organization and interpretation of sensation. Receiving sensory stimuli and perceiving such information is necessary for an individual to comprehend and adapt to his environment.

A person receives environmental information through his senses; he sees objects, he smells odors, he hears sounds, he feels textures and he feels bodily movement or position. As the nervous system assimilates the sensory information, schemas are formed. Schemas are labeled by the behavior sequence to which they refer (i.e., sucking schema, movement schema, etc.). With added information judgments are made; thus, the fire feels hot, the ice cold, the object appears round or square. This perceptual behavior is a process of assimilating sensory information received from the senses and making a judgment about this sensation. The judgment can be made only because of the past sensory information that has previously been assimilated to form schemas. In the process of assimilating sensory information the body accommodates to the information it is trying to assimilate.[29] This assimilation-accommodation process is perceptual-motor behavior. The following is an illustration of this process.

A baby, for the first time, comes in contact with a spoon. He makes a series of bodily or motor accommodations; he looks at it, touches it, grasps it, sucks it, and so on. These accommodations can take place because of the past interactions with other objects that the child has previously assimilated to form schemas, and thus he can direct his body accommodations. This assimilation-accommodation process is termed adaptation.[31] For example, the baby has already adapted to a nipple (sucking schema), and thus he can direct his body to suck the spoon. He has previously adapted to a rattle (movement-noise schema), and thus he can direct his body to bang the spoon up and down. As the child sucks the spoon he receives different sensations from the spoon than from the nipple, and as he moves his arm he receives different sensations from the spoon than from the rattle. He has thus acquired new information about sucking and about arm movement.

In the process of adapting to the spoon, the child assimilates the fact that when his arm moves up and down he may get a noise from the spoon as it bangs on the tray, whereas when the arm goes to the mouth he gets a spoon to suck. Thus, the child accommodates his body or motor behavior to the schema he wants. He can only adapt to the present environment because of the past interactions to which he has already adapted.

Each new environmental experience adds new information to

CHART 14-1

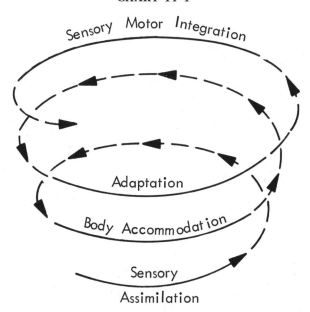

schemas, and cognitive structures are formed.[29] This process of environmental functioning exists throughout our developmental life span. The assimilation of sensory information, the formation of schemas, and the body accommodations produce the adaptation to the environment or the Cognitive-Perceptual-Motor process. (see Chart 14-1)

Sensory-motor integration is the result of organizing the assimilated information and the body accommodations. Through the integration of the isolated schemas a cognitive structure is either revised or produced from isolated schemas.[2,29,40]

In the description of CPM behavior, the hypothesis of the development of this behavior is presented (see Chart 14-2). The diagram, a spiralling continuum of development, illustrates the concept that higher level behavior is dependent upon the ontogenetically earlier development. The spiralling continuum further illustrates that the accomplishment of a behavioral skill, or the CPM process, is dependent upon the introduction and development of new behaviors.

In summary, it is suggested that CPM behavior has four characteristics: (1) physiological and psychological integration; (2) the mode of behavior is the adaptation-assimilation-accommodation process; (3) the behavior imposes changes upon the schema structures — sensory motor integration and maturation results; (4) with resultant maturation there are changes in behavior.

CHART 14–2   HYPOTHESIZED DEVELOPMENT

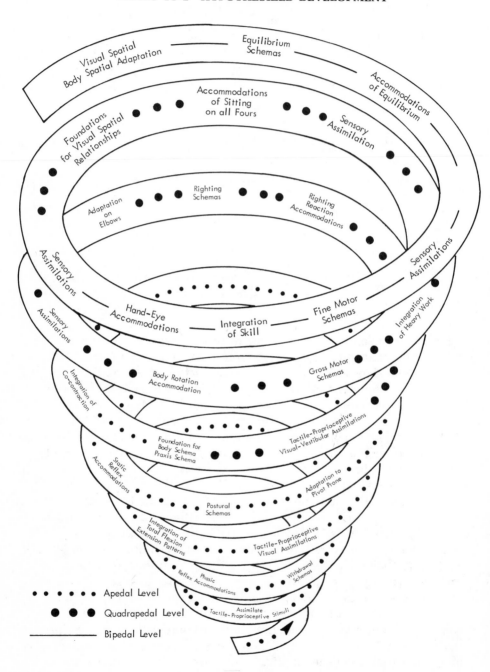

Visual Spatial
Body Spatial Adaptation

Equilibrium
Schemas

Accommodations
of Equilibrium

Foundations
for Visual Spatial
Relationships

Accommodations
of Sitting
on all Fours

Sensory
Assimilation

Adaptation
on
Elbows

Righting
Schemas

Righting
Reaction
Accommodations

Sensory
Assimilations

Sensory
Assimilations

Sensory
Assimilations

Hand–Eye
Accommodations

Integration
of Skill

Fine Motor
Schemas

Integration
of Heavy Work

Integration of
Co-contraction

Body Rotation
Accommodation

Gross Motor
Schemas

Foundation for
Body Schema
Praxis Schema

Tactile-Proprioceptive
Visual-Vestibular Assimilations

Static
Reflex
Accommodations

Adaptation to
Pivot Prone

Postural
Schemas

Integration of
Total Flexion
Extension Patterns

Tactile-Proprioceptive
Visual Assimilations

Phasic
Reflex Accommodations

Withdrawal
Schemas

Assimilate
Tactile-Proprioceptive Stimuli

• • • • • •   Apedal Level

● ● ●   Quadrapedal Level

————   Bipedal Level

In order to discuss the aspects of sensory motor integration related most directly to the CPM process and to the occupational therapist's evaluation and treatment of this dysfunction, emphasis will be placed on the following areas:

1. Reflexes and reactions that occur as accommodations to tactile, proprioceptive, vestibular and visual assimilations.
2. Adaptations of these accommodations to righting and equilibrium reactions.
3. Levels of muscle development in postural adjustment to space that occur with these accommodations-adaptations.
4. Sequential gross and fine motor development integrating tactile discrimination, body integration and visual-spatial relationships.

The specific components of each area are presented in Charts 14–3,4,5. Some examples will be chosen to integrate the levels as illustrations of the CPM process.

DEVELOPMENT OF THE COGNITIVE-PERCEPTUAL-MOTOR PROCESS

According to Piaget, the behavior repertoire of the newborn consists of a few reflex-like activities: rooting, sucking, tongue movements, gross body activity.[29] The first three are essentially the only responses of going toward the stimulus (i.e., the environment). The gross body movements are protective reactions of avoiding or "withdrawing from"; for example, the Moro reflex. These protective reactions soon undergo specific accommodations by integrating the proprioceptive extensor stretch reflex. This allows the baby to reach out to the environment.[47] This period is of extreme importance because it is the crucible from which CPM behavior emerges.

The reflexes of the infant undergo definite accommodations as a result of their environmental contact.[28] In the newborn a relatively simple stimulus, usually a tactile or proprioceptive assimilation or the infant's position in space, results in a widespread body accommodation with a motor response of the whole body or a total response of a whole segment of the body.[20,25,26,41,45,46] This assimilation-accommodation provides the foundation for the baby to move. It also initiates the levels of muscle development and provides all the elements necessary for the baby to integrate the visual, tactile, proprioceptive and adjustment to space (vestibular) assimilations. Completely new reactions are not added as the CNS develops, but more primitive reactions are adapted and elaborated as the encounters with space become more demanding and the tactile-proprioceptive responses become more discriminating.[46,47] As a result, the observable assimilation-accommodation-adaptation of the whole body in a voluntary movement, such as

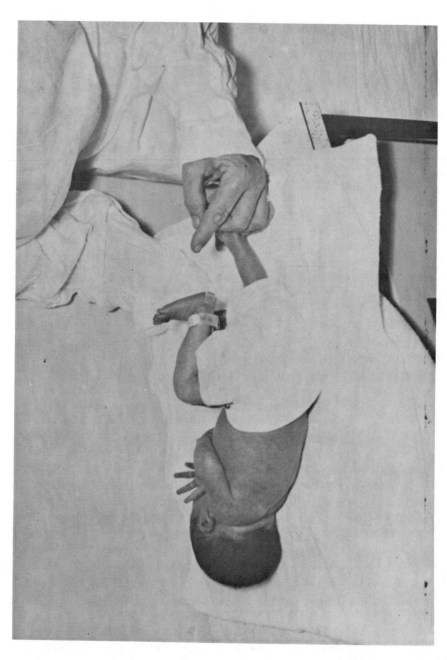

Fig. 14–1   Flexor withdrawal.

picking up a pencil, may be almost imperceivable as compared to the total body response of the newborn to a relatively simple stimulus.

The phylogenetically older reflexes and reactions mediated in sub-cortical centers are accommodated to higher integrated automatic adaptations to space and the visual tactile-proprioceptive assimilations, such as are seen in righting and equilibrium reactions. These form the background to perform voluntary gross and fine motor adaptations.[17,18,19] This process is responsible for, and the result of, the development of the CNS, and is basic to the CPM process.

The child is born on the apedal level. Reflexes and reactions can be observed when he is prone or supine lying and when he is held upright or inverted.[27,39]

The newborn is dominated by spinal and brain stem reflexes which are mediated at the sub-cortical level. The spinal reflexes, elicited up to two months of age, are phasic or movement reactions integrated at the spinal cord level in response to tactile stimulation. The response is observed in a part of the body and the result is a total flexing or extending of the part.[20,27,39] This first level of muscle activity is complete shortening of agonists and lengthening of antagonists.[34,42] The flexor withdrawal reflex (Fig. 14–1) is seen in the infant as a response to tactile stimulation.[20,27] Stimulation on the sole of the foot with the leg extended produces a complete flexion of the extremity. This total response of withdrawal is a form of protection from environmental contact. The infant is assimilating the tactile stimulus and he directs his body accommodations to withdrawal, which produces a total flexion pattern of the extremity. As an adult we must be able to perceive dangerous stimulation, such as fire, and withdraw from it. At this level the withdrawal is a highly integrated discriminatory response, but this response had its beginnings with the protective schema.

The crossed extension reflex (Fig. 14–2) involves the lower extremities bilaterally. This appears to be the beginning of integration of the two sides of the body. The stimulus which causes the reflexive flexion of one leg also causes extension of the opposite leg.[20] At this level the reflexes are a total non-discriminating reaction to the tactile stimulation. As the child develops, these reflexes are accommodated into a reflexive schema controlled by higher central nervous system centers and the response becomes adapted and more discriminating. For example, stepping on an object such as a pebble causes the foot to dorsiflex with minimal knee and hip flexion, and at the same time the extensors of the opposite leg are stimulated to maintain balance. This response resembles the crossed extension reflex which has been assimilated into the system, and thus the body accommodates with an appropriate motor response. The person adapts to his environment.

Tactile stimulation of the hand of the newborn first results in an avoiding response. This response is not completely adapted until 5 or 6

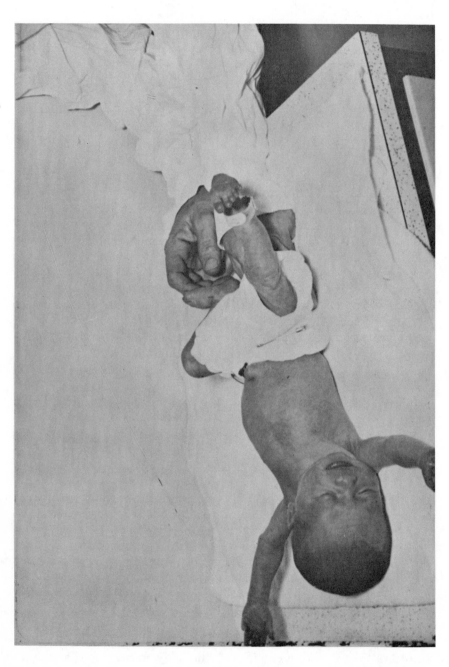

Fig. 14-2 Crossed extension.

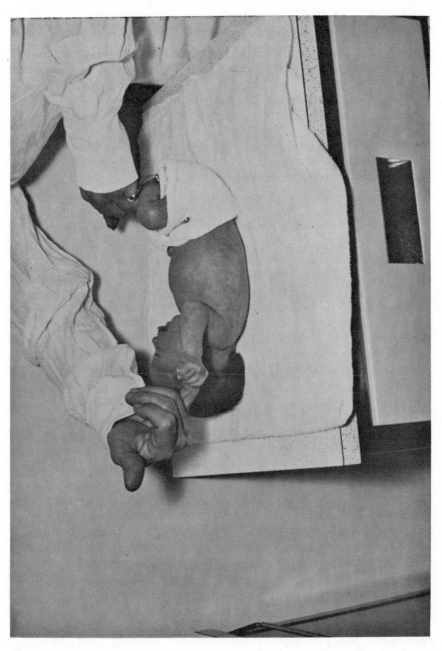

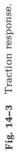

Fig. 14-3   Traction response.

years of age, as evidenced by the pre-school child who is noted to demonstrate over-abduction of the fingers and exaggerated dorsiflexion of the hand as it approaches an object.[46,47] However, the adaptation of avoidance begins shortly after birth and leads ultimately to prehension. It begins with the traction response which can be elicited by pulling on the infant's upper extremity, which induces strong flexion in all joints. By 1 month of age, tactile stimulation on the hand will cause this same traction response (Fig. 14–3). This is the assimilation of a new stimulus to a prior response. By 2 months stimulation between the thumb and index finger will cause flexion and adduction of these digits. It is the beginning of the grasp reflex, the accommodation of a prior motor adaptation to a new stimulus.[45,46]

Although these early reflex and motor schemas involve flexion patterns primarily, it is noted that the assimilation-accommodation process is present. The appearance of the extension reflexes results in increased resistance to passive flexion of the extremities involved. It is the beginning of the proprioceptive stretch reflex and a forerunner to the extensor tone necessary for sitting and standing.[45,46] These flexion-extension reflexes of the lower extremity also provide the basis of reciprocal innervation for walking on the bipedal level. Early automatic walking, the accommodation to tactile-proprioceptive assimilation, is observed in the newborn held in the upright position.[1] The newborn makes other postural accommodations to space with primary standing in the upright position, increased flexion in the inverted position, and by the tonic labyrinthine reaction in prone and supine lying.[18]

As the reflexes are repeated, due to the fundamental tendency for nerve cells to repeat an activity, the reaction is consolidated and stabilized. However, this repetition also provides the necessary condition for change. For example, Spitz describes the rooting reflex and its relation to the transition from tactile to proprioceptive response.[43] The rooting reflex is elicited by tactile stimulation of the external part of the mouth, and the response is rotation of the head toward the stimulus, followed by a snapping of the mouth. In the nursing infant, this response leads to taking the nipple into the mouth. Repetition of this tactile stimulus-response mechanism also continually stimulates the neck proprioceptors, providing a condition for change so that head rotation is accommodated to respond to proprioceptive stimuli from the neck and elicit the postural responses that are assimilated at the brain stem level (Fig. 14–4).[17,43,45]

The brain stem reactions are static postural reactions.[27] The response to a stimulus is a change in the distribution of muscle tone throughout the body as the result of a change in the position of the head or of the body in space.[20,27,45] It is this proprioceptive stimulus and response that is of greatest importance. These reactions are normal in many children up to 4 to 6 months of age.[20]

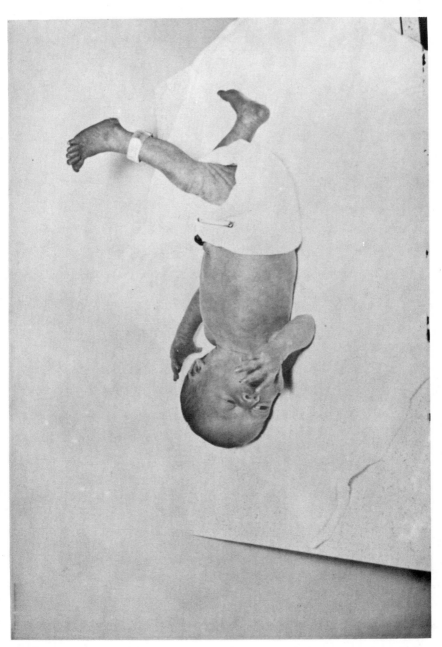

Fig. 14–4 Rooting accommodating to elicit a postural response.

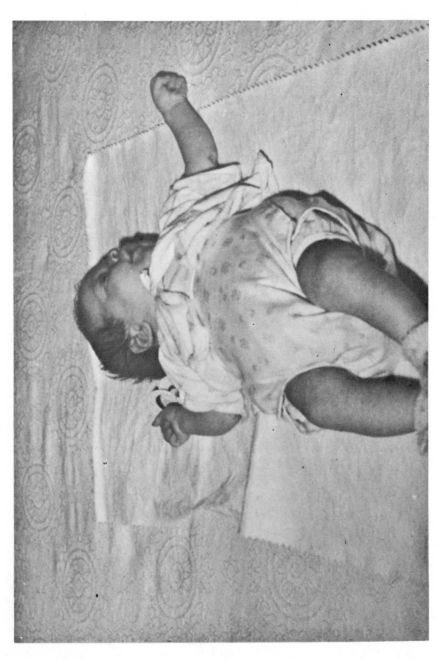

Fig. 14-5 Asymmetrical tonic neck.

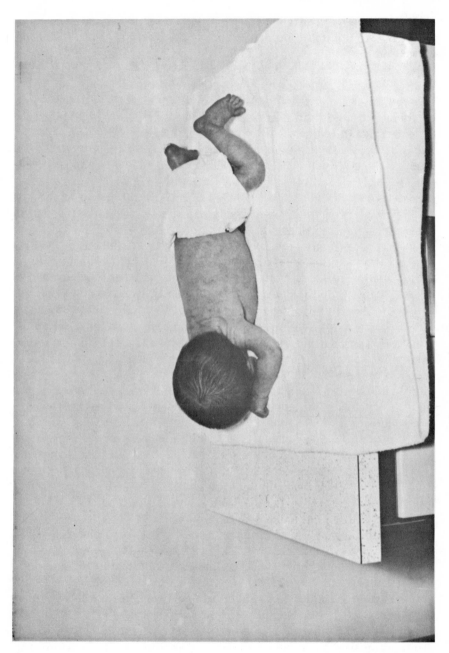

Fig. 14-6   Tonic labyrinthine – prone.

First is the asymmetrical tonic neck reaction (Fig. 14–5); turning the head and stimulating the neck proprioceptors results in extension of the extremities on the face side and flexion of the limbs on the skull side. The symmetrical tonic neck reaction is demonstrated by flexing the neck. The result is flexion of upper extremities and extension of the lower extremities. Extension of the neck elicits the opposite extension of upper extremities and flexion of lower extremities. The tonic labyrinthine reaction is the result of the position of the body in space. The stimulus is to the vestibular mechanism and the response is extensor tone in the supine position and flexor tone in the prone position (Fig. 14–6).[20,27]

Also included among the brainstem reactions are the negative and positive supporting reactions.[20,27] These reactions are adapted from the segmental spinal responses to stimulation on the sole of the foot, but now encompass a more total body response. The infant held in the upright position and lowered toward the floor will demonstrate more controlled flexion of the lower extremities — the shortening range of the flexors. This is modified by the appearance of extension or positive supporting reaction (Fig. 14–7). The child is held in the same position, but now, when the forefoot touches the supporting surface, stimulation to the proprioceptors from stretch of intrinsic foot musculature results in extension of the hips, knees and ankles and the infant "stands" on his toes.[20,27] Again, the stretch reflex becomes evident to inhibit the flexion and facilitate total extension in a gross pattern. This is a precursor to the normal extension for bipedal activities. In later development a minimal stimulus on the foot will produce appropriate extension for balance and interact with flexion for reciprocation.

Throughout the brain stem level, it is evident that the proprioceptive stimulus facilitates the extensor stretch reflex and inhibits the primitive flexor patterns; the extended limbs in the asymmetrical tonic neck reflex, the lower extremities in the positive supporting reaction, and the whole body in the tonic labyrinthine reflex.[20,27]

The infant begins to reach out reflexively into space. The true grasp reflex has developed so that a distally moving contact stimulus to the medial part of the palm produces a flexion and adduction of the fingers which is sustained when they are pulled on (Fig. 14–8). As this reflex becomes fully developed, the traction response can no longer be obtained.[46,47] The predominant muscle activity is still shortening of the agonists and lengthening of the antagonists. The gross motor pattern of withdrawal is accommodated by the postural reflexive extension. Head raising in the prone position begins to appear. It is evidence of early cephalocaudal development and inhibition of the tonic labyrinthine flexion in prone position by intermittent neck extension.

It is suggested that at this level of development the child is assimilating his environmental contacts and his body is accommodating with

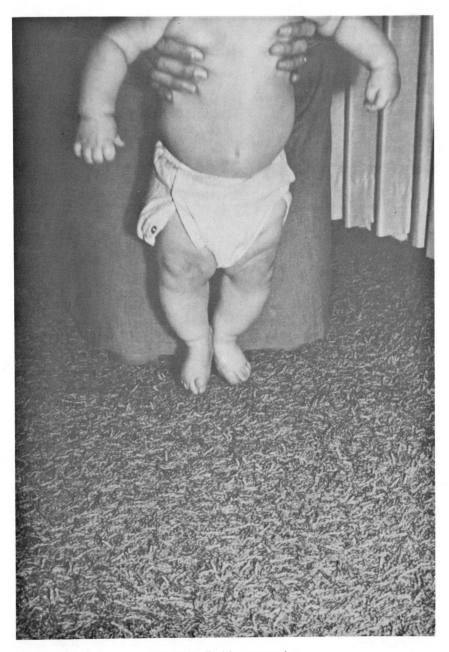

Fig. 14–7   Positive supporting.

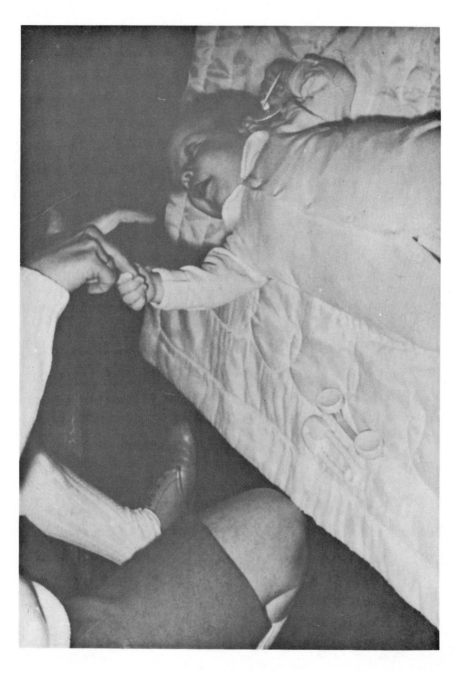

Fig. 14-8 Grasp reflex.

certain motor acts. This level of adaptation must be completely assimilated into the system to the point of losing its original identity, in order to allow the body to accommodate voluntarily to the environment it is attempting to assimilate. If not, the child cannot formulate new cognitive structures. For example, if the traction response has not lost its original identity a child will accommodate to a spoon placed in his hand by flexing his entire arm, or flexor tone will predominate resulting in poor motor accommodations. When the TNR has not been incorporated into the system the child will extend his arm or extensor tone will predominate each time his head turns. This mode of body accommodation would not permit a hand to mouth pattern necessary for self feeding.

It is necessary to assess the presence or absence of these reflexes and reactions and their control over body movement in order to effectively treat a CPM dysfunction. If residual effects of these spinal and brain stem patterns influence the body accommodations, treatment must focus on aiding the person to adapt to the tactile and proprioceptive environment by inhibiting the response of the reflex, and facilitating a higher level of response.

Before a meaningful response can be made from the tactile stimulation, a person must discriminate stimuli. Discrimination develops as the primitive protective responses become inhibited. The work of Ayres, Rood and others, stresses that this inhibition comes about as a result of touch-pressure.[5,7,42] In essence, the adaptation of touch-pressure leads to discriminatory structures. If a body surface cannot discriminate tactile stimulation, a person will continue with a form of the protective response as opposed to a discriminatory one; he withdraws from the stimuli, protects himself, as seen in the flight-like behavior in hyperactivity.[57] When the protective response is present in the older child or adult, it may indicate that his tactile perception is influenced by primitive behavior. The presence of the protective schema will interfere with higher level skills. Thus, the development of discrimination would be indicated before the child could be expected to accomplish higher level skills.

The tactile and proprioceptive receptors are active in the prenatal period, and at birth the neonate experiences a "complete separation" from his mother's body. The baby indicates a "need to feel"; this is best gratified through the baby's relationship with his mother. This contact is a form of touch-pressure which is necessary for the inhibition of protection. The baby receives the touch-pressure contact with the mother's body when he is held, wrapped in a blanket, being fed and generally tended by the mother. This form of inhibition is associated with a constant visual stimuli for the baby (that of the mother's face). The baby is adapting to his environment and the integration of tactile, proprioceptive, and visual assimilation with motor accommodations is present.

The newborn displays anxiety when his clothes are removed. He cries with discomfort and his clutched hands wave frantically in the air. This is an anxiety created by the baby's first experience of space. The baby learns to cope with space as he begins his conscious awareness of the body.[43] The adaptation of the sensory stimuli and co-contraction of the muscles lead to the beginnings of body awareness. The proprioceptive messages arising from the muscles, joints and from the labyrinth give the baby the assimilation of joint position, movement and balance. In the neonatal period the static postural reactions effect changes of muscle tone in the body by stimulating the labyrinths (change position of head and body in space as described in the tonic labyrinthine and supporting reactions) or by stimulating the proprioceptors of the neck (head in relation to body as described in the asymmetrical and symmetrical tonic neck reactions). It is suggested that

CHART 14-3

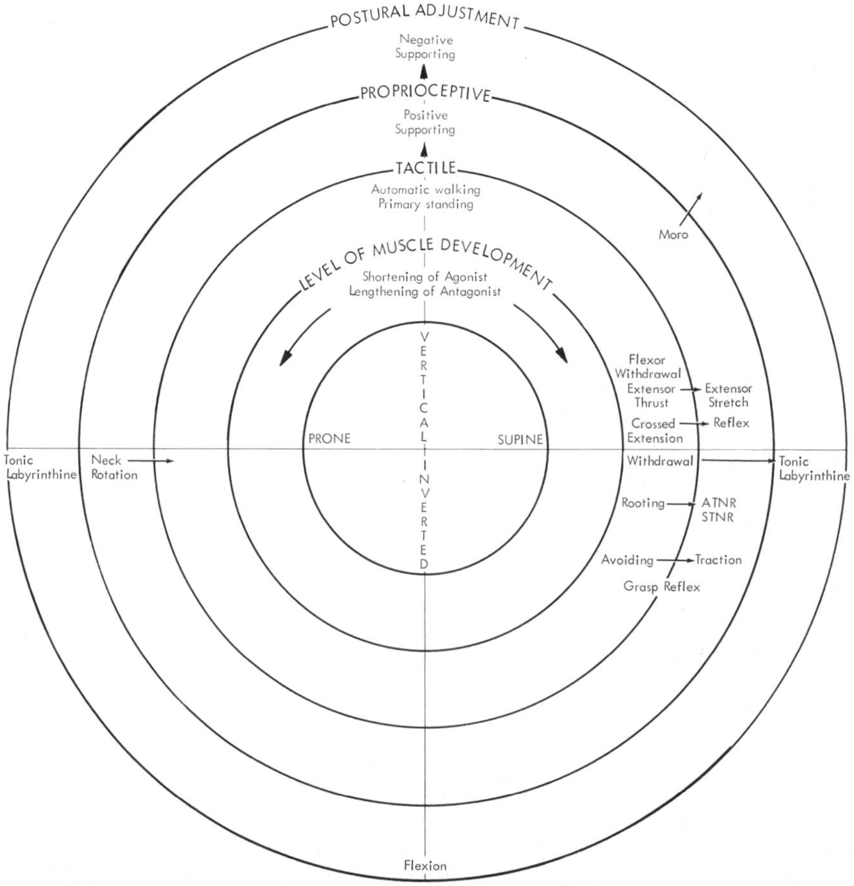

POSTURAL ADJUSTMENT

Negative
Supporting

PROPRIOCEPTIVE

Positive
Supporting

TACTILE

Automatic walking
Primary standing

Moro

LEVEL OF MUSCLE DEVELOPMENT

Shortening of Agonist
Lengthening of Antagonist

VERTICAL INVERTED

PRONE   SUPINE

Flexor
Withdrawal
Extensor ——► Extensor
Thrust   Stretch

Crossed ——► Reflex
Extension

Tonic
Labyrinthine | Neck —► Rotation

Withdrawal ———► Tonic Labyrinthine

Rooting —► ATNR STNR

Avoiding —► Traction

Grasp Reflex

Flexion

these tonic neck and tonic labyrinthine reactions are basic to proprioceptive perception, and the foundation for the formation of the body schema.

Body schema is a neurophysiological function resulting in a cognitive structure of the different anatomical parts of the body and their relationship to space.[5] In order to cope with the anxiety producing element of space, an infant depends upon the knowledge of his body. The body serves as the reference point from which one interacts with the environment. The interaction with the environment is also dependent upon praxis or the ability to motor plan, which is defined as the determination of the type and sequence of motor accommodations.[5] Praxis and body schema are closely associated and dependent upon each other.

As the spiralling continuum progresses, assimilation of new stimuli and body accommodation continues to add new information, and cognitive structures of body and praxis schema emerge until motor skill is present.

In summary, the apedal level evolves into the development of body schema and praxis which results from the adaptation of tactile, proprioceptive, vestibular and visual impulses arising from reflexive and purposeful motor accommodations (Chart 14–3).

The development of righting reactions is necessary for the child to attain the quadrupedal level. These reactions are mediated in the midbrain and interact with each other toward establishing the normal relation of head and body to each other and to space.[20,27] They begin as the adaptation of the earlier tactile and proprioceptive assimilation-accommodation and reach maximum effect at about 10 to 12 months of age. At this level tactile stimulation again assumes importance in the form of body contact with the environment and the interdependent relationship between tactile and proprioceptive assimilation-accommodation becomes more apparent.

The infant first raises his head momentarily in the prone position (Fig. 14–9).[20,27] On the brain stem level, the postural tonic labyrinthine reflex was elicited from the infant in prone position. This increasing stimulation of the upper chest, the tactile body contact with the environment, causes body righting, acting on the head and the head is raised to assume a new position in space.[17]

During the same stage of development, the infant in supine position has previously responded to head rotation with an asymmetrical tonic neck reflex. Repetition of this schema increases the tactile body contact on the upper back on the face side, and the former asymmetrical postural response is accommodated to neck righting so that rotation of the head causes the infant to roll over as his whole body follows the head (Fig. 14–10). The gross motor schema expands from this cephalic initiation. As the infant receives increasing tactile stimulation in prone,

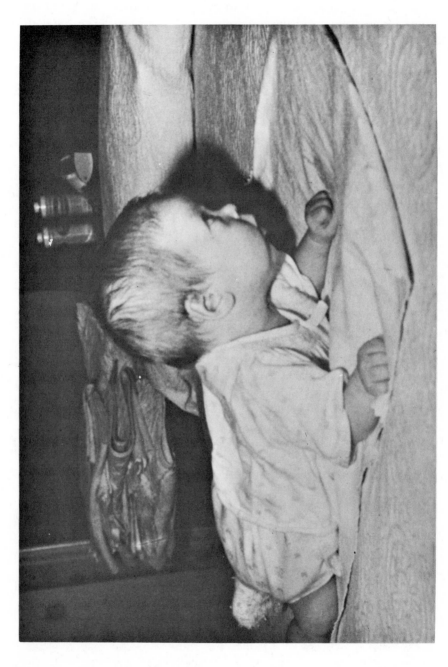

Fig. 14-9   Head raising, prone

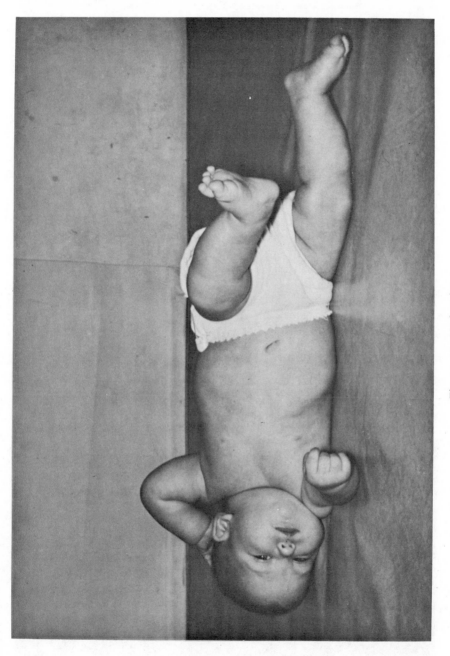

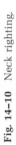

Fig. 14-10   Neck righting.

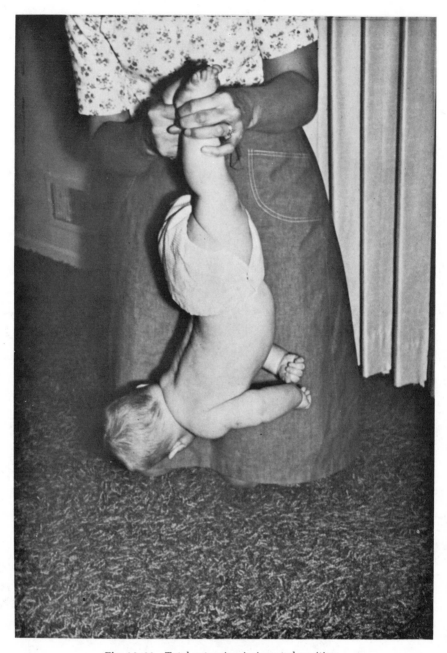

Fig. 14–11   Total extension in inverted position.

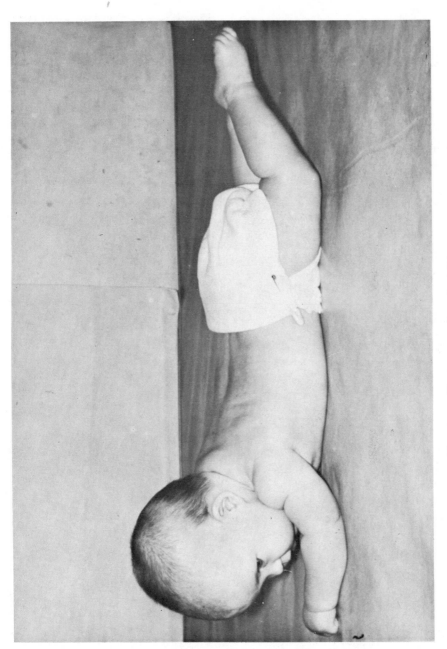

Fig. 14-12 Pivot prone motor adaptation.

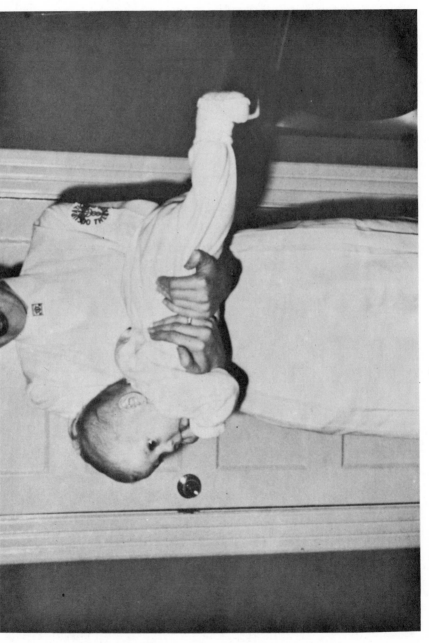

Fig. 14-12. Landau reflex

he raises his head for longer periods of time and lifts his upper trunk off the supporting surface and the body attempts to align itself with the new head position.[17]

Increasing activation of the extensors on the first level of muscle activity is further facilitated as the child is suspended in the inverted position (Fig. 14-11). He assumes this extended position of the neck, trunk, and hips and the characteristic gross motor schema is the pivot prone position (Fig. 14-12). Pivot prone is similar to the Laudau reflex which is not completely adapted until 2 years of age (Fig. 14-13). The response is elicited by holding the child suspended in the prone position and extension of the neck activates the proprioceptors and causes extension of the trunk and lower extremities. The pivot prone is modified by the second level of muscle activity — co-contraction.[33-42]

Co-contraction begins with the neck muscles, and can only emerge after complete adaptation of the labyrinthine reflex acting on the head, which began in prone head raising.

The blindfolded child is suspended in prone, or supine, or tipped laterally and will right his head to a vertical position in relation to the floor. All muscles of the neck are activated in shortening and lengthening. They are now prepared to act simultaneously and contract around the joint to stabilize it. In the prone position, the infant can adapt the head to align with the extended trunk. His head is free to move in all directions without going through the complete range of motion. As the co-contraction schema progresses to include the shoulders, he maintains the on-elbows position. In this position, he develops a new gross motor schema and the initiation of the third level of muscle activity; heavy work motion superimposed on co-contraction. The infant uses his upper extremities to pull his body forward and push it back, thereby projecting his whole body into space (Fig. 14-14). The distal ends, in this case the elbows, are fixed and the shoulders move from the co-contracted position. When co-contraction of the trunk develops, he reacts to the inverted suspension with deliberate flexion of the neck, trunk and hips, in an attempt to hold his thighs with his hands.[39] This is an adaptation of the earlier total flexion pattern.

The infant's rolling pattern is also accommodating. Previously, the stimulation on the body caused it to turn as a whole. Now the stimulus causes one segment to reach at a time in the body-righting-on-body reaction (Fig. 14-15).[27] The important element is the rotation between body parts and the proprioceptive effect upon each other. The head and body constantly strive to maintain their normal alignment through adaptations to all the stimuli received. This rotation also precedes the amphibian reaction which is preliminary to assuming the quadrupedal level. The amphibian (Fig. 14-16) is elicited by stimulating the pelvic area of a prone lying child. He will react by lifting his head and flexing

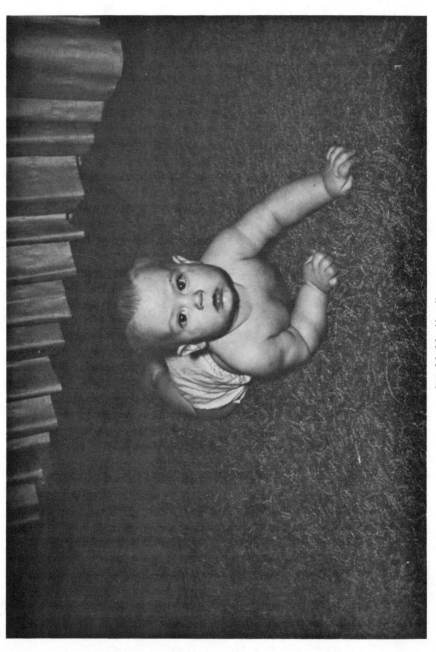

Fig. 14-14   On-elbows.

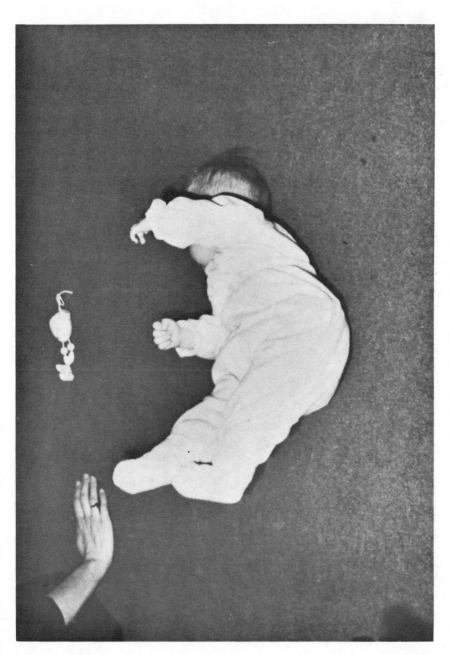

Fig. 14-15 Body-righting-on-body reaction.

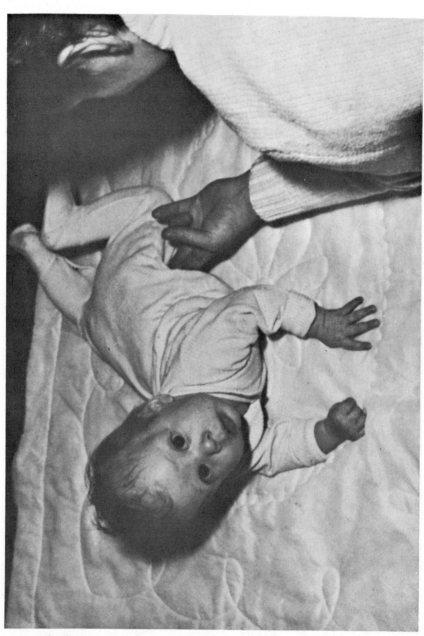

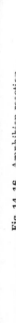

Fig. 14-16. Amphibian reaction.

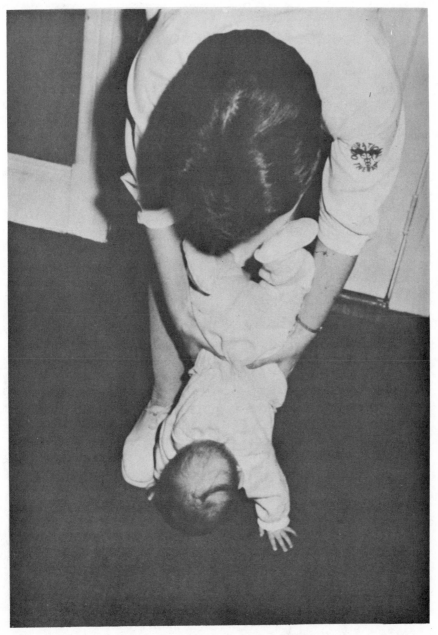

Fig. 14–17   Protective extensor thrust.

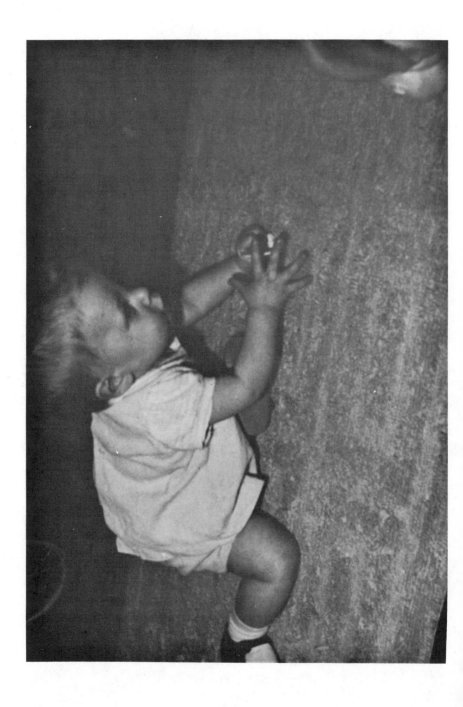

the arm and flexing and abducting the leg on the side stimulated.[27] Some children will adapt this amphibian reaction to moving back and forth in prone and begin to facilitate reciprocal, coordinated movements in all four extremities. In all children, it precedes assuming the all-fours position, and some adapt it to the rotation pattern in body righting so that turning supine to prone and assuming crawling become one coordinated schema.

Another reaction is also developing (Fig. 14–17), the protective extensor thrust.[17,25,26,27] The child suspended in the inverted position immediately extends his arms toward the floor to protect himself. This reaction is accommodated to the crawling position as the child now supports himself with upper extremities extended. Once the child assumes the quadrupedal position, he frequently rocks back and forth, re-emphasizing and expanding the heavy work motion superimposed on co-contraction.[34,42] This time the distal fixed ends are the hands and knees. The neck, trunk and elbows are reinforcing their co-contraction schema in this new position.

Throughout these stages of rapid development, the child is perceiving more and more of the stimuli from the environment and attempts to move toward it. In attempting to move, he begins to develop the last level of muscle activity, that of skill.[34,42] The beginning of skill occurs when the distal end is free to move because all the more proximal joints are stabilized. The child who wishes to project himself into space can lift his hand to initiate it and the reciprocal motion develops (Fig. 14–18).

From the all-fours position, the child can rotate body parts in sequence and assume the sitting position. At this level, he must use complete rotation in prone, up on all fours and then into sitting; he cannot yet assume sitting from a supine position (Figs. 14–19 through 14–23).[14-19,20,21,22,23]

The child at this level of rapid development has the opportunity to view his environment from different positions and is beginning to explore it. His righting reactions in response to position in space assimilate the new visual perceptions and his adjustment to space accommodates both labyrinth and visual stimuli. The optical righting reaction is elicited by the same positions as the labyrinthine righting reaction, but no blindfold is used.[27] The visual orientation represents cortical participation and becomes more significant at this level.

Throughout this period when the child projects himself more into space and is more affected by visual perceptions, his hand activity changes significantly. The grasp reflex is adapted to the crude palmar grasp by 4 to 5 months of age (Fig. 14–24). Further adaptation occurs as tactile stimulation on the medial side of the hand causes some supination and initiates an orienting response (Fig. 14–25). It is the instinctive

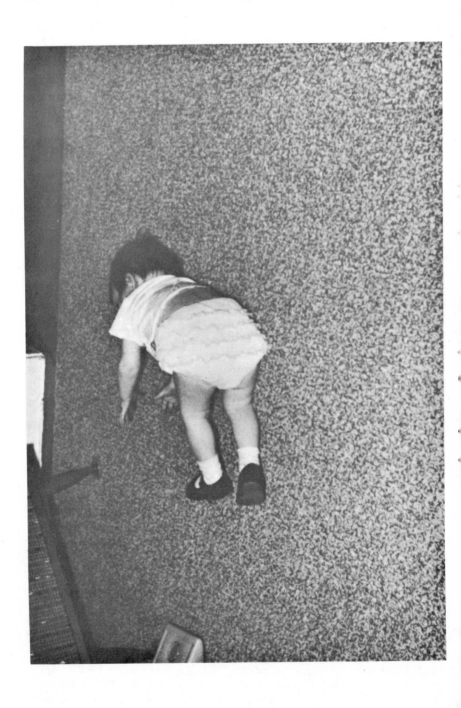

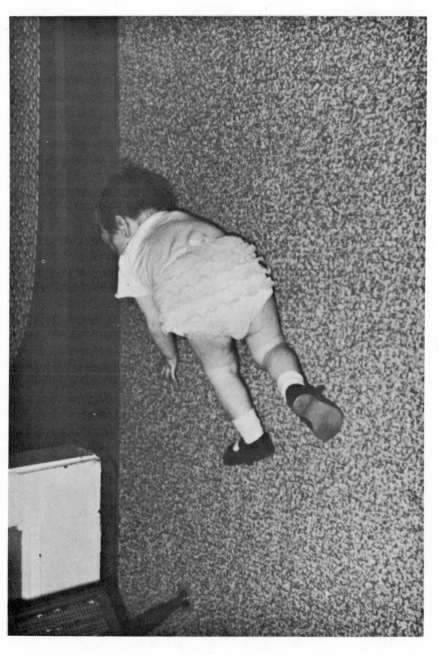

Fig. 14–20

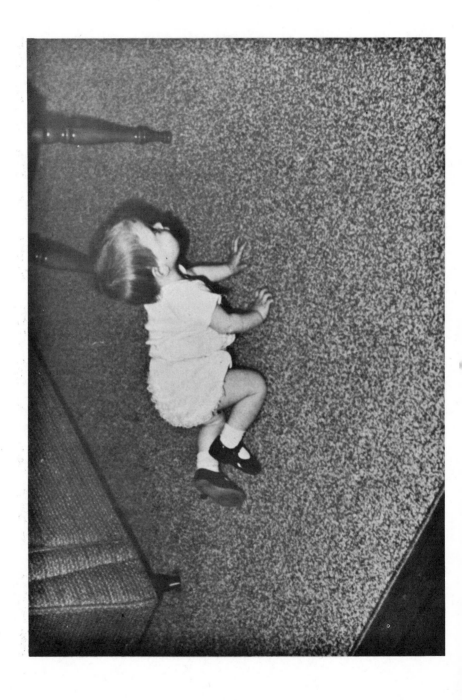

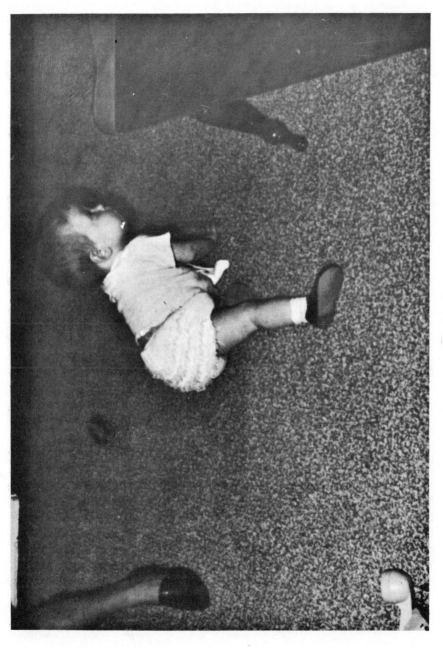

Fig. 14-22

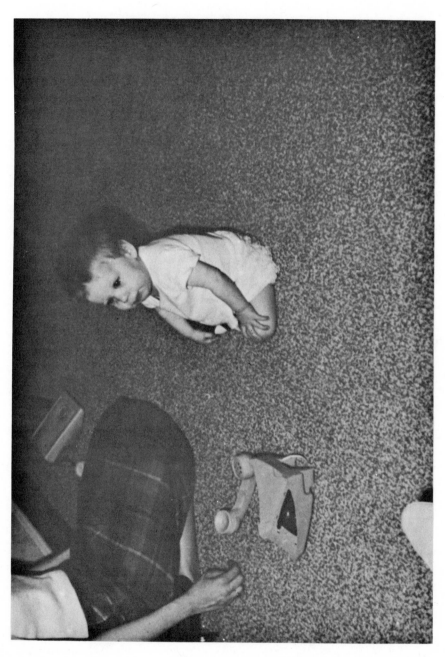

Fig. 14-23

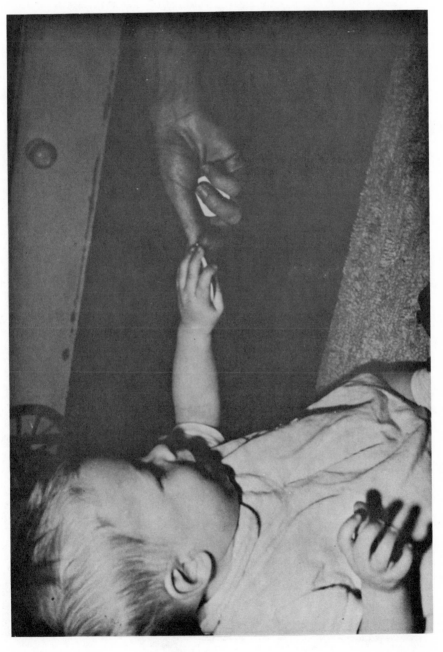

Fig. 14-24 Crude palmar grasp.

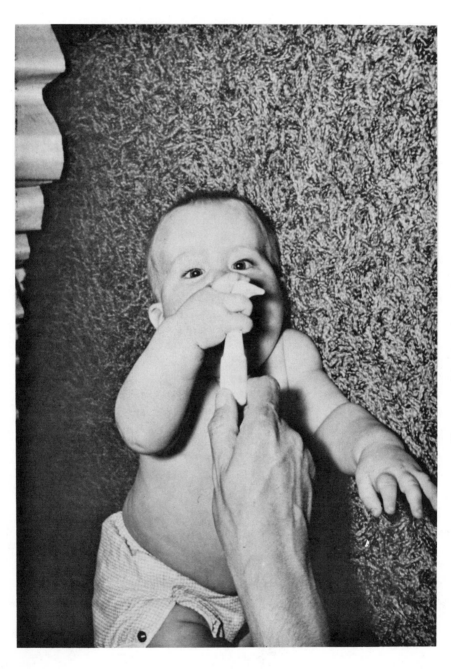

Fig. 14-25 Initiation of orienting response.

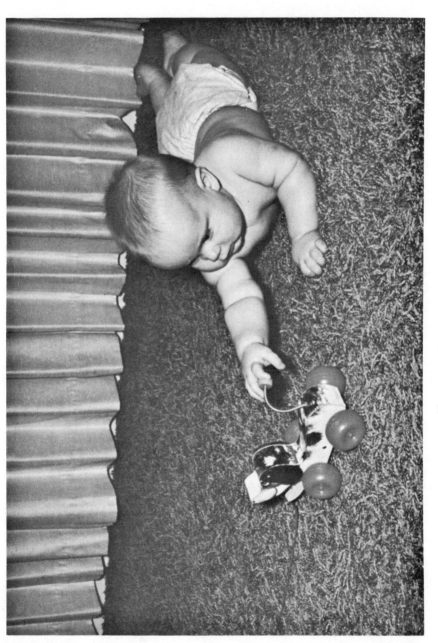

Fig. 14–26 Groping after stimulus.

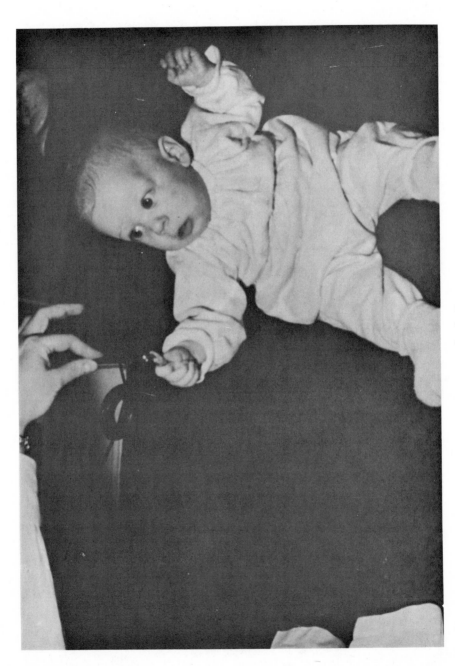

Fig. 14-27   Instinctive grasp.

grasp reaction. The child begins to grope after a retreating stimulus (Fig. 14-26). By 8 to 10 months of age, he not only gropes after the stimulus, but orients to it and grasps it (Fig. 14-27). The instinctive grasp reaction accommodates the palmar grasp toward the development of supination. The child at this midbrain level has further enhanced his adaptation to space.

During the quadrupedal level, the child's occupations are concerned with continuing the development of body schema and praxis and the development of visual-spatial relationships. This phase is an important step in the development of form perception. The integration of proprioceptive and visual perception has new meaning. At this point in development, the child has built a foundation of information gained during the apedal phase. He calls upon these past experiences and integrates them with the adaptation-integration of righting. This total integration allows the child certain feelings and assumptions about his own body—how it relates to itself and how it relates to space. These experiences give the child the adaptation and integration needed for making sensory judgments about spatial relationships (i.e., up-down, on one side or the other, in front or behind). These concepts begin during his apedal days, but with the emergence of righting reactions he applies these concepts beyond himself. He can now relate to space by moving himself and objects within his environment.

Development of visual perception allows the visualization of objects as they are in motion and moved to a different position. Progression in the development of proprioception and tactile perception allows the child the experience of integrating his own body in motion and moving to a different position. This adds new dimensions of knowledge for form perception.

Perception of form relates to the assumptions we make about the tangible environment, the similarities and differences of the objects within the environment. This perception develops as the child manipulates objects, the tactile proprioceptive and visual impulses give him information about the shape, size, and texture of the object. As the object is in motion or moved to another position, the child perceives these changes by relating the object in space to himself (Fig. 14-28).

As the development of body to space is progressing, so is the development of the relationship of the body parts. This is the schema of body integration, the ability to integrate the right side of the body with the left side. In the sequential development of body integration, the adaptation of righting reactions, motor accommodations, and heavy work muscle activity leads to a schema of gross motor activity and the resultant bilateral body integration.

Sensory-motor accommodations of bilateral body integration such as patty-cake, pushing up on the elbows, rolling over, pivot prone,

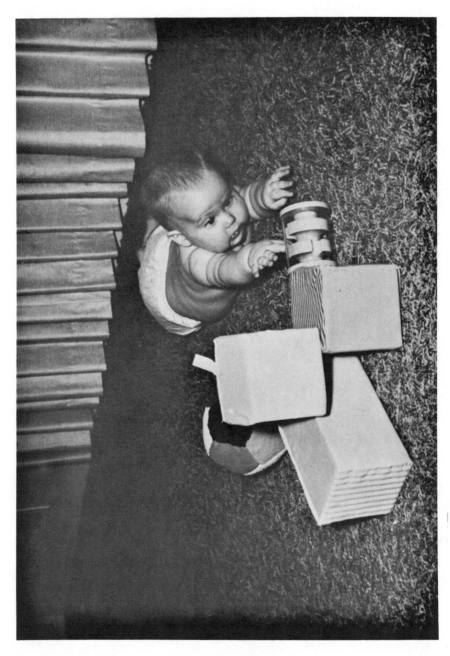

Fig. 14-28   Tactile, proprioceptive, and visual perception of the tangible environment.

CHART 14-4

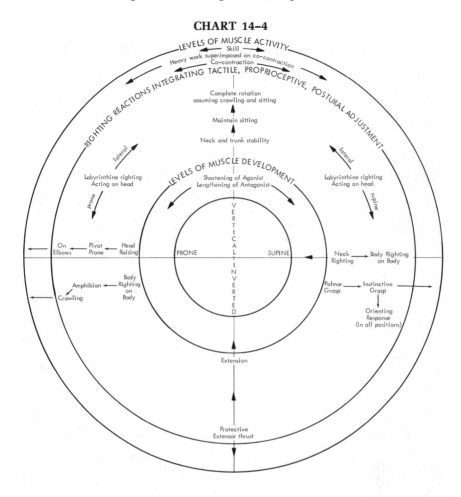

plus the manipulation and visual perception of objects gives the baby the necessary experience for establishing the perception of form and position in space.

In summary, the quadrupedal phase of development finds the emergence of righting reactions enabling the motor tasks of rolling, sitting, and getting on all fours. These righting reactions are likewise the precursor to the perceptual phenomenon of praxis, body integration, and the perception of form and spatial relationships (Chart 14-4).

Final adaptation-integration of reflex assimilation and motor accommodations occurs on the cortical level. The demands made upon any organism are in direct relationship to the response that organism makes to its environment. If the demands are simple, the behavior is simple; if the demands are complex, the behavior is correspondingly complex.

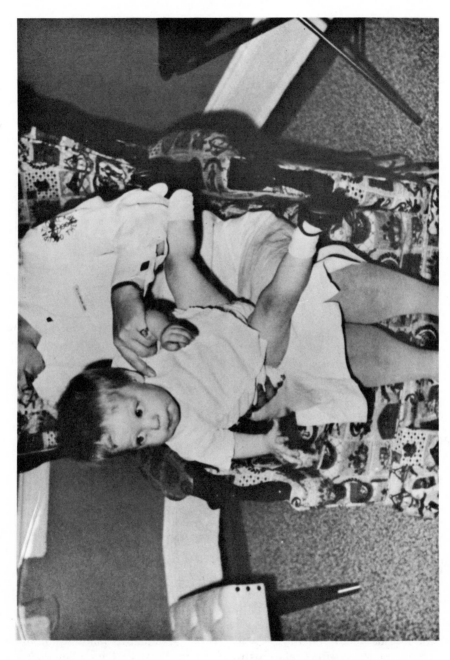

Fig. 14-29 Equilibrium reaction in sitting. (Note head and trunk righting, extended

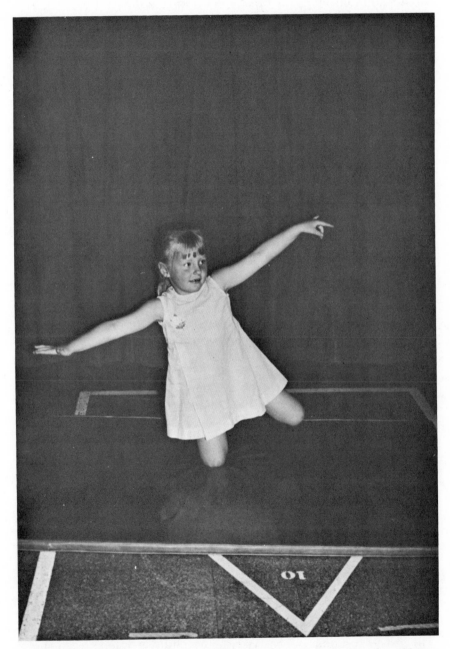

Fig. 14–30   Equilibrium reaction in kneel standing. (Note fully developed equilibrium reaction.)

As the child develops the bipedal level of standing and walking, running and jumping, the demands of a constantly changing environment require complex and flexible behavior. He must maintain his body alignment and balance against the forces of gravity as he moves about in space. To accomplish this he must develop equilibrium reactions.

Equilibrium reactions are responsible for body adaptation in response to a change in the center of gravity. They appear normally at about 6 months of age and continue throughout life.[27] The development of these reactions at each level is indicative of cortical accommodation of the phylogenetically older reactions (already described) and assimilation of new stimuli from the environment. They provide the balance necessary for the child to maintain each motor level and prepare him to proceed to the next motor level.[17,19]

Just as the stimuli that elicited brain-stem reactions were accommodated to righting reactions at the midbrain level, the stimulus that elicits righting reactions is accommodated to equilibrium reactions at the cortical level. It was noted in the discussion of midbrain development that when the tactile receptors and proprioceptors on one side of the body received increased stimulation and the vestibular mechanism was activated, a righting reaction occurred. The whole body usually responded by turning, sitting, or crawling. In order for the child to maintain these positions, it is not appropriate for a complete change of position to occur with each stimulus. The response must be accommodated into a more discriminatory reaction by the body and extremities so that the position can be maintained in spite of changes in the center of gravity. As the child maintains each position, he reinforces the appropriate level of muscle activity and is ready for the next step in sequential development.

An equilibrium reaction occurs when the center of gravity is changed, resulting in increased stimulation to the tactile receptors and proprioceptors on one side or area of the body, stimulation to the vestibular mechanism, as well as a change in the visual orientation to the environment. All these stimuli are mediated at the sub-cortical and cortical levels and the body responds not by turning toward the stimuli, but by pulling back to the original center of gravity and maintaining that position. The head and trunk right themselves toward vertical body alignment; the extremities toward the center extend and abduct to assist the trunk and bring more weight to the center; the opposite extremities may extend and abduct to prevent the midbrain righting reaction from emerging and to protect if the stimulus is strong (Fig. 14–29). This basic reaction is observed as the child maintains each motor schema: prone lying, supine lying, four-foot kneeling, and sitting.[17]

As he approaches the bipedal level, the reactions become more intricate because the area for stimulation and balance is more confined.

He assumes kneel-standing. With this, co-contraction and heavy work muscle patterns in the upright position begin to develop. An equilibrium reaction in this position provides the first experience in maintaining body weight on just one extremity—a necessity in walking (Fig. 14–30).[17] Kneeling-walking initiates reciprocation on the bipedal level.

The child stands, holds on, and bounces up and down. He experiments with rocking back and forth. He is developing a heavy work pattern superimposed on co-contraction. He sits down abruptly and gets up again. He is constantly assimilating this new body position to the environment. When the heavy work pattern is established, he is ready for skill movements forward into space. He is visually stimulated to move his body to another place and as he propels forward, he reciprocates in hopping steps similar to the earlier initiation of crawling, but this time to maintain upright body alignment. Now when he leans backward, a hopping step keeps him from sitting down, and sideways motion elicits a typical equilibrium reaction, or with increased stimulation, a cross-over hopping step.[17] The forerunner to hopping reactions is observed on the apedal level when the child is held upright and the tactile stimulation is over a wide area on the foot. On that level, the reaction is non-functional stepping. At the cortical level, the slightest stimulus on the foot from a change in position, integrated with the vestibular and visual stimuli, results in an accurate hopping step or balance reaction.[45,46,47]

Repetition of these reactions increases skill in the volitional walking pattern. The child develops intricate reciprocal innervation of all the musculature involved through the accommodation of the primitive spinal and brain stem reflexes that first facilitated these muscles and the adaptation of righting reactions that involved the body as a whole.

Skill is further developed in the upper extremity, too. Acquisition of the instinctive grasp reaction provided accurate projected movement of the hand in space. It accommodated with repetition into a pincer grasp: tactile stimulation to one digit causes flexion of that digit without inducing flexion of all digits (Fig. 14–31). Voluntary prehension and eye-hand coordination progress.[45,46,47]

Further adaptation-organization continues for many years; eye-hand coordination becomes more skillful; assuming a sitting position progresses from complete rotation (Fig. 14–32), to partial rotation (Fig. 14–33), to symmetrical sitting (Fig. 14–34) at 6 years of age. Jumping, skipping, running and hopping are added to the motor activities. The individual is flexible in his ever-changing environment. The basis for his responses began at birth.

In the bipedal stage, the child is expanding his motor planning skills and refining his body schema. Purposeful motor experiences are

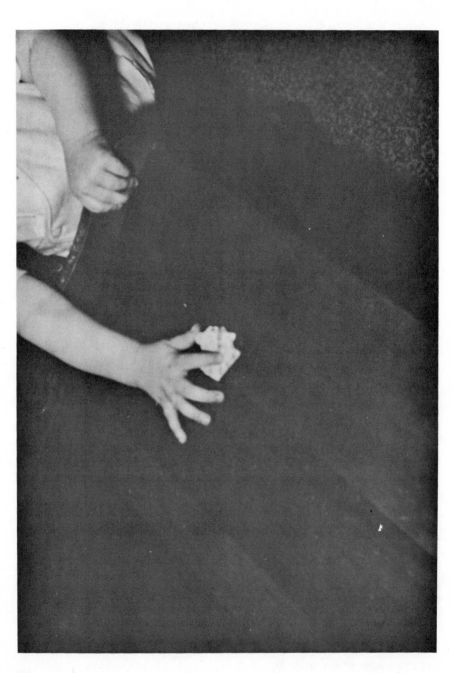

Fig. 14-31   Pincer grasp.

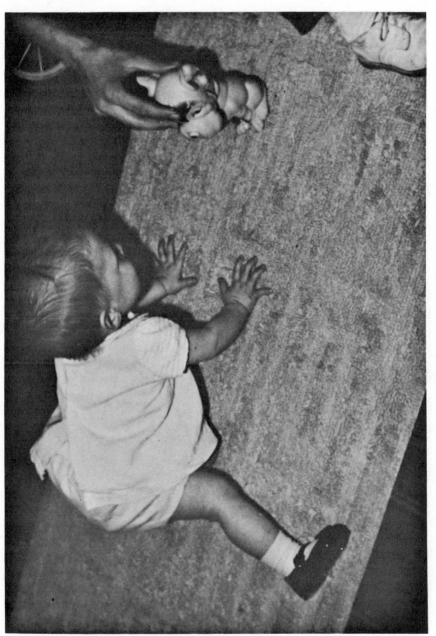

Fig. 14-32   Complete rotation.

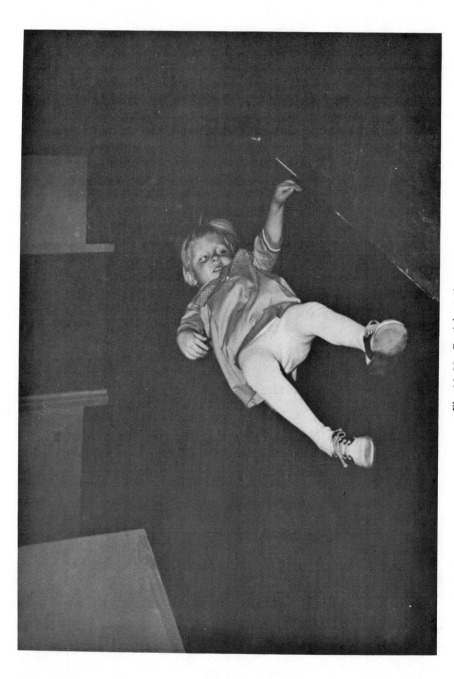

Fig. 14-33   Partial rotation.

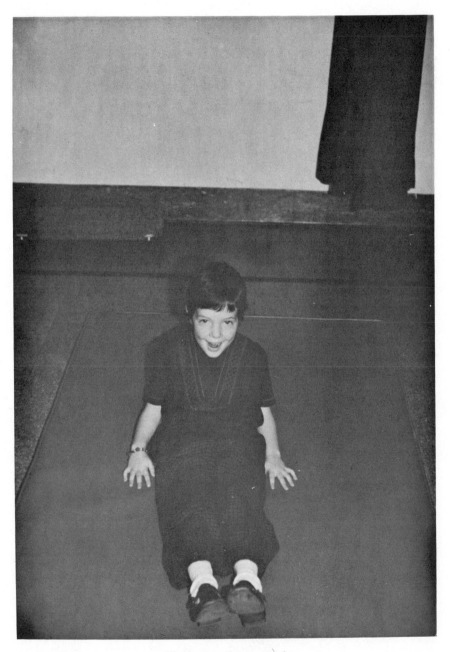

Fig. 14–34 Symmetrical.

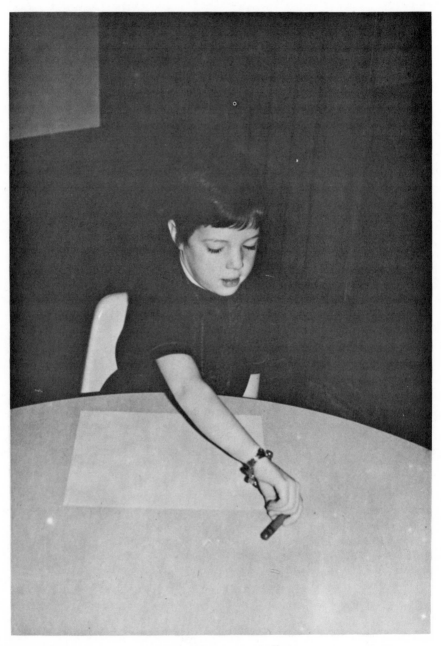

Fig. 14–35   Crossing midline.

amplified requiring further extension of the body in space. The body adapts to the change of the center of gravity and visuo-spatial perception takes on new meaning.

The motor tasks accomplished in the first two levels require simple motor planning. As the child learns to stand and walk, gross motor planning becomes more difficult. He jumps, hops, climbs, walks on rails, curbs, and joins in group games. These tasks require complicated gross motor planning and a well defined body schema which is the result of sensory-motor integration. The equilibrium reactions are the precursor to complicated motor planning and body integration. The forces of the right and left side of the body counteract each other in reciprocal motion and the body can maintain balance by the sensory-motor integration at the cortical and sub-cortical levels. Through this adaptation-integration a schema of reciprocal body integration evolves.

Although simple body integration is developing in the earlier stages, it is with the emergence of equilibrium reactions that man becomes coordinated in his reciprocation. With the scope of motor planning expanding, the equilibrium responses are refined and the child discovers that he can cross the midline of the body, function on the opposite side and still maintain balance (Fig. 14–35). It is with these experiences of balancing that the child confirms which side is dominant and which is recessive. There is no objective evidence to indicate the developmental sequence of dominance. It is hypothesized that with equilibrium reactions, dominance evolves in this sequence: (1) bilateral body integration; (2) reciprocal body integration; (3) body integration across the midline; (4) dominance and recessive body integration.

Equilibrium reactions have contributed to the refinement of gross motor skills and the child begins to focus upon fine motor planning. Prehension occupations begin to develop, such as small peg toys, crayons, scissors, pencils. The development of prehension occupations are dependent upon the adaptation-integration of tactile, proprioceptive, vestibular and visual stimuli, with the motor accommodation while manipulating objects.

Just as gross motor skills are dependent upon ontogenetically earlier adaptation-integration at the apedal level, so in fine motor skill, the grasp reflex being the foundation for the development of fine motor planning. Eye-hand skill requires fine motor planning and is the result of sensory-motor integration, assimilating and accommodating to the past experiences of tactile, proprioceptive, vestibular and visual stimuli.

In summary, the bipedal level adds new dimensions to praxis, visuospatial relationships, postural and body integration. Gross and fine motor skills become evident (Chart 14–5). The reflex and reaction accommodations that occur as a result of tactile, proprioceptive, vestib-

CHART 14-5

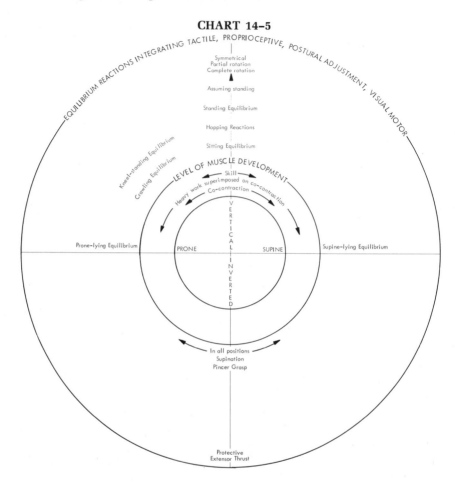

ular and visual assimilations provide the adaptations for sensory-motor integration. This spiralling process of (1) tactile assimilation and phasic accommodation with (2) proprioceptive assimilation and static accommodation with (3) vestibular-visual assimilation and postural-accommodations with (4) sensory-motor integration is summarized in Chart 14-6. In addition the corresponding muscle development is illustrated. Gross and fine motor skills are a result of this CPM sequential development.

The knowledge of the reflexes and reactions enables the occupational therapist to evaluate the adaptation process of his patients by analyzing the influence that each reflex and reaction has upon his patient's postural and movement accommodations.

CHART 14-6

LEVELS	REFLEX-REACTION	MUSCLE DEVELOPMENT
Tactile assimilation with phasic accommodation	1. Rooting 2. Sucking 3. Avoidance 4. Flexor withdrawal 5. Crossed extension 6. Automatic walking 7. Extensor thrust 8. Traction	Complete lengthening and shortening of agonist and antagonist
Proprioceptive assimilation with static accommodation	9. Grasp 10. Postural inversion-flexion 11. Asymmetrical tonic neck 12. Symmetrical tonic neck 13. Tonic labyrinthine 14. Postural inversion-extension	Co-contraction
Vestibular assimilation with postural accommodation	15. Supporting reactions 16. Righting reactions 17. Orienting response 18. Equilibrium reactions	Heavy work superimposed on Co-contraction
Sensory-motor integration	← →	Skill

The motor accommodations seen are a result of the combination of reflexes and reactions occurring simultaneously. Therefore, isolated reflexes and reactions are generally not seen with CPM patients, but patterns of the adaptation process which reoccur in the same circumstances can be traced to the influence of specific reflexes and reactions. With CPM dysfunction the therapist may identify only traces of the typical reflex or reaction by their influence upon the muscle tone and the motor planning patterns.[18]

In the discussion of CPM development emphasis thus far has been placed on the sensory-motor period from infancy, where all seems to be protective and is total body responses, to 5 to 6 years of life, when the child is managing his environment with greater adaptation and organization.

With the maturation of the CNS there is additional control, but not substitute control for integration. The cerebral hemispheres continue to maintain a dependence upon lower structures; the spinal cord, brain stem, and midbrain.[3,40] There can be efficient cortical integration only when the adaptations of the lower structures are well organized. This is a basic principle underlying occupational therapy for motor accommodation.

A second principle stressed in the above discussion is that of inter-sensory integration. This is the process of associating the sensory information from different senses.[15] Of particular significance is the integration of the visual assimilations with tactile, proprioceptive and vestibular stimuli[3] which becomes so evident in the quadrupedal level.

The developmental trends seen during this sensory-motor period (0 to 6 years) are important for the occupational therapist's contribution to the evaluation-treatment of patients with CPM dysfunction. It is on the sensory-motor process that the occupational therapist can best focus his attention. Deviations in development during this period influence the CPM performance in the post sensory-motor period, ages 6 to 11.[16,29]

It is this period in which a large body of research regarding perception and theories of the CPM process has been established.[1,36,38] However, factual knowledge regarding development must still be considered provisional.

The work of Ayres has given the occupational therapist scientific data on which to base his evaluation and treatment procedures.[4,5,6] Her factor analytic study revealed five significant factors associated with perceptual-motor dysfunction: (1) Apraxia—the inability to motor plan; (2) Dysfunction of postural and body integration—the inability to integrate the parts of the body and their relationships; (3) Dysfunction of visual form and spatial relationships—the inability to perceive visually forms and their spatial relationships, such as up, down, right, left; (4) Dysfunction of visual figure ground—the inability to distinguish and identify superimposed and embedded figures; (5) Tactile defensiveness—inability to discriminate tactile stimuli and hence the body accommodates with a protective response.[4]

The factors of apraxia, postural and body integration and tactile defensiveness are directly related to the sensory-motor period; the other factors are highly influenced by the integration of the tactile, proprioceptive, vestibular and visual assimilation and the motor accommodations. Ayres suggests that a change in neurological integration may aid a person to respond to educational procedures.[3]

Studies have indicated the necessity to consider the individual perceptual modalities and not to consider the combined modalities as one gross conglomerate perceptual picture.[38] The perceptual modalities with which the occupational therapist must be concerned are (1) tactile, (2) proprioceptive-vestibular, and (3) visual. Although auditory perception is an important modality in the CPM process the occupational therapist is not trained in this area. He must, however, have an understanding of the auditory process and its influence upon CPM behavior.

Throughout the post sensory-motor period the development of these modalities is not at the same rate with any given age span. There is a divergence of performance of the perceptual modalities with normal children.[38] For example, the 5 and 6 year old may be concerned with the development of his tactile-proprioceptive and vestibular perception, where the rate of development may be rapid. In contrast, there may be less growth in the visual and auditory areas. From 7 to 11 there appears to be more growth with the visual and auditory modalities and less growth with the somesthetic perceptions.[38]

During this post sensory-motor period the child continues to develop and refine his perceptual and motor skills and to integrate these with the formation of cognitive structures. The development of standardized tests has indicated the child's growth with tactile discrimination of finger gnosis, two point discrimination, identification of a moving stimulus on the skin (graphesthesia) and the identification of forms placed in the hand.[10,19,38]

The identification of proprioceptive development has been assessed primarily by the proprioceptive use in body movements, such as is seen in the imitation of body gestures,[11,14,38] with the manipulation of forms and with kinesthetic memory.[9,38] There are no standardized instruments that have stressed the development of vestibular functions during the post sensory-motor period. The result of vestibular influence is seen with the child's imitation of body gestures, postural adjustments and acquisition of equilibrium reactions.[26]

It is suggested that the child first visually recognizes shapes, sizes and forms. He then analyzes the spatial relationships of the components and the superimposed and embedded figures. Thirdly, he develops an ability to synthesize the visual stimuli (putting the parts together to form a total gestalt).[38]

Frostig has developed a classification for visual perceptions. Her work indicates an ability for: (1) form constancy or the identification of a form regardless of its size or placement within symbols; (2) figure ground — the recognition of forms hidden within a gestalt; (3) position in space — the identification of a position of a form (up, down; right side, left side); (4) spatial relations — the recognition of form relationships in the spatial areas; (5) eye-motor coordination — the visual-motor ability of directing the motor planning of the arm when using a pencil.[30]

Tests of Ayres,[9] Beery,[13] and Bender[14] have also contributed to our knowledge of the development of visual-motor integration. These test batteries clearly indicate the continued growth process of visual-motor integration during the 7 to 11 year age span.

Although the occupational therapist is usually not responsible for the assessment and treatment of auditory perception it is important to have some understanding of this phenomenon. Wepman[51] and Kirk[36] have developed instruments that have suggested developmental trends for auditory perceptions. A child must develop an ability to discriminate sounds: the bell from the drum, the "b" from the "d", pen from pin; in order to comprehend his auditory environment. He must not only be aware of the sound, but he must also be able to focus on a sound that is pertinent to a given situation. This ability is likened to figure-ground or being able to pick out and focus on the pertinent sound from all the background sounds, regardless of the volume or intensity of the sound. To illustrate, a child must focus on what the teacher is saying and inhibit the background sounds such as street noises, the hum of the lights, or the tick of the clock. Auditory memory is also crucial to the CPM process. A person must be able to remember all of the sentence that is said, and not just part of it. This developmental trend is easily seen with the younger child who can remember only one instruction at a time as compared to the older child who can remember complex instructions, such as "John, take this paper to the living room, put it on the table next to the sofa and turn out the lights."

Although the development of auditory perception begins during infancy, it is in the post sensory-motor period that refinement of these skills becomes evident.[38]

There appears to be no difference in the perceptual development of boys as compared to girls. However, the incidence of dysfunction with learning disorders, reading disabilities, and minimal brain dysfunction is higher in males than females. There is no evidence to indicate that the male's physiology is less mature, which makes one hypothesize that the male's adaptability to environmental stresses may be the basis for the dysfunction, rather than the difference in normal development.[38]

It is further suggested that the socio-cultural background has an influence upon CPM behavior.[38] One's experiences play an important role in the acquisition of skills. Therefore, it is imperative for the occupational therapist to be aware of the patient's history, in order to assess whether the CPM dysfunction may be a result of, or influenced by a lack of environmental experiences.

During this post sensory-motor period the child continues the assimilation-accommodation process, but at this level the behavior is more complex and integrated. He has a wealth of past information which he must recall and organize in order to make a judgment about his present environment. This must be done in one temporary, brief organized act.

Evidence seems to indicate that perceptual-motor development begins to plateau at about age 11 and the cognitive process takes on new meanings.[29] Perceptual-motor functions are so integrated into the cognitive structure that they are not easily recognizable as a pure perceptual-motor act. The emphasis upon cognitive development continues through adolescence and adulthood.

As reported by Welford,[48,49] the normal aging process involves changes in functional abilities that affect the CPM process. This is suggestive of a general decline of previously acquired functions. Taylor[44] reports on the CPM dysfunction seen with older stroke victims.

The development process of adaptation-integration continues throughout one's life span. This mode of functioning provides the basis for the occupational therapist's treatment procedures. The infancy pre-school period with its maturation of reflexive and reaction schemas and structures provides the foundation for cortical integration (Chart 14–2). With the post sensory-motor period of 7 to 11 years there is continued growth of the various perceptual modalities and motor accommodations. During the adolescence-adult years the perceptual-motor acts are so integrated in the formation of cognitive development that they lose their specific identification. Cognition takes on new meaning. In later years there is a suggestion of decline with sensory-perceptual-motor functioning.

The knowledge of this developmental process is imperative and basic to the occupational therapist's evaluation and treatment of CPM dysfunction.

DEFINITION OF COGNITIVE-PERCEPTUAL-MOTOR DYSFUNCTION

A CPM dysfunction may be defined as the inability to adapt and to integrate environmental experiences. The nervous system does not assimilate sensory stimuli, thus the body cannot direct or sustain appropriate and effective motor accommodations. Instead, there are isolated schemas and insufficient sensory-motor integration. This inability leads to inaccurate adaptations and fails to provide sound information for the formation of cognitive structures.

To illustrate, assume that the baby in the previous example has CNS pathology. When he comes in contact with a spoon, he may receive sensory stimuli through his eyes, ears, tongue and bodily movements. He fails to integrate what he sees, feels, or hears from this experience. Nor does he integrate this experience with the past schemas of the nipple and rattle. Without this integration the baby cannot utilize the past experiences; hence he cannot make judgments. The baby has sensory reception, but no sensory perception of the spoon.

Without this integration and organization he does not build onto his sucking schema. Thus, his cognitive structures are incomplete. In essence, he is left with isolated schemas of a spoon, a rattle, and a nipple. He does not integrate the experiences in order to form structures. He fails to perceive the spoon, thus he cannot direct effective motor accommodations. The following example is used to further illustrate CPM dysfunction.

A child is shown the letters "b" and "d". These symbols consist of two forms, a circle and a vertical line. Their form relationship constitutes the specific symbol (i.e., forms connected at the bottom of the line, "b" on the right and "d" on the left).

In the process of adapting to what he is shown it is necessary to rely upon past experiences. Because of CNS pathology, this child was unable to develop form structures from playing with toys, such as balls, blocks, and puzzles. Instead, he may have developed a schema of blocks, balls, and puzzles. His body schema could not be integrated into a right-left structure. There was a lack of organization and integration of forms and spatial directions. Therefore, the child fails to perceive the "b" and the "d".

This child may continue to misperceive symbols and fail to learn to read and write. A remedial program of reading and writing may not benefit a child of this type. In essence, practice with letters and reading only exposes the child to something he has already failed. A more effective approach would be: (1) to find out "why" he cannot perceive a "b" and "d"; (2) to begin his treatment at this developmental level.

As a simplified example, the evaluation may indicate that this child cannot make tactile discriminations. In his process of assimilating tactile sensations his body accommodates with a withdrawal. Without the ability to discriminate this child could not have adapted and formulated structures regarding forms when he was playing with blocks, nor could he be expected to perceive visually a letter and to utilize form concepts. The evaluation further indicated the child's poor body schema. His postural adjustments to space gave him no basis for the development of spatial concepts of up and down, right and left. Hence, this child could not make form relationships. Treatment then must begin by helping the child to develop tactile discrimination and appropriate postural accommodations.

Although the dysfunction is usually associated with children, it is not limited to the pediatric age group. Adult patients, notably post CVA, have been found to have characteristics of CPM dysfunction similar to those found in children.[44]

Cognitive-Perceptual-Motor dysfunction is not a single diagnosis nor a disease, but a pathological condition which may result from a variety of etiological factors. It is important for the occupational therapist to be aware of the many varied etiological factors which may contribute to deviations in this behavior. Chart 14–7 lists a sampling of diagnostic categories that have been classically seen by the occupational therapist for CPM evaluation and treatment. This does not mean that other diagnostic categories not mentioned will not need CPM treatment nor (does it mean) that when a specific diagnosis exists CPM treatment is always indicated.

CHART 14-7

SOME PATHOLOGICAL CATEGORIES

CONGENITAL-DEVELOPMENTAL DEVIATIONS	ACQUIRED-REGRESSED DEVELOPMENT AND/OR DEVELOPMENTAL DEVIATIONS
Turner's Syndrome	Encephalitis
Down's Syndrome	Meningitis
Tay-Sachs Syndrome	Neoplasms of Brain
Infantile Autism	Organic Brain Syndrome with Psychosis
Childhood Aphasia	Schizophrenia
Cerebral Palsy	Autism
Epilepsy	Ego Deviations
Minimal Brain Dysfunction	Behavior Disorders of Childhood
Spina Bifida	and Adolescence
Ego Deviations	Aphasia
Hydrocephalus	Multiple Sclerosis
	Spinal Cord Injuries
	Arteriosclerosis
	Cerebrovascular Disease
	Asthma
	Arthritis
	Muscular Dystrophy

A CPM dysfunction manifests itself with varied symptomatology. With some patients, influences of primitive reactions and poor sensory-motor integration can be noted; with others this may not be seen. Deviations with any one of the perceptual modalities may be delineated by standardized testing. There can be visual dysfunction with no tactile or proprioceptive difficulties. Auditory perceptual functions may manifest themselves as entities.

Persons with deviations in CPM behavior present many problems which usually require a team of specialists to assess and treat. The occupational therapist must remember that he is concerned with a person, a total personality with special emotional, social, intellectual and physical needs. He must consider the person, his place in the family and community, as well as the measurement of his CPM development. At times certain needs are more urgent for other therapeutic attention than the occupational therapist's program for sensory-motor integration. Sometimes the occupational therapy program must be directed toward other needs before a CPM program begins. The occupational therapist must consider several factors in determining the efficacy of CPM training. These will be discussed in the section on evaluation-treatment.

In general, it can be said that the occupational therapy evaluation, together with the case history and evaluations by other disciplines will determine the efficacy and immediate goals for a treatment program. The purpose for an occupational therapy CPM program is to provide a person with the most effective adaptation to his environment, but it cannot do more than develop the person's potentialities.

EVALUATION

The Cognitive-Perceptual-Motor evaluation is the foundation upon which the occupational therapist builds his approach, decides upon the occupational media and sets expectations. This evaluation is the analysis, interpretation and synthesis of the person's CPM behavior. It is the foundation without which treatment cannot, nor should not proceed.

Although the occupational therapist's CPM evaluation is primarily done as the beginning step to treatment, it can be utilized by a physician in his determination of the diagnosis. This evaluation is only one part of the process which determines a diagnosis, but it is a valuable one, as it: (1) evaluates the integration of the sensory-motor process; (2) describes the person's adaptation process; (3) describes the effect of this process upon maturation and behavior; (4) describes the developmental profile.

The occupational therapist, with his concern for human developmental behavior, needs as much information as can be obtained about the person's process of adaptation. The CPM assessment should describe visual, auditory, tactile, proprioceptive and vestibular perceptions and the postural and movement accommodations.

The occupational therapist analyzes, interprets, and synthesizes the material gathered by observing situations; by interviewing the patient, his family, or teacher; by reviewing the patient's history, which takes into account the life situation of the patient; and by testing for objective and reliable data.[32]

The CPM evaluation can be grouped into three categories: (1) that dependent upon special tests; (2) that dependent upon observing behavior; and (3) that dependent upon the interview and developmental history.

Special Tests

Standardized tests will aid in determining what tasks a person can accomplish as compared to the expected performance for persons of a given age. The tests will yield a performance score. However, the score will not reveal the method or approach the person took to the solution, nor will the score describe the basis for failure. This is gained by supplementing material gained in observations and by the therapist's interpretation of what the test items may reveal. The scores give a skeletal overview while the observations provide the "flesh," which enables the person to be seen as a true human being.[32]

A test is an extension of the examiner. It provides him with a systemized and standardized method of observing behavior. One important value of a test is the opportunity it gives the examiner to observe how a person functions.[32]

Any examiner must be trained and supervised in the use of standardized test materials. Without proper training and supervision an examiner might administer the test in an improper manner, misinterpret test items, score the test improperly and fail to observe pertinent behavior.

Chart 14–8 includes a listing of available testing materials as they relate to the perceptual modalities and motor accommodations.

Observations

A person comes to an evaluation with varied symptomatology. The examiner's goal is to learn as much as he can about the behavior of this person. He needs to know what the behavior is, how it is accomplished, or why it cannot be accomplished, and why it exists. He can determine whether occupational therapy is indicated, as well as the appropriate goals and methods of treatment. In this process of assessment there is no substitute for observations gained during the evaluation periods.

The observations begin the moment the examiner first sees his client. Does the person show anxiety? Does he speak softly, slowly, or is he explosive? Is he neatly dressed? Does he follow conversation? How does he approach a test item? How does he handle material? Is he rigid? Does he recover from failure? The list of questions and observations is endless. The skilled and experienced examiner makes use of his observations.

During the evaluation, patterns of behavior may emerge and spontaneous situations occur that will affect the course of the evaluation. The examiner must call upon his own resources. He may not be able to utilize a test in its standardized method (and must note that in reporting) and he may need to create his own methods to analyze the situation. One does not create methods and situations just for the sake of creation. Improvised situations must pertain to assessing behavior in order to plan a treatment program and to contribute to a diagnosis.[32]

Interview and History

An important part of a comprehensive evaluation is gained by the interview and history of the therapist's client. The interview can give information about the family's reaction to the client, clues about the nature of the involvement, and the client's reaction to his problem. It can provide insight into his feelings about the evaluation, and his feelings about his environment. The history indicates the types of experiences and stimulation the client may have encountered. It can reveal his likes and dislikes. In the case of a child, the history takes into ac-

CHART 14-8
EVALUATION INSTRUMENTS

Author	Reference Number	Test	COGNITIVE-PERCEPTUAL-MOTOR MODALITIES					
			Visual	Tactile	Proprioceptive	Vestibular	Auditory	Visual-Motor Accommodation
Ayres	8	Ayres Space Test	X					
Ayres	9	Southern California Motor Accuracy Test						X
Ayres	10	Southern California Kinesthesia and Tactile Perception		X	X			X
Ayres	11	Southern California Figure-Ground Test	X					
Ayres	12	Perceptual-Motor Tests	X		X	X		X
Beery	16	Developmental Test of Visual-Motor Integration						X
Bender	17	Bender-Gestalt						X
Berges	18	Imitation of Gestures			X			X
Denhoff	24	Meeting Street School Screening Test	X	X	X		X	X
Egan	25	Developmental Screening				X	X	X
Fiorentino	27	Reflex Testing		X	X	X		X
Frostig	30	Developmental Test of Visual Perception	X					X
Gesell	31	Gesell Developmental					X	X
Kephart	35	Purdue Perceptual-Motor Survey						X
Kirk	36	I.T.P.A.					X	X
Prechtl	42	Neurological Examination of Full Term Newborn		X	X	X		X
Weschler	50	W.I.S.C.						X

count the toys the child does like, and does not like, how he plays with toys, what is he allowed to do at home, what constitutes his typical day. It gives insight into his behavior by considering the outstanding developmental landmarks, such as when he sat, stood, walked, talked and rode a tricycle. It is helpful to know if anything occurred before the evaluation to affect the performance; for example, a spanking, a threat, or a bribe. In addition, cultural, emotional or socioeconomic deprivation may have relevance to the performance during the evaluation. In the case of an adult, it is helpful to know about his typical day, as well as his cultural, emotional, or socioeconomic history.[32]

The examiner analyzes, interprets and synthesizes all the material gained from tests, observations, interviews and history. These sources provide the comprehensive information upon which the occupational therapist will build the treatment plan. The information gained by assessment is communicated by reporting the significant behavior and deviations noted, the interpretations of the examiner and the recommendations for treatment. This report is a permanent part of the client's record and must be shared with all persons concerned with the client. The report must be in intelligible and meaningful language for the reader or listener, whether it be to a physician, a psychologist, teacher or another therapist. The report must be as concise as possible, yet the significant and essential findings must not be left out.[32]

The method of reporting is determined by the situation and the people with whom the occupational therapist communicates. The following examples of reporting the findings of an evaluation are included to give the reader one method of reporting. In addition, these case findings should be used for discussions regarding the interpretation of data.

Example 1

Occupational Therapy

Evaluation Report

Name: J. Jones   Date: 7/27/70

Birthdate: 1/10/65

Date of Eval.: 7/20/70

Chronological Age: 5 years 7 months

Referral Information: J. was referred by his pediatrician for a perceptual-motor evaluation. Dr. B. reported that J. had completed 9 months in a private pre-school which he attended 3 hours daily. The teacher reported to Dr. B. that J. appeared to have emotional problems and did not function in group activities. He was hyperactive, explosive and fearful. Pre-school recommended that the child should not start kindergarten this fall. The developmental exam given by Dr. B. showed difficulties with gross motor and adaptive behavior. Dr. B. reported the child to be clumsy and awkward with his motor pursuits. He could not accomplish motor skills beyond the 3 year level.

History: Information by mother indicated a normal pregnancy and birth. However, J. was an AB-O blood incompatibility. He was referred to the newborn center for the first 3 weeks of life, but no transfusion was done. No record of early development available. Child has been in good physical health. Mother stated J. was a fussy baby who did not nurse well and did not like to be held. He is the first of three children and mother states that after her other two, she now realizes something was wrong that first year, as J. was a different and difficult baby to handle. J. was not as active and did not respond to her or her husband. Because he cried when they held him, they did not play with him as much as with the other children. She reported his early developmental landmarks to be within slow normal limits, however, she stated that J. did not sit independently until 11 months. When he did motor tasks they were different from the way her other two did them. She stated, "he did things with great effort and never seemed to enjoy life." He learned to ride a tricycle at 3½ years and presently has a bicycle with training wheels which he cannot ride independently. He likes to play in the sand box with his trucks and loves to swing on a glider. He is destructive with his toys, breaking them while playing. He does not play with any one thing for long periods except swinging which he will do for 30 minutes to an hour. He has difficulty climbing, running, jumping and keeping up with his playmates. He falls easily and frequently. The mother described him as being overly active at home, but his activity had no purpose; he goes from one thing to another and never sits still. Dinner time is described as a "nightmare." He always spills things, wiggles in his seat, and usually leaves the table in tears. Mother feels father is too strict with him and expects too much of him. However, she states that the father does spend a lot of time with him trying to teach him to ride his bike, climb and play ball and usually has a lot of patience with him. Mother tries to reason with him when he has misbehaved, but says no form of discipline seems to work. Mother feels sorry for him because he has no friends. There are neighborhood children with whom he can play, but they have stopped coming to the house as J. usually hits them. Because of the poor peer relationships his parents felt pre-school experience would benefit him, but she does not feel he socializes any better. In pre-school he did begin to show interest in coloring and painting. He does not take care of his dressing activities; needs help at the dinner table with pouring and cutting. He still wets the bed at night and has frequent accidents during the day. The parents started being concerned about his behavior when he was 4 years old, as his speech was slow and he cried so frequently.

Tests Administered & Scores
1. Ayres Space Test   −1-03
2. Southern California Figure Ground: −0.5
3. Southern California Motor Accuracy:
   Left Hand — Accuracy Score: −1.7   Adjusted Score: −2.6
   Right Hand — Accuracy Score: −1.9   Adjusted Score: −2.4
4. Southern California Kinesthesia and Tactile Perception:

Subtest	Standard Score	More Accurate Hand
Kinesthesia	−1.9	Left
Manual Form Perception	−0.9	Right
Finger Identification	−2.9	Left
Graphesthesia	−2.3	Left
Localization of Tactile Stim.	−0.7	Left
Double Tactile Stimuli	−2.0	Left

5. Southern California Perceptual-Motor Test:
   Imitation of Postures: −2.3
   Crossing Midline of Body: −2.6
   Bilateral Motor Coordination: −2.5
   Right-Left Discrimination: −2.4
   Standing Balance — Eyes Open: −1.1
   Standing Balance — Eyes Closed: Fell down — could not assume.
6. Frostig Developmental Test of Visual Perception:

Subtest	Age Equivalents
Eye-Hand Coordination	3 yrs. 9 mos.
Figure-Ground	4 yrs. 0 mos.
Form Constancy	4 yrs. 6 mos.
Position in Space	4 yrs. 0 mos.
Spatial Relations	4 yrs. 0 mos.

Observations: J. was reluctant to come to the evaluation. He cried when he separated from mother, but as soon as he entered the testing room he stopped crying. He socialized passively. His voice was explosive and high pitched. He had many articulation errors and appeared to misperceive many words. He could follow only one-step directions and was distracted by background sounds. He wiggled in the chair, shuffled his feet and scratched at his arms and face throughout testing periods. He was less hyperactive during free play periods, but could not stay with any self chosen activity for longer than 2 minutes. J. displayed negative behavior during the testing situation; he frequently said, "I won't do this," and on three occasions knocked the test items onto the floor. He would attempt to manipulate the examiner, particularly when he could not succeed with test items. He drooled and had tongue overflow when concentrating on an activity.

J. chose to use the right hand for most activities. He used a gross grasp with crayon and pencil. When cutting with scissors there was increased extensor tone in the right upper extremity. Influence of the ASTNR was also noted with other fine motor tasks, such as using crayon, pencils and pegs. With table top activities the child leaned to the left and kept his head close to the table and his neck rotated to the right. He was able to assume a pivot prone position, but could maintain this for only 3 seconds. Poor co-contraction of the scapulae and shoulder girdle musculature was noted. He rolled using a neck righting pattern. The age appropriate body-righting-on-body was absent. He was able to right his head in space with visual cues, but demonstrated slow head righting reactions with vision occluded. He could assume the sitting position from supine using a partial rotation pattern. He crawled with frequent interruption of the reciprocal sequence. He assumed the standing position from supine by using a partial rotation pattern to crawling, assuming kneel standing, and then to standing using one hand on the wall for support. Equilibrium reactions were slow in sitting position; in kneel-standing he resorted to righting reaction by going into the crawling position. He demonstrated hopping reactions, but no equilibrium reactions were noted in lower extremities in standing position. He could not hop, skip, tandem walk, nor jump down from a 6″ step.

Tests of kinesthesia and tactile perception presented J. with constant failure. His hyperactivity and anxiety increased. He scratched at his hands and frequently said, "I don't like this game" or "It's time to go now." He wanted to resort to visual clues and became negative when not allowed to do so. Although J. preferred to use his right hand, the perceptual abilities on the left are more accurate. His approach to imitation of gestures indicated inefficient body accommodations. He seemed to perceive visually the examiner's body gestures, but was unable to imitate without frequently looking at his own extremities. Influence of the ASTNR was noted while assuming some postures. This was also evident with the motor accuracy tests. He frequently attempted to switch hands and showed some body rotation to right and left sides. With the Ayres Space Test, J. gave impulsive choices at the beginning, which lowered his score. The more difficult items presented a challenge and he indicated motivation to succeed. He has difficulty perceiving visual rotations in space. Manipulating the test items was difficult for J., and at times he refused to place the blocks. He was concerned about the time factor and said, he could do better if I would put that watch away. He enjoyed the figure-ground test items. His difficulty with Frostig's figure-ground is more related to his inability to trace the item than to his visual misperception. He had more difficulty perceiving forms such as squares and triangles, than circles.

Interpretations: J.'s tactile, proprioceptive and vestibular misperceptions contribute to his poor postural and motor accommodations. The influences of the primitive ASTNR and righting reactions interfere with his accomplishment of age appropriate skills. He has a protective defensive reaction to tactile stimulation. His visual perceptions appear to be poorly integrated with somesthetic stimuli contributing to his difficulty with spatial relationships. His visual abilities are not age adequate. He can recognize shapes, colors, and size, but cannot effectively analyze visual stimuli. There are signs of poor auditory perception.

Recommendations: J. would benefit from an occupational therapy program. He should be seen for individual treatment 3 times weekly, once weekly group sessions and a supervised home treatment program. J. should be seen by a speech pathologist to rule out auditory perceptual problems. Because of the child's behavior and the history presented by the mother, it is recommended that J. and his family be seen by psychologist for projective testing, as well as cognitive development. The results of this evaluation will be discussed with the family on 8/7/70.

Example 2

Occupational Therapy
Evaluation Report

Name: S. Smith   Date: 7/1/70

Birthdate: 2/19/63

Date of Eval.: 6/16/70 & 6/26/70 & 6/27/70

Chronological Age: 7 years 4 months

Referral Information: S. was referred by Dr. L., resident psychiatrist, for a perceptual-motor evaluation, as a part of the total work up at the Child Development Center. S. has had severe learning problems in school. She has just completed her second year in first grade and the school does not feel she should be advanced to 2nd grade nor can they maintain her in a regular classroom. Because of her normal I.Q. she is not a candidate for the special education program and the school requests some advice from the Child Development Center for appropriate placement for S.

History: S. has been seen by Dr. L. for 12 months. The diagnosis was childhood schizophrenia with autistic tendencies. Both parents are receiving psychotherapy (history not known at this time). S. attends class, but does not participate. In the classroom she shuffles her feet, makes animal-like noises and spends most of the day painting or watching the aquarium that is in the classroom. S. likes to look at books, but will not join in the small reading groups. She does not participate in games and stands by the door and watches her classmates during recess. She frequently resorts to fantasy when engaged in conversation.

Tests Administered & Results:
1. Southern California Motor Accuracy Test:
   (Preferred Hand)   Right Hand: Accuracy Score: +1.3
                                     Adjusted Score: +1.8
2. Ayres Space Test: +1.97
3. Southern California Figure – Ground Visual Perception: +1.9
4. Southern California Kinesthesia and Tactile Perception:

Subtest	Standard Score	More Accurate Hand
Kinesthesia	+0.6	Right
Manual Form Perception	+0.4	Same
Finger Identification	+1.7	Right
Graphesthesia	+0.5	Same
Localization of Tactile Stim.	−0.8	Right
Double Tactile Stimuli	+0.5	Right

5. Southern California Perceptual-Motor Test:

Imitation of Postures:	+1.3
Crossing Midline of Body:	+1.1
Bilateral Motor Coordination:	+1.2
Right-Left Discrimination:	+1.9
Standing Balance – Eyes Open:	+0.4
Standing Balance – Eyes Closed:	−0.9

6. Frostig Developmental Test of Visual Perception:

Subtest	Age Equivalent
Eye-Hand Coordination	8 yrs. 6 mos.
Figure-Ground	7 yrs. 11 mos.
Form Constancy	8 yrs. 3 mos.
Position in Space	7 yrs. 3 mos.
Spatial Relations	7 yrs. 11 mos.

Observations: S. came to the evaluation with her aunt. She was reluctant to go with the examiner, and hung onto her aunt. She agreed to go when her aunt suggested that she would walk along to the room. No testing could be done the first visit. S. withdrew and sat in a chair

.and shuffled her feet. She looked around the room. After 10 minutes she quickly ran to the cupboard and found some puzzles and said, "I like puzzles, this is what I'll do." She sat quietly for 10 minutes working with several puzzles. The examiner took a book and started reading to herself; S. pulled her chair next to examiner and looked on. When the examiner started to read aloud S. said, "I can read that, don't read to me." Many attempts were made to engage S. in social activity with examiner, but S. remained actively detached from the situation. On several occasions she made eye contact with examiner, but no change in facial expression. At the end of 30 minutes the examiner suggested she and S. go get an ice cream cone. S. came along, but walked two to three steps behind examiner. Upon returning to the center, S. and examiner went to the playground. Examiner sat down in glider swing. S. came up and also sat down to swing with examiner.

There was no further conversation during the first hour; however, S. let examiner hold her hand when returning to her aunt.

During the next two visits testing could be carried out in the standardized manner. There was no conversation by S., but at times she did smile. She made appropriate object relationships with test items, and toys. No fantasy was observed. When the items represented a challenge to her she was more motivated to cooperate. Her gross motor accommodations appeared age adequate, as well as her performance with test items.

Interpretation: No evidence of perceptual-motor dysfunction was indicated. S. might benefit from a play therapy program to encourage personal relationships. This examiner would like to continue to see her once weekly during the summer. This would be done with the direction and supervision of S.'s psychotherapist.

TREATMENT PRINCIPLES FOR COGNITIVE-PERCEPTUAL-MOTOR DYSFUNCTION

The occupational therapy program for the treatment of CPM dysfunction is based on these postulates: (1) that a change in sensory-motor integration will enable a person with deviant CPM behavior to adapt more effectively to the environment; and (2) that this change is brought about by controlled sensory input preceding purposeful motor output.

The theoretical procedures are in the early exploratory phase, and a great deal of behavioral research by the occupational therapist will need to take place before procedures can be applied with predicted success.[2]

Basic to the treatment procedures for sensory assimilation-body accommodation is the knowledge the occupational therapists possess concerning neurophysiology and its effect upon functioning.[33,40] Comprehension of neurophysiological structures is a must before the occupational therapist can effectively treat CPM dysfunction.

Emphasis is placed upon understanding the concepts of CPM behavior and the neurophysiological premises upon which these developmental concepts are based. This approach will provide the therapist with the best judgment to understand and utilize the theoretical procedures for changing CPM behavior.

There are four major treatment principles for occupational therapists which will be discussed: (1) Treatment begins with a thorough evaluation. (2) Treatment takes into account and, wherever possible, follows the sequence of normal development. This approach considers that high level skill controlled by cortical integration is dependent upon organized and efficient maturation of the lower structures. (3) Treatment is based and dependent upon the process of intersensory integration; that is, the assimilation of sensory experiences, followed by the motor accommodations. (4) Treatment considers the importance of the patient's, parents' and of the family's counseling and guidance, home care, and education for a satisfactory emotional and social adjustment.

Principle 1

Treatment begins with a thorough evaluation. The evaluations of sensory assimilation, motor accommodations, and environmental adaptations are necessary to establish: (a) the efficacy of treatment; (b) the approach for treatment procedures; (c) the immediate therapeutic goals, and an overview of the long range goals.

It is the responsibility of the occupational therapist to accept or reject a patient for treatment as determined by the results of the evaluation. Re-evaluations can determine future goals and the time when the patient has received maximum benefit from an occupational therapy program.

In the recommendation for occupational therapy the therapist answers certain questions in order to formulate a treatment plan. (1) Is the patient's level of functioning (presented by the interview and history) plus the present problem, a result of CPM dysfunction? Is there, in fact, sufficient dysfunction in the CPM process to affect and retard the patient's functioning level? Is this dysfunction amenable to occupational therapy, or would another discipline's treatment program better benefit this patient? Is the examiner equipped to treat the dysfunction, or is it advisable to refer the patient to another therapist for treatment?
(2) What is the developmental profile of the patient's CPM process? What perceptual modalities are giving the patient the most difficulty and how do they affect his adaptation? What perceptual modalities are

functioning best for the patient, and how do they affect his adaptation? Which aspects of perception are normal for the person's chronological age and which are abnormal? Which aspects of the CPM behavior are grouped around a specific level of development? Which aspects are scattered over several levels of development?

(3) What are the immediate goals for treatment? What long range goals can be established? What treatment procedures will be used and why?

(4) How frequently should the patient be seen for treatment? What home care program can be initiated? What is the family's understanding and acceptance of the problem? How long will treatment be continued? Is there financial ability to cover treatment costs, or will financial assistance be required? Can the patient come into the clinic or will home treatment be necessary? If the patient lives in an outlying community where therapists are not available, can the family come in periodically for supervised home care? Is there public health personnel in the community who could be used for supervision?

(5) What other disciplines are seeing the child? Can, and how, will the occupational therapy program be coordinated with other services?

Principle 2

Treatment takes into account and, wherever possible, follows the sequence of normal development which considers that high level skill controlled by cortical integration is dependent upon organized and efficient maturation of the lower structures. The hypothesized development (Chart 14–2) is a means for guiding the therapist's plan for treatment progression. When a person is accomplishing high level behaviors, such as running, jumping, writing and reading he is still improving and enlarging upon the assimilation-accommodation process of visual, tactile, proprioceptive and vestibular stimuli. However, the accomplishment of skilled behavior is dependent upon earlier development.

Although the recapitulation of the developmental sequence has been stressed, it should not be assumed that the occupational therapy program must mirror each developmental step of the infant. Once the therapist has determined the areas of poor integration of lower level responses to higher adaptive behavior, he can provide activities that are age and sex appropriate. By the nature of the activity, sensory-motor integration will be enhanced on an automatic level. This would then parallel the process of development in the infant at higher level reactions inhibiting or integrating the lower responses until adaptive and voluntary activities are performed with a background of sensory-motor integration.

The following example illustrates the above principle: When the response to tactile stimulation is one of avoidance or withdrawal for protection, the immediate therapeutic goal would be to inhibit this primitive response and facilitate discrimination. It has been suggested that inhibition of the protective response is a result of touch-pressure stimulation of the cutaneous receptors.[5] Treatment procedures of Rood can be applied by the therapist who has full knowledge of the theoretical basis and specific application of this technic.[34,42] When these sensory stimulation technics are utilized, tactile discrimination is further enhanced by the proprioceptive feedback from the body accommodation. These motor responses may also require facilitation from the therapist by positioning, movement, application of resistance and choice of activity. This assimilation-accommodation process contributes to the development of body schema and motor planning.

Principle 3

Treatment is based and dependent upon the process of intersensory integration (i.e., the assimilation of sensory experience followed by the motor accommodations). The sensory integrative process of organizing the assimilated sensory stimuli with the body accommodations is the most basic step to treatment. Although the visual and auditory perceptions are important to sensory integration and the CPM process, it is on the critical steps of the development of tactile, proprioceptive and vestibular assimilation, and the motor, postural and movement accommodation that the occupational therapist can best focus his attention.

The following illustrates the above principle. When an 8 year old child has not learned to cut with scissors by repetition and the trial and error method of learning, a therapist must look back through the learning progression of that skill until the child's proper sequence of development is identified. When this child is evaluated, it is identified that he cannot use scissors because he has no pincer grasp and supination accommodation. These accommodations are absent because he has no orienting response. The lack of orienting response is a result of poor tactile, proprioceptive and visual discrimination and integration; therefore, this child maintains a crude palmar grasp. The immediate treatment procedures will incorporate controlled tactile and proprioceptive input followed by age appropriate motor behaviors to accommodate the instinctive grasp.

Principle 4

Treatment considers the importance of the parents', family's, and patient's counseling and guidance; home care; and education for a satisfactory emotional and social adjustment. The occupational therapist cannot treat in isolation. The success of the patient's case management depends upon the communication and coordination of the occupational therapist's treatment program with the other disciplines concerned with the patient and his family.

CHART 14–9
SUGGESTED OCCUPATIONAL MEDIA

Sensory Assimilation	Gross Motor Accommodation	Adaptation toward Development of:
Controlled tactile input Controlled vestibular input Proprioceptive feedback	*Gross postures and patterns of motion as described by Rood (withdrawal and rolling pivot prone, on elbows, all fours, standing)	Body schema and praxis Postural and body integration
Controlled tactile input Controlled vestibular input Proprioceptive feedback	*Righting and equilibrium reactions Integrative patterns of assuming and maintaining positions (complete rotation, partial rotation, symmetrical) by Bobath	Body schema and praxis Postural and body integration
Controlled tactile, vestibular input Proprioceptive feedback integrating with visual stimuli	*Activities for Apedal-Quadrupedal Positions* Skooter board activities Obstacle courses; Bean bag; Ball playing; Charades; Rolling; Crawling; Relays; Follow-the-Leader; Rhythm bands	Body schema and praxis Postural and body integration Visual-spatial relationships
Controlled tactile, vestibular input Proprioceptive feedback integrating with visual stimuli	*Activities for Bipedal Positions* Running; Jumping; Skipping; Hopping games Playground equipment (swings, barrels, slide, climbing bars) Obstacle courses; Ball playing; Musical games	Refinement of body schema, praxis Postural and body integration Visual-spatial relationships
Controlled tactile input Proprioceptive feedback integrating with visual stimuli	*Fine Motor Accommodations* Puzzles; Finger plays; Educational toys; Origami; Crafts; Coloring; Writing; Cutting; Peg boards	Visual-motor integration

*Do not use unless trained in principles and technics of Rood and Bobath.

The occupational therapy program for sensory-motor adaptation can only provide so much toward integration. There are many other structures, particularly psychological, social, and genetic which influence each person's integration.

The occupational media chosen for specific treatment programs depend upon the patient's sex, age, deficits, capabilities, interests, the therapist's training and skilled ability with specific procedures. The activities in Chart 14–9 are included as suggestions to guide the reader's thinking in the utilization of media.

The occupational therapy program for the treatment of CPM behavior is based upon neurophysiological principles and follows the progression of human development. Treatment procedures are in the exploratory stage and must be considered highly provisional. At this time the best approach to the treatment of CPM dysfunction is the knowledge and understanding of this behavioral phenomenon.

SUMMARY

The content of this chapter constitutes a theory regarding the characteristics of Cognitive-Perceptual-Motor behavior. This behavior has a neurophysiological substratum which underlies growth and development. The functional invariants of sensory assimilation and motor accommodations enhance environmental adaptations which form behavior schemas. With intersensory integration new experiences form a network of schemas to establish a Cognitive-Perceptual-Motor behavior. These invariants occur within and between the three levels of the sensory-motor period and are critical in determining the maturation of the post sensory motor periods.

The occupational therapist concerned with the habilitation of CPM dysfunction must begin the program with a thorough understanding of the patient's deviations in behavior and levels of functioning. This evaluation is the foundation upon which the therapist builds his treatment program.

The treatment procedures are based upon principles of normal development progression and controlled sensory-motor adaptations to build a background cortical integrative process.

BIBLIOGRAPHY

1. Andre, T., and Autgaerden S.: Locomotion from Pre- to Post-Natal Life. Clinics in Dev. Med., 24, London, W. Heinemann Books Ltd., 1966.
2. Ayres, A. J.: Sensory Integrative Processes and Neuropsychological Learning Disability. Learning Disorders. 3. Seattle, Special Child Publications, 1969.

3. ———: Deficits in sensory integration in educationally handicapped children. J. of Learning Disabilities, 2:160-168, 1969.
4. ———: Patterns of Perceptual-Motor Dysfunction in Children—A Factor Analytic Study. Percept. Motor Skills, 20:335-368, 1965.
5. ———: Perceptual-Motor Training for Children. Approaches to the Treatment of Patients with Neuromuscular Dysfunction, 6:17-21, Dubuque, Iowa. William C. Brown, 1964.
6. ———: The development of perceptual-motor abilities: a theoretical basis for treatment of dysfunction. Am. J. Occup. Therapy, 17:221-225, 1963.
7. ———: Tactile functions; their relation to hyperactive and perceptual-motor behavior. Am. J. Occup. Therapy, 18:6-11, 1964.
8. ———: Ayres Space Test. Los Angeles, Western Psychological Services, 1962.
9. ———: Southern California Motor Accuracy Test. Los Angeles, Western Psychological Services, 1966.
10. ———: Southern California Kinesthesia and Tactile Perception Tests. Los Angeles, Western Psychological Services, 1966.
11. ———: Southern California Figure-Ground Visual Perception Tests. Los Angeles, Western Psychological Services, 1966.
12. ———: Southern California Perceptual-Motor Tests. Los Angeles, Western Psychological Services, 1968.
13. Beery, K., and Buktenica, N.: Developmental Test of Visual-Motor Integration. Chicago, Follett, 1967.
14. Bender, L.: Bender Visual Motor Gestalt Test, New York, The Psychological Corp.
15. Berges, J., and Lezine, I.: The Imitation of Gestures. Clinics in Developmental Medicine No. 18, London, W. Heinemann Books Ltd., 1965.
16. Birch, H., and Lefford, A.: Intersensory Development in Children, Monographs of the Society for Research in Child Development, 28, serial no. 89, 1963.
17. Bobath, B.: The very early treatment of cerebral palsy. Dev. Med. Child Neurol. 9:373-390, 1967.
18. ———: Abnormal Postural Reflex caused by Brain Lesions. London, W. Heinemann Books Ltd., 1965.
19. Bobath, B., and Cotton, E.: A Patient with Residual Hemiplegia. J. Am. Phy. Therapy Assoc., 45:849-864, 1965.
20. Bobath, K.: The Motor Deficit in Patients with Cerebral Palsy. Clinics in Dev. Med. No. 23, London, W. Heinemann Books Ltd., 1966.
21. ———: The neuropathology of cerebral palsy and its importance in treatment and diagnosis. Cereb. Palsy Bull., 1:13-33, 1959.
22. ———: The neuro-developmental treatment of cerebral palsy, J. Am. Phys. Therapy Assoc. 47:11, 1967.
23. Bobath, K., and Bobath B.: An assessment of the motor handicap of children with cerebral palsy and of their response to treatment. Am. J. Occup. Therapy, 22:1-14, 1958.
24. Denhoff, E., et al.: Developmental and predictive characteristics of items from the Meeting Street School screening test. Dev. Med. Child Neurol., 10:220, 1969.

25. Egan, D., et al.: Developmental Screening 0-5 Years. Clinics in Dev. Med. No. *30*, London, W. Heinemann Books Ltd., 1969.
26. Ellis, E.: The Physical Management of Developmental Disorders. Clinics in Dev. Med., No. *26*, London, W. Heinemann Books Ltd., 1967.
27. Fiorentino, M.: Reflex Testing Methods for Evaluating C.N.S. Development. ed. 2, Springfield, Charles C Thomas, 1965.
28. ——: Reflex Therapy, in Approaches to the Treatment of Patients with Neuromuscular Dysfunction, 6:38-43, Dubuque, Iowa. William C. Brown, 1964.
29. Flavell, J.: The Developmental Psychology of Jean Piaget. Princeton, Van Nostrand, 1963.
30. Frostig, M.: Developmental Test of Visual Perception. ed. 3, Palo Alto, Consulting Psychologists Press, 1964.
31. Gesell, A., and Armatruda, C. S.: Developmental Diagnosis, New York, Halber, 1947.
32. Gilfoyle, E.: The Three Faces of Ev., in Perceptual-Motor Dysfunction Evaluation and Training, proceedings of Occupational Therapy Seminar. 55–70, Madison, Univ. of Wisc., 1966.
33. Harris, F.: Control of gamma efferents through the reticular activating system. Am. J. Occup. Therapy, *23*: 397–408, 1969.
34. Huss, J.: Application of the Rood Techniques to Treatment of the Physically Handicapped Child, Occupational Therapy for the Multiply Handicapped Child. 86–96, Chicago, Univ. of Ill. Press, 1965.
35. Kephart, N., and Roach, E.: Purdue Perceptual-Motor Survey. Columbus, Merrill Dodds, 1966.
36. Kirk, S., and Mc Carthy, J.: Illinois Test of Psycholinguistic Abilities. Urban, Illinois Institute for Research and Exceptional Children, 1968.
37. Llorens, L., and Ruben E.: Developing Ego Functions in Disturbed Children: Occupational Therapy in Milieu. Detroit, Wayne State Univ. Press, 1969.
38. Martin, H., and Gilfoyle, E.: Assessment of Perceptual Development. Am. J. Occup. Therapy, *23*:387–395, 1969.
39. McGraw, M.: The Neuromuscular Maturation of the Human Infant, New York, Hafner, 1966.
40. Moore, J.: Neuroanatomy Simplified. Dubuque, Iowa, Kendall Hunt, 1969.
41. Prechtl, H., and Beintema, D.: The Neurological Examination of the Full Term Newborn Infant. Clinics in Dev. Med. no. *12*, London, W. Heinemann Books Ltd., 1964.
42. Rood, M.: The Use of Sensory Receptors to Activate, Facilitate, and Inhibit Motor Response, Autonomic and Somatic, in Developmental Sequence, Approaches to the Treatment of Patients with Neuromuscular Dysfunction. 6:26–32, Dubuque, Iowa. William C. Brown, 1962.
43. Spitz, R.: The First Year of Life, New York, International Univ. Press, 1965.
44. Taylor, M.: Controlled Evaluation of Percept-Concept-Motor Training Therapy After Stroke Resulting in Left Hemiplegia. Final Report of Rehabilitation Institute, Inc., Detroit, Social and Rehabilitation Service, Grant #RD-2215-M, 1969.

45. Twitchell, T.: Attitudinal Reflexes: The Child with Central Nervous System Deficit. U.S. Dept. of Health, Education and Welfare, Children's Bureau, Pub. No. 432, 1965.
46. ———: Normal Motor Development: The Child with Central Nervous System Deficit. U.S. Dept. of Health, Education and Welfare, Children's Bureau, Pub. No. 432, 1965.
47. ———: Variations and Abnormalities of Motor Development: The Child with Central Nervous System Deficit. U.S. Dept. of Health, Education and Welfare, Children's Bureau, Pub. No. 432, 1965.
48. Welford, A., and Birren, J.: Behavior, Aging and Nervous System. Springfield, Charles C Thomas, 1965.
49. Welford, A.: On changes of performance with age. Lancet, 1:335–339, 1962.
50. Wechsler, D.: Wechsler Intelligence Scale for Children. New York, Psychological Corp., 1949.
51. Wepman, J.: Wepman Test of Auditory Discrimination. Chicago, Language Research Assoc., 1958.

15

Home Health Care—A New Frontier for Occupational Therapy

M. ARLENE MELLINGER, M.A., O.T.R.

The concept of home health care is not really new. Nursing care of the sick at home, on a visiting basis, has been provided for years by official health departments and voluntary agencies such as visiting nurse associations. Some agencies began to add other health care services such as physical therapy, medical social work and homemaker home health aides. In some instances, occupational therapy was also included.

The past decade witnessed an increasing awareness of the benefits of multi-service home care programs in reducing the length of the hospital stay for patients of all ages and in assuring continuation of appropriate health care services to these patients within their respective homes.

In the United States, the advent of Medicare and its Conditions of Participation for Home Health Agencies, effective July 1, 1966, gave impetus to the growth and development of comprehensive home care programs. The conditions are, in effect, regulations which must be met by agencies seeking certification as home health agencies. These regulations require the provision of skilled nursing care plus at least one other therapeutic service on a visiting basis to patients in their respective homes. Other therapeutic services are identified as occupational, physical and speech therapy, medical social services and home health aide services.

PREVALENCE OF OCCUPATIONAL THERAPY AS A HOME HEALTH AGENCY SERVICE

As of January 1969, Social Security Administration data revealed that 352 out of 2161 certified home health agencies provided occupational therapy. Physical therapy was provided by 1571 of these agencies, home health aide service by 1042 agencies; speech therapy by 477 agencies and medical social service by 393 agencies.

A comparison of the number and types of home health agencies reporting provision of occupational therapy with the number of certified agencies included in the report, furnishes a significant clue to the concentration of occupational therapy service at that time.

Number Certified Home Health Agencies Compared to Number Providing Occupational Therapy as of January 1969

Number and Type of Agencies (2161)	Number Providing Occupational Therapy (352)
1,294 Official Health Departments	129 or 10%
541 Visiting Nurse Associations	112 or 20.7%
172 Hospital based	62 or 36%
107 Combined government and voluntary agencies	25 or 23.4%
20 Proprietary	8 or 40 %
15 Extended care facility based	5 or 33.3%
12 Rehabilitation facility based	11 or 91.7%

The unavailability of qualified occupational therapists is one reason why many community agencies such as health departments and visiting nurse associations do not provide occupational therapy as one of their home health services. Equally significant is the fact that occupational therapy has been traditionally associated with treatment centers such as hospitals and rehabilitation facilities. Occupational therapy as a community agency based home health service is an unfamiliar area of practice for many occupational therapists; consequently they have difficulty in identifying the role of occupational therapy in a public health agency's home care program.

TYPES OF PATIENTS ADMITTED TO HOME CARE PROGRAMS

Home health agencies provide care for patients of various ages and economic levels. The cost of care may be covered by Federal Health Insurance For the Aged, in the case of a Medicare patient. An increasing number of non-governmental health insurance plans will pay for home care services. In other instances, the patient or his family may pay for the care.

Diagnoses of patients admitted to home care programs include:

Cerebral vascular accidents	Arthritis
Cardiac conditions	Cancer
Respiratory conditions	Fractures
Neuromuscular conditions	Amputations
Parkinson's disease	Multiple sclerosis

The home health agency's considerations for accepting patients for home care include:

1. The agency's ability to provide the services required for the patient in accordance with the physician's orders and plan of care.
2. Attitudes of the patient and family toward his care at home.
3. Availability of family or substitute family member able and willing to participate in the patient's care.
4. Adequacy, in terms of physical facilities, of the patient's residence for his proper care.

As far as occupational therapy services are concerned, the occupational therapist must be capable of adapting his treatment procedures to the patient's home environment. The occupational therapist who has always been accustomed to treating patients within a hospital or rehabilitation facility may be dismayed to discover that some types of treatment activities which can be used effectively within the treatment center will not be successful within the patient's home. For example, metal hammering may be appropriate for increasing range of motion and muscle strength in a patient's wrist when used within the structured environment of a hospital or rehabilitation facility. However, if the occupational therapist decides to use this treatment activity within the patient's home, it may prove to be totally inappropriate in that the patient's family cannot tolerate the noise. If the patient is an apartment dweller, speedy repercussions may be forthcoming from the neighbors. In such an incident, the occupational therapist's error would be failure to consider the environment within which the treatment activity was utilized.

DEVELOPING OCCUPATIONAL THERAPY SERVICES IN A HOME HEALTH AGENCY

Because occupational therapy has been traditionally associated with hospitals, rehabilitation centers and other patient care facilities, many home health agencies are unfamiliar with its role as a home health service. There is a tendency to confuse occupational therapy with physical therapy since both are concerned with the restoration of physical function and similar terminology is often used on their referral and evaluation forms.

Occupational therapists find themselves faced with the challenge of assisting home health agencies to identify those areas in which occupational therapy can be effectively utilized as a home health service. The occupational therapist who serves on a home health agency's advisory committee is in a key position to interpret occupational therapy's role as a health care profession, and to assist the agency with policies concerning its use.

An effective method of interpretation is to translate occupational therapy's role into simple statements of purpose. For example, occupational therapy can be effectively utilized as a home health service to:

1. Remedy or reduce disability through the use of activities designed to increase joint motion, muscle strength and coordination.
2. Enable the patient to overcome the handicapping effects of a physically or visually disabling condition through the selective use of assistive devices, adapted equipment, clothing adaptations, and special self help technics.
3. Assist the disabled homemaker to perform successfully customary household tasks through instruction in work simplification, use of assistive devices and adapted household equipment.
4. Provide instruction in energy saving technics for cardiac patients and others with limited physical reserve.
5. Provide prevocational evaluation of patient's interests, skills and capabilities when the possibility of referral for vocational rehabilitation or selective job placement is considered medically feasible.
6. Assist the chronically ill and disabled patient to determine and to constructively use his remaining capabilities so that he may retain a sense of purposeful living.

It is possible to condense these statements into succinct categories for medical referral purposes. They can then be included on the agency's medical order form which is completed and signed by the patient's physician. Some occupational therapists have found the following format to be effective:

Orders For Occupational Therapy

Check purpose:
( ) Aid in restoring useful function
( ) Compensate for permanent loss of useful function
( ) Prevocational rehabilitation evaluation
( ) Assist patient to determine and constructively use remaining capabilities

---

Upon receipt of the initial order and completion of evaluation of the patient's disability problem, the occupational therapist prepares his recommended treatment plan for the physician's approval.

This procedure for procuring orders for occupational therapy provides a basic interpretation of the unique range of occupational therapy services. It also enables both the occupational therapist and the agency to ascertain quickly the purposes for which occupational therapy is primarily utilized.

RESPONSIBILITIES OF THE OCCUPATIONAL THERAPIST EMPLOYED BY A HOME HEALTH AGENCY

1. *Education*
   a. Orients home health agency personnel to occupational therapy and the purposes for which it can be effectively utilized as a home health service.
   b. Participates in the agency's in-service education program.
2. *Consultation*
   a. Provides consultation to, or serves as a member of the agency's advisory group of professional personnel.
   b. Provides consultation and guidance to other health agency personnel, or others directly concerned with the patient's care, regarding technics to promote optimal use of his remaining capabilities and/or rehabilitation gains.
   c. Provides consultation to the administrator regarding employment of additional occupational therapy personnel when the need for such is indicated and assists with formulation of appropriate job descriptions.
   d. Consults with the administrator concerning the occupational therapy budget.
3. *Conference Participation*
   a. Participates in conferences with the home health agency's staff concerning evaluation of the patient's needs, and development of the total plan of care for the patient.
   b. Participates in other staff conferences as requested.
4. *Treatment*
   a. Makes home visits to evaluate patients' disability problems.
   b. Determines treatment goals; develops treatment plan based upon evaluation results and the physician's orders.
   c. Consults with other health care disciplines concerned with the patient's care and integrates occupational therapy treatment into the total patient care plan.
   d. Personally administers or supervises the occupational therapy program.

e. Instructs the patient's family, or substitute family member, concerning those aspects of treatment in which they may work with the patient.

f. Provides instruction and supervision to other health team personnel who will assist with treatment and follow up.

g. Conducts ongoing evaluation of the patient's progress in cooperation with other health team personnel.

h. Reports patient's treatment response to his physician and changes treatment plans and goals in accordance with the physician's orders.

5. *Records and Reports*

a. Records, dates and signs into the patient's medical record (which is maintained by the agency):

1. Evaluation report.
2. Treatment goal and plan.
3. Report of each treatment visit.
4. Patient's response to treatment and follow up recommendations. If treatment is to be discontinued, the reasons should be included along with follow up recommendations when advisable.

b. Provides the home health agency administrator with periodic reports as required. One such report may pertain to:

1. Number of referrals received.
2. Number of patients evaluated.
3. Number of patients treated and number of treatment visits per patient.
4. Number of patients discharged from occupational therapy.
5. Number of patients for whom treatment is continued.

SUMMARY

Within the past decade the number of home health agencies in the United States has tripled and continues to grow. A steadily increasing number are interested in providing occupational therapy services. Employment by a home health agency can be a highly stimulating experience for the resourceful occupational therapist who enjoys the challenge this new frontier provides. It requires an occupational therapist who is thoroughly knowledgeable in the treatment of physically disabled patients, one who is versatile in adapting procedures for use within the patient's home environment.

Goals shared by the home health agency's professional staff include:

1. Helping the patient to help himself.
2. Reducing the patient's dependency on others for personal assistance.

3. Enabling the patient to function as a participating member of his home and community.

The occupational therapist who can demonstrate occupational therapy's effectiveness in assisting with the achievement of these goals soon comes to be recognized as a valuable member of the home health care team.

BIBLIOGRAPHY

Bernd, J. R.: Occupational therapy for the homebound. J. Rehab., 32:21, 1966.

Colt, A. M.: Public policy and planning criteria in public health. Am. J. Public Health, 59:1678, 1969.

Conditions of Participation Home Health Agency, Federal Insurance for the Aged. HIR-12(9–68), U.S. Dept. of Health, Education and Welfare, Social Security Administration.

Mellinger, M. A.: Guidelines for Occupational Therapists Regarding Home Health Agencies in New York State. New York State Dept. of Health, Albany, New York, 1969.

Ryder, C. F., Stilt, P. G., and Elkin, W. F.: Home health agencies past, present, future. Am. J. Public Health, 59:1720, 1969.

Standards for Occupational Therapy Service Programs. Am. Occup. Therapy Assoc., New York, New York, 1968.

West, W. L.: The occupational therapist's changing responsibility to the community. Am. J. Occup. Therapy; 21:312, 1967.

———: Occupational Therapy—Philosophy and Perspective. Am. J. Nurs., 68:1708, 1968.

16

Occupational Therapy for the Blind and Partially Sighted

ELIZABETH L. HUTCHINSON, O.T.R.
and
ELIZABETH M. WAGNER, O.T.R.

BLINDNESS

From the earliest times and throughout the entire world, people have had trouble relating to those individuals who were blind. This anxiety has been manifest in various practices, ranging all the way from brutal and inhuman treatment to over-solicitude and a tendency to force blind people into a role of dependency. Most of the writing on the subject has been done by sighted people. Only within the last few years have we seen any quantity of studies and autobiographies designed to reveal how blind people feel about themselves, and their reaction to the help they have been offered.

Although necessarily subjective, and in some cases controversial, this particular body of literature can provide an important orientation to the field of blindness. The occupational therapist who intends to work with blind patients would do well to become familiar with the thinking of some of the more articulate authors of such books.

The two most important factors for the occupational therapist to consider regarding blindness are *attitudes* and *perspective*. Blindness is undeniably a sensory impairment of the first magnitude, and it is natural that the word "blind" carries an emotional overtone. To be isolated from one's environment by lack of vision obviously hampers the development and education of a child, and imposes a social and vocational burden on an adult. To what degree the visual *impairment* is transposed into a *handicap* will depend largely on the attitudes of the blind individual himself, his family, the professional people with whom he comes in contact, and society in general.

Occupational therapy is a means of offering encouragement and the opportunity for developing abilities, for attaining an objective outlook and for learning how to do things independently. What steps the occupational therapist takes to refer blind patients to services furnished by others, and what types of assistance he himself provides, will depend on the therapist's familiarity with resources, his professional knowledge and judgment, and above all on his perspective.

Definition of Blindness

Not all those who are classed as blind have a total absence of sight. The term blind is loosely used to describe anyone with a visual impairment severe enough to affect his normal performance and way of life. Definitions of blindness can be expressed either in terms of ophthalmic measurements or in terms of visual function.

In the United States, blindness is generally defined as visual acuity for distant vision of 20/200 or less in the better eye, with the best possible optical correction; or visual acuity of more than 20/200 if the widest diameter of the field of vision is restricted to an angle no greater than 20 degrees. A measure of 20/200 visual acuity means that a person can see no more at a distance of 20 feet than a person with "normal" vision can see at a distance of 200 feet. This measurement is customarily determined by testing with the Snellen chart, or with the "E chart," which can be used for illiterates, and pre-school children as young as four years of age. "Restricted field" means roughly that vision is clear straight ahead, but not to either side, like looking through a tube.

The above definition, derived from the Social Security Act of 1935, is based on the definition of economic blindness adopted by the American Medical Association in 1934. It is used in most states in establishing eligibility for the federal-state program of aid to the blind. Persons whose sight falls within these limits are generally referred to as "legally blind."

The National Health Survey and some other groups have used a functional definition such as: inability to read ordinary newsprint even with the aid of glasses. Ordinary newsprint is usually 8-point type. This implies visual acuity of 20/50, considerably more vision than allowed for under the definition of legal blindness.

Visual acuity is not entirely dependent on the structure of the visual apparatus. The occupational therapist must be aware that psychological and environmental factors also play an important part in functional vision. The normal changes in the eye, due to age, must also be considered. Among the factors not related to the eye itself are: the amount and type of illumination, reflection and glare, contrast between the object being observed and its surroundings, fatigue, motivation, and problems of perception such as are found in individuals with brain damage.

Whether couched in anatomical or functional terms, the perfect definition for "the blind" has not yet been found. It has been suggested that the term "blind" be reserved for the 20 per cent of the legally blind, with total lack of vision, and that further efforts be made to develop appropriate definitions for the remaining 80 per cent who have various degrees and types of partial vision.

Incidence of Blindness

The number of blind people in the United States can only be estimated. Each state maintains a register of its blind citizens, with mandatory reporting, but minor differences in definition, and under-reporting, have hindered valid findings and rendered statistics unreliable.

In 1962, the Model Reporting Area for Blindness Statistics was organized under the sponsorship of the National Institute of Neurological Diseases and Blindness of the U.S. Public Health Service. This is a great step forward, as it represents a team approach to the problem of reporting and compiling information. The cooperating states must subscribe to the stated objectives of the program, and maintain certain basic standards for uniform registration and the production of comparable data. It is expected that the state registers will be improved in accuracy and completeness, and that a reliable base line for blindness statistics will eventually be forthcoming.

For 1970, the best estimates available indicate a population of some 447,000 persons who are legally blind, with an increase to about 519,000 expected by 1980. If we include those who would come under a broad definition of the partially sighted, these figures can be more than doubled.

Principal Causes of Blindness

Any occupational therapist who plans to work with those having visual disability should study the anatomy of the eye, and be conversant with the main causes of blindness. It is important to think in terms of age groups, since prenatal factors and conditions associated with the aging process account for a large proportion of blindness.

The leading causes of blindness are senile cataract and glaucoma. Cataract is an opacity of the crystalline lens of the eye which prevents light from entering the eye and thus limits vision. It can be corrected by surgery, which in the vast majority of cases is safe and successful. Glaucoma results from excessive pressure within the eyeball. Peripheral vision is usually affected first, followed by loss of central visual acuity unless the disease is diagnosed early and treatment followed.

Although progress of the disease can be halted, lost vision cannot be restored. Almost 50 per cent of all blind persons are in the 65 and over age group, and almost 30 per cent of all blindness is due to these 2 causes. Diabetes and vascular disease also may cause blindness, especially among older people.

Prenatal conditions, both hereditary and congenital (present at birth), comprise another segment of the causes of blindness, as do conditions brought about by prenatal infections. Among the former are congenital malformations of the eye, congenital cataracts and glaucoma, albinism, and retinitis pigmentosa. Among the latter are visual impairment due to toxoplasmosis and maternal rubella. The incidence of retrolental fibroplasia (RLF) has been decreased by controlling the amount of oxygen given to premature infants, but it is still a major cause of blindness among school-age children. Among all age groups, the problem of accidental eye injuries calls for continuous attack.

NEWLY BLINDED PERSONS

Occupational therapy can be used to advantage in several branches of work with blind or visually handicapped persons, but in no field can the therapy be applied to greater advantage than with the newly blinded person. His adjustment to his handicap usually begins in the hospital. The patient's ultimate success in life depends largely on early training and on the intelligence and the attitude of those who first come in contact with him.

An effort must be made to convince the newly blinded patient that, in spite of his handicap, his individuality is not lost and that if he is otherwise physically and mentally fit, he is capable of leading an independent, active life. It is also necessary to prove this fact to his family and friends and to hospital personnel whose routine duties leave little time to study the problems of the individual. From the start he should be encouraged to be independent and should be helped to regain self-confidence by being shown how to care for his personal needs, how to use his hands and how to sharpen his perception through his other senses, for these do not automatically become keener. He can be told of the existing aids for the blind or partially blind, such as braille, the talking book machine, orientation and mobility training (including use of the long cane and the dog guide) and special techniques for personal management (ADL). He also should be informed of existing facilities established to help him to reorganize his way of living, and should be told where information may be obtained regarding vocational training and job placement. The achievements of successful blind persons can also be an inspiration to the patient.

Those working with blind persons must have the proper concept of blindness and must think of it as an inconvenience rather than as an affliction. It must be recognized that although the shock of blindness undoubtedly has its emotional effect on the patient, the reaction is not the same in all persons, and the needs of the individual patient must always be foremost in planning an approach. After the initial shock, loss of sight to most persons is not so disturbing as the loss of freedom of motion, the dependence upon others and often the feeling of economic insecurity.

Occupational therapy for the newly blinded patient should begin as soon as possible during his hospitalization and for the best results should be coordinated closely with other departments in the hospital — especially medical, nursing and social service.

Some patients may not know how serious the eye condition is, and others may be well aware that there is no hope of improvement. Whether it is a permanent or a temporary disability, the individual must be encouraged to do things for himself, for with few exceptions he will be able to carry on most of his former activities. Learning to help himself in the hospital is the beginning of his return to normal living, so that he can meet his family and friends at home in an easy natural way. If it is possible for the patient to return to his former employment or to one closely allied, he should be encouraged to do so.

Tact and resourcefulness are essential in approaching the newly blinded person. The impression made on the first visit to the patient is perhaps more important to those with visual handicaps than to those with other disabilities. The voice of the therapist is one means by which the patient forms his picture of the individual. Therefore, it should be natural, friendly, sincere and devoid of sentimentality. A blind person is quick to notice impatience in the voice or in the attitude of those working with him. The manner should be natural and free without forced cheerfulness or maudlin sentimentality, characterized by sympathetic understanding and sincerity. In working with persons who depend upon others for impressions of things, frankness and truthfulness are essential. Give praise when praise is due, but do not be afraid to inform the individual of errors made. Criticism always should be followed by constructive suggestions.

Selection of Activities

It is advisable to progress slowly in encouraging the patient to make something with his hands. If his interest is not aroused on the second or even the third visit, this is not to be regarded as a failure. Great care must be exercised in selecting an activity. It should not be so difficult that the patient will not succeed in accomplishing it. An early failure for the blind person may so discourage him that he will never make another attempt. Patience is essential, and the person should be allowed to complete a project regardless of the time required. As with all patients, resistance to fatigue must be watched and work stopped at the first sign. In addition to the type of handwork that can be taught to the bed patient, there are other activities for him, such as writing, lighting his own pipe and cigarettes and feeding himself. If after the first two or three visits the patient has begun to realize that his manner of life will be changed very little, he has achieved the first step forward in the reorganization process. The goal of occupational therapy with the visually handicapped patient is to help to restore his self-confidence and independence.

The simplest and perhaps the most effective means of interesting the patient is to teach him to tell time (for time seems to be an eternity with nothing to do). He may learn to do this by removing the crystal of a clock or of his own watch and placing his fingers on the hands of the time-piece. Special watches with raised dots may be purchased, or the patient's own watch may be converted by a jeweler who places dots or patches on the face at the quarter, the half and the full hour numerals. He can also be shown how to detect differences in coins and how to use the telephone dial.

Early in convalescence, the patient can be encouraged to take an interest in his personal appearance; he can be taught how to care completely for his own needs and later to dress himself. While he is still in bed he can wash his face and hands and comb his hair; later he may shave, bathe and clothe himself. He should be impressed with the great necessity for being well-groomed; for if his shoes are unpolished and his hair and nails are unkempt, it is attributed to his blindness. Psychologically, this is not good because it produces pity. The handicapped person should strive to live so that his conduct and attitudes merit respect and praise, which are far stronger stimulants for him than pity. An attractive appearance wins the approval of others and gives the individual the satisfaction of a sense of accomplishment. He should learn to be systematic in all things and especially so in the care of his clothing. In so doing he may devise methods for selecting matching ties, suits, and shirts as he dresses each day.

Women patients may be approached in the same way, and in addition, can learn how to apply make-up if they are accustomed to using it. Interest in personal appearance cannot be aroused too soon since it is so valuable in building morale.

By introducing the patient to the manual arts and selecting those appropriate to his temperament and background, he can prove to himself that although he lacks sight he is able to use his hands. The work should be interesting to him and should not be limited to those skills that are commonly thought of as the only types of work blind people can do.

If the patient is interested in flowers, he can plant the bulb of a flower with a fragrant odor, so that he will have the pleasure of tending it as it grows. This interest can be extended to growing herbs in a window box or tending a garden after the patient is at home. Offering opportunities to develop manual dexterity is the first step in helping the patient to develop his sense of touch, which becomes so important to him. Handling articles of various shapes, materials and weights may help to enhance this sense. This is not necessarily the time to suggest the study of braille, as it may be too tedious for the average person to undertake in the early stage of his adjustment, but the patient should know what it is and that it is one of the aids to becoming independent.

If there is an occupational therapy clinic in the hospital, the patient should be encouraged to attend. He should not be segregated but should take part in whatever activities are carried on. If he can help other patients, he should be encouraged to do so in order to show him that he is still capable of being useful. In the clinic he gains additional self-confidence as he undertakes more difficult work and is given the opportunity to acquire greater independence and to develop work tolerance. He can learn typing, assembly or machine work with the use of special guides if necessary, sandpapering and furniture finishing, as well as many other activities.

Activities of Daily Living

The remaining senses can compensate to a degree for loss of sight, and they can become more acute if the individual does all within his power to develop them. Hearing is of great importance because it is an aid in helping the individual to orient himself. Research is now being carried on to develop and to test methods for raising the hearing of blind persons to a greater degree of usefulness. Occupational therapy can be applied by helping the patient to develop his hearing to the utmost, by listening to various sounds in relation to the direction from which they are coming. These may be the tick of a clock, the sound of a typewriter, of faucets dripping or any small sound that is enough to give him an idea of his location.

The sense of feeling can be developed not only with the hands but also with the feet. A patient can be taught to notice the difference between a thick and a thin rug or to note the absence of a rug or the location of a rough place in the floor or on a step. When he is able to be outdoors he can use the sun as it shines on his face to help to orient himself.

The use of the sense of smell as an aid to orientation can be brought to the attention of the patient while he is in the hospital. He can learn later to notice the various odors when outside the bakeshop, the tobacco store, the leather shop, the candy store or the butcher shop.

When the patient is able to be up and around his room or ward, he can gain a mental image of the room by placing his hands on the various objects and observing their relationship to each other. Many blind persons may be self-conscious when walking with a sighted person, and they should be taught how to walk properly. The blind person should touch the elbow of his guide lightly so that he follows the guide, who is the first to come to the curb or an obstacle. After the patient becomes accustomed to walking in this way, it is unnecessary to say "step up" or "step down" because the blind person can follow the slightest movement of the guide's arm.

The art of training a blind person's remaining senses for optimum orientation and mobility has been given the name "peripatology." Several universities are now offering a curriculum for training peripatologists. Graduates of these courses can be found in many localities, employed in agencies for the blind, rehabilitation centers, and schools for the blind. This new profession includes among its functions teaching the long cane technique, which is enabling many blind people to broaden their range of travel without a guide.

A number of adjustment centers for the visually handicapped have been established in various sections of the country where orientation and mobility are taught, and other aids which will help the individual to adjust to his handicap are made available. Aptitude tests especially designed for blind persons also are given. Occupational therapy can be used to advantage in these centers.

The dog guide is a valuable aid to blind persons who desire and can use one. It should be thought of as an appliance which makes a blind person more independent and efficient, in the same way an artificial limb or a hearing aid helps those in need of them. The freedom of motion afforded by a dog guide broadens the scope of activities of the individual, improves his morale and health, and gives him confidence and a feeling of equality with those who see. Learning to walk with a dog is a highly technical process, and it can be taught only by specialists in that field. Its use is valuable for the man or the woman who is physically and mentally fit, neither too young nor too old, who has purpose in life and the desire to be active in remunerative employment or to participate in community activities.

Newly blinded persons should avoid developing the characteristic shuffling gait or groping hands. Good posture and a normal gait in walking should be stressed. Going up and down stairs becomes a nightmare to some newly blinded persons, but they should be encouraged to use the stairs before phobias develop.

The fact that a visually handicapped person, because of his inability to move about freely, may not be able to take as much exercise as he needs is frequently overlooked. If the physician approves, a program of daily exercises can be outlined and the patient encouraged to take them after leaving the hospital so that he will have good muscle tone. It is important for him to engage in as many of his former activities as possible and to continue contacts with old friends. There is no reason for him to give up old friends and to seek new companions with a similar disability.

In occupational therapy with visually handicapped persons, the benefit of recreation should be kept in mind. Recreation is essential to a rounded life, and this is especially true for the person with a visual handicap. He should become acquainted with the games that are especially adaptable for his use, such as dominoes and checkers. Braille playing cards offer an excellent way to awaken the interest of a newly blinded person in braille. Cribbage and chess can also be enjoyed. If the patient likes to dance, to swim, to bowl, to hike or to garden, he should be encouraged to do so if that appeals to him. Many blind persons take complete charge of their gardens.

If a patient likes to be read to, arrangements can be made through his state library for him to have a talking-book machine, which is supplied by the Library of Congress on a free loan basis. These machines are similar to a portable record player. Any phonograph which has a speed of 16⅔ r.p.m. can also be used. The American Foundation for the Blind, under contract to the Library of Congress, records talking books, and it also publishes "Talking Book Topics," a periodical from which reading material can be selected. A large number of books in a variety of topics have been recorded, and also a number of monthly magazines including *The Reader's Digest*. These records are available in designated libraries for circulation and are mailed without cost.

Braille is an indispensable tool in the education of the blind child, and may be equally necessary for the adult. As for those who become blind late in life, some may be able to learn and use braille to advantage, while for others the skill or the motivation, or both, may be lacking. In the latter cases, perspective is needed to determine the right time to introduce the idea of learning braille, and to advise the patient about studying it. When learning braille is clearly indicated, the therapist should know where a competent teacher can be obtained.

Any occupational therapist who works with blind children or adults should be familiar with braille himself. Patient's clothes can be marked with tiny metal tags with braille letters indicating color. Canned goods, phonograph records, projects in craft classes all can be identified in braille, and the therapist should be able to read these labels in order to assist the patient in using them.

If the therapist wishes to learn to transcribe braille, the Library of Congress offers a basic course by mail, and some local agencies for the blind can help. Braille can be transcribed by hand with a slate and

498 Occupational Therapy for the Blind and Partially Sighted

stylus, or with a machine, such as the Perkins brailler, obtainable from Howe Press, Perkins School for the Blind, Watertown, Mass. Braille should be transcribed on one side of the paper only if a sighted person is to read it. Such books are hand-produced by volunteer transcribers. Books and periodicals produced in large numbers on braille presses are embossed on both sides of the page.

The "Braille Book Review" is published bi-monthly by the American Foundation for the Blind. From it, blind persons can select classics and up-to-date reading material which is available from regional libraries for the blind (under the Federal program) without charge.

Tape recorders have become very popular as well as useful for visually handicapped persons and they serve many purposes. In addition to talking books and books in braille, the Library of Congress also has a tape collection for blind persons who furnish their own listening equipment.

Research for developing and testing aids and appliances used by blind men and women in the home and elsewhere is being conducted in many places. A selection of aids and appliances is available from The American Foundation for the Blind and from local blind agencies. Among the classifications of equipment are: writing devices, games, kitchen aids, mathematical aids, medical aids (some of which are available only to physicians or registered nurses), music aids, tools and instruments, and time-pieces.

A discussion of occupational therapy for a newly blinded person cannot be complete without considering the family. Often the emotional reaction of the family is as great as, if not greater than, that of the patient himself, and the relatives should be taught how to treat the patient when he returns home. The importance of maintaining a normal attitude cannot be overstressed. Sentimentality is to be avoided, but sympathetic understanding is needed. The family should realize that it is kinder and more advantageous to the individual to allow him to do all that he can for himself, in order to help him to develop self-confidence and independence. The more he takes part in family activities, the sooner he becomes accustomed to his handicap.

Home teachers are available, from the state division or commission for the blind, who visit the home to teach the visually handicapped member how to do household chores and other things if he so desires.

THE BLIND CHILD

A considerable amount of research has been carried on in the area of the preschool blind child, and it is advisable for the occupational therapist to be informed of the latest procedures. Parents can be taught the principles of elementary training for the blind child, who should be taught how to feed and dress himself, the use of toys, how to use his hands and how to play with other children. Extra care is needed in training the blind child who, unlike the sighted child, cannot learn through imitation.

Since many of the babies and children the therapist may come in contact with will be partially sighted, he should have a clear understanding of the differences between the vision of infants and children and adults. The visual acuity of the normal baby is approximately 20/200 at six months, 20/60 at two years, and does not reach 20/20 until the child is somewhere between the fourth and fifth years. Furthermore, children have great powers of accommodation — the ability to bring into focus objects at varying distances from the eye. Children can read small print by holding the page close to their eyes without hurting them. As the child becomes an adult, he gradually loses his power of accommodation and needs "longer arms." Whether "normal" or partially sighted, the child or adult who wants to read or to examine any object will usually hold the book or the article at the distance where he can see it most clearly. If this distance happens to be 2 in. from the eye itself, the therapist should not be disturbed.

Furthermore, children do not need as much light for close work as do adults. The need for stronger and stronger illumination develops with age. It should be born in mind that poor lighting does not cause eye disease, but that enough light to see by, at whatever age, minimizes eyestrain, and increases the speed and efficiency of reading. Occupational therapists working in the geriatric field should be particularly aware of the illumination requirements of their patients.

Occupational therapists are being called on more and more to serve as part of the evaluation and treatment team for the blind child who functions on a retarded level, emotionally disturbed blind children, multiply-handicapped blind children and deaf-blind children. Each of these categories is a specialty in itself, and training in addition to the basic occupational therapy curriculum is important. The newly blinded child may also be referred to occupational therapy.

Almost 10 per cent of the blind population is under 20 years of age. In the United States more than 20,000 blind children are enrolled in school. The majority are in public schools, although blind children can still attend residential school facilities. Low-vision optical aids, large print material, braille books, and material on records or tape all have their place in the education of partially sighted and blind children.

Fortunately, there is an increasing tendency to provide programs in the residential schools for the blind for exceptional blind children — such as the gifted, those with multiple-handicaps, children with the rubella syndrome and the deaf-blind.

In 1968, Title VI of the Elementary and Secondary Education Act was amended to include provision in Part C for the development of comprehensive regional centers for deaf-blind children, including those affected by the 1963–1965 rubella epidemics. These centers are authorized to provide services to deaf-blind children and their parents, their teachers, and others who work with them. Programs will include comprehensive diagnostic and evaluative services and adjustment, orientation and education for the deaf-blind infants or children; as well as consultative and educational services for their parents and personnel. The occupational therapist skilled in child development has a key role to play in this program.

THE ELDERLY BLIND

At the other extreme, the aging blind (particularly those 65 years of age and over) need the services that the occupational therapist can provide. Elderly men and women who are blind, those who have a severe visual handicap, and those whose visual impairment is accompanied by a hearing loss of greater or lesser degree are found not only in hospitals, but in convalescent and nursing homes, home-care programs, and "golden age clubs." This, too, is a specialized field, and those who work with geriatric patients need innate skills and special training.

Communication with the Deaf-Blind Adult

Occasionally, the occupational therapist may be called upon to work with a deaf-blind adult. In this case, some means of communication with the patient is the first necessity. The American Foundation for the Blind can supply information concerning methods of communication; simple aids such as "conversation cards" which combine block letters and braille; and the "Tellatouch," a device which provides a simple means of communication with a deaf-blind person who knows braille. Another resource for information concerning the deaf-blind is the recently organized National Center for Deaf-Blind Youth and Adults, located in New Hyde Park, Long Island, New York. This facility and program is sponsored financially by the Federal Government, and operated by the Industrial Home for the Blind.

SPECIAL WORKSHOPS

Not only have there been changes in work with visually handicapped persons in the educational field, but also in the field of sheltered employment. Formerly, workshops were designed to provide employment for blind persons, some of whom were capable of being employed in regular industry but were unable to obtain employment other than in a subsidized shop. Through special training programs and a change in employer attitudes, many of these persons are now absorbed in industry and the service trades. However, the workshop remains for those incapable of competing with sighted persons, especially those with multiple handicaps.

Workshops are also used for evaluating the potentials of blind individuals seeking employment. Occupational therapists interested in working with visually handicapped adults should be able to apply their training and find employment in these workshops.

VOCATIONAL REHABILITATION

From the beginning of occupational therapy with newly blinded persons, the work with the patient should be planned and directed so that each step advances him toward the ultimate goal of independence and return to his established place in society. If it is not possible for him to return to his former employment, plans should be made for vocational training. The occupation should be chosen because it suits the educational and social background as well as the desire and the abilities of the individual, rather than because it is something a visually handicapped person can do. Occupations in which persons with such a handicap have excelled are the law, the ministry, massage, teaching, social work, music, business management, ownership of stores and hotels, politics, the operation of vending stands, salesmanship (insurance, real estate and numerous commodities), farming, poultry raising and dairy operating.

State agencies for the rehabilitation of blind persons are found in all fifty states, the District of Columbia, Guam, Puerto Rico, and the Virgin Islands. Among the services provided are: counseling, physical examination, vocational diagnosis, medical services, personal adjustment, vocational training, job placement, and job adjustment. The occupational therapist should be familiar with the scope of these programs and how to arrange for procuring those needed by his patients.

NEED FOR OCCUPATIONAL THERAPY

Occupational therapy in the field of the visually handicapped has kept pace with the general expansion of the profession. Recently the American Foundation for the Blind in conjunction with the American Occupational Therapy Association sent a questionnaire to the approximately 5,000 practicing registered occupational therapists, asking about service to blind patients. Of the approximately 2,500 who responded, 85 per cent were treating one or more blind patients, or had within the past twelve months. An outgrowth of this study is expected to be the presentation of courses in various parts of the country to increase the practicing therapists' knowledge about blindness. A special interest group on blindness is being organized within the American Occupational Therapy Association, and a *Blindness Newsletter* is being started on a trial basis.

These developments all indicate progress in the field of occupational therapy for the visually impaired. The profession can make an even greater contribution as more occupational therapists become interested in the many facets of the work. Surely there can be no greater purpose than that of helping a blind child toward the best possible educational program or a newly blinded individual to reorganize his manner of doing things, so that he will have faith in himself as a human being and will maintain the desire to be a contributing member of society.

BIBLIOGRAPHY

Books and Pamphlets

Asenjo, A.: A Step-by-Step Guide to Personal Management for Blind Persons. New York, Am. Found. for the Blind, 1970.

Bourgeault, S. E.: Glossary of Professional Terms for Use in the Area of Service to the Visually Impaired in Asia. New York, Am. Found. for Overseas Blind, 1969.

Brodey, W. M.: Human Enhancement: Its Application to Perception. In Proceedings of the National Seminar on Services to Young Children with Visual Impairment, June 17-19, 1968. New York, Am. Found. for the Blind, 1969.

Carroll, T. J.: Blindness: What It Is, What It Does, and How to Live with It. Boston, Little Brown and Company, 1961.

Chevigny, H., and Braverman, S.: The Adjustment of the Blind. New Haven, Yale University Press, 1950.

Cholden, L. A.: A Psychiatrist Works with Blindness. New York, Am. Found. for the Blind, 1958.

Contemporary Papers. Volume II. Am. Assoc. of Workers for the Blind, Washington, D.C., December 1967.

Cooper, L. Z., and Krugman, S.: The Rubella Problem, In Disease-a-Month, February 1969. Chicago, Year Book Medical Publishers, February 1969.

Curtis, W. S., Donlon, E. T., and Wagner, E. M., eds: Deaf-Blind Children: Evaluating their Multiple Handicaps. New York, Am. Found. for the Blind, 1970.

Dinsmore, A. B.: Methods of Communication with Deaf-Blind People. New York, Am. Found. for the Blind, 1959.

Directory of Agencies Serving Blind Persons in the United States. ed. 15. New York, Am. Found. for the Blind, 1967.

Fellendorf, G. W.: Bibliography on Deafness. A Selected Index. The Volta Review 1899–1965. The American Annals of the Deaf 1847–1965. Washington, D.C., 1966.

Graham, M. D.: Toward a Functional Definition of Blindness. In Research Bulletin, No. 3, pp 120-133. New York, Am. Found. for the Blind, 1963.

Halliday, C.: The Visually Impaired Child – Growth, Learning, Development – Infancy to School Age. Louisville, Kentucky, Instructional Materials Reference Center, Am. Printing House for the Blind, 1970.

Home Teachers of the Adult Blind: What They Do; What They Could Do; What Will Enable Them to Do It. Washington, D.C., Am. Association of Workers for the Blind, Inc., 1961.

Hutchinson, E. L.: The visually handicapped person in his community. In American Association of Workers for the Blind, Proceedings. Washington, D.C., Am. Association of Workers for the Blind, 1961.

If Blindness Occurs. Morristown, New Jersey, Seeing Eye, Inc., rev. 1970.

Klinger, J. L., Frieden, F. H. and Sullivan, R. A.: Mealtime Manual for the Aged and Handicapped. New York, Simon and Schuster, 1970.

Löwe, A., and Westerman, B.: Bibliography on Deaf-Blindness. Dortmund, Prof. Dr. Beschel, 1969.

The Model Reporting Area for Blindness Statistics. Washington, D.C., National Institute of Neurological Diseases and Blindness, 1966.

N.S.P.B. Fact Book: Estimated Statistics on Blindness and Vision Problems. New York, The National Society for the Prevention of Blindness, Inc., 1966.

Rehabilitation of Deaf-Blind Persons. Volumes 1-7. New York, The Industrial Home for the Blind, 1958.

Robbins, N.: Speech beginnings for the deaf-blind child: a guide for parents. Perkins Publication No. 22. Watertown, Massachusetts, Perkins School for the Blind, 1963.

Rusalem, H. et al.: New Frontiers for Research on Deaf-Blindness. Brooklyn, New York, Anne Sullivan Macy Service for Deaf-Blind Persons, The Industrial Home for the Blind, 1966.

Scott, R. A.: The Making of Blind Men: A Study of Adult Socialization. New York, Russell Sage Foundation, 1969.

Shaffer, R. N., and Weiss, D. I.: Congenital and Pediatric Glaucomas. St. Louis, C. V. Mosby Co., 1970.

Understanding Braille. New York, Am. Found. for the Blind (undated).

Vaughan, D., Cook, R., and Asbury, T.: General Ophthalmology. ed. 5. Los Altos, California, Lange Medical Publications, 1968.

Journals

Alkan, H.: Occupational therapy for eye patients. Am. J. Occup. Therapy 17:190, 1963.

Berkow, J. W., Shugarman, R. G., Maumenee, A. E., and Patz, A.: Retrospective study of blind diabetic patients. J.A.M.A., 193:867, 1965.

Burns, D. J., and Stenquist, G. M.: The deaf-blind in the United States—their care, education, and guidance. Rehab. Lit. Nov. 1960. pages 334-344.

Clark, G.: The need for occupational therapy in retinal detachments. Am. J. Occup. Therapy 17:19, 1963.

Dinsmore, A. B.: Unmet needs of deaf-blind children. The New Outlook for the Blind, Oct. 1967 (reprint).

Fox, J. vanD.: Improving tactile discrimination of the blind: a neurological approach. Am. J. Occup. Therapy 19:6, 1965.

Goodman, W.: When you meet a blind person. The New Outlook for the Blind, 64:186, 1970.

Moor, P. M.: What teachers are saying about the young blind child. J. Nurs. Educ., Vol. 15, No. 2, Winter 1960. (unpaged).

Sevel, D., and Hart, J. A.: Occupational therapy for the hospitalized eye patient. Am. J. Occup. Therapy 23:339, 1969.

Voorhees, A. L.: Counseling the Blind. Vocational Guidance Quarterly, 3:55, Winter 1954–55.

Wagner, E. M.: Maternal rubella, a general orientation to the disease. The New Outlook for the Blind, 61:97, 1967.

Special Issues

American Journal of Occupational Therapy:

Auditory Field	7:1	1953
Geriatric Field	15:139	1961
Visual Field	5:137	1951

The New Outlook for the Blind

Anne Sullivan Macy, 1866–1936 and Services for the deaf-blind. 60:101, 1966.

The Blind Child Who Functions on a Retarded Level. 63:289, 1969.

Films

Communicating with Deaf-Blind People. 16 mm-sound – color. Available from American Foundation for the Blind.

Happy, Forward. 16 mm-sound – color. Available from The Seeing Eye.

What a Blind Man Sees. 16 mm-sound – black and white. Produced by the Industrial Home for the Blind, Brooklyn, New York. Available from Am. Found. for the Blind.

LIST OF RESOURCES

American Foundation for the Blind, Inc.
15 West 16th Street
New York, New York 10011

American Foundation for Overseas Blind
22 West 17th Street
New York, New York 10011

American Printing House for the Blind, Inc.
1839 Frankfort Avenue
Louisville, Kentucky 40206

Industrial Home for the Blind
57 Willoughby Street
Brooklyn, New York 11205

International Association of Rehabilitation Facilities
7979 Old Georgetown Road, Suite 600
Washington, D.C. 20014

National Accreditation Council for Agencies
  Serving the Blind and Visually Handicapped
79 Madison Avenue, Suite 1406
New York, New York 10016

National Industries for the Blind
50 West 44th Street
New York, New York 10036

National Society for the Prevention of Blindness, Inc.
70 Madison Avenue
New York, N.Y. 10016

Recording for the Blind, Inc.
215 East 58th Street
New York, New York 10022

The Seeing Eye, Inc.
Morristown, New Jersey 07960

U.S. Department of Health, Education and Welfare
Washington, D.C.

U.S. Library of Congress
Division for the Blind and Physically Handicapped
Washington, D.C.

Matilda Ziegler Magazine for the Blind
20 West 17th Street
New York, N.Y. 10011

ACKNOWLEDGEMENT

The authors wish to express their appreciation to Daniel I. Weiss, M.D.,
Clinical Assistant Professor of Ophthalmology, New York University School of
Medicine, who graciously consented to review this manuscript.

17

Occupational Therapy in Geriatrics

ALBERTA D. WALKER, PH.D., O.T.R.

INTRODUCTION

The term *geriatrics* refers to that branch of medicine which is concerned with the diseases and hygiene of old age. The diseases and their treatments will not be discussed in this chapter. The use of occupational therapy for specific diseases and dysfunctions will be covered elsewhere in this text. Instead emphasis will be placed on the following areas: first, on the social conditions of the aged in the past, present and future, which have or will have an influence on the kind of treatment, including occupational therapy, which the aged receive in our society; secondly, on the role of the patient, and the role of the therapist involved in the treatment program.

Since both participants, patient and therapist, are products of their social environment, it is imperative that some rapport be established initially for the treatment to be effective. A meaningful approach in establishing rapport with the aged is to be keenly aware of and to appreciate the patient's social dilemma. With this knowledge the therapist is in a better position to change an attitude which might otherwise seriously affect the success of the treatment. No other specialty area in occupational therapy tests the therapist's maturity and sincerity more rigorously than the field of geriatrics.

An overall approach to this chapter will be one of social gerontology — the process of aging. The individual is not a product of one generation — his own — but of the generations prior to his. Furthermore, each stage of his life influences the next stage. Thus, a person does not suddenly or automatically become aged at 65, but instead is in the process of aging from birth to death. Therefore, today a great deal of stress is placed on flexibility of roles; that is, the individual receives greater satisfaction in his social environment if he has the capacity to adjust to his surroundings. Consequently, the following discussion will center around the aged and aging concomitantly.

PART I

SOCIAL TREATMENT OF THE AGED IN THE PAST

The aged have received various kinds of social treatment throughout recorded history. A brief discussion will follow of the approaches used by the ancient Hebrews, Greeks, Romans, medieval Europeans and colonial Americans.

The Hebraic treatment of the aged, as in all other cultures, must be understood against the background of their changing social conditions. The status of the aged is deduced chiefly from the figure of the desert patriarch, who dominated his extended household, which ranged from wives to servants who attached themselves to his enclave for protection. Respect for the aged, especially for the patriarch, was essential, based on experience in surviving a forbidding environment. The husband or master had considerable power over his household, and aging did not diminish his authority. Age was inseparably linked with respect, power and mysticism among the ancient Hebrews. Long life was viewed as a blessing rather than a burden. Aging was equated with wisdom; youth with inexperience and making hasty, ill-conceived decisions.

The idealization of the aged and of aging was perpetuated in Greece. But attitudes in ancient Greece differed sharply from Hebraic conceptions. The former turned to greater glorification of youth. Although differing from the ancient Hebrews in their perceptions and social treatment of the aged and aging, the ancient Greeks were similar with respect to interest in life in the present. They sought to enjoy life to the fullest and mourned its slipping away. Their literature reflected their dread of old age.

Men of power could count on losing it to ambitious youth as the passage of years eroded their capacities. Women could anticipate successive husbands, neglect or abandonment. Parents could hope that their children would support them in old age, but this could be accomplished only against great odds. In fact, to the ancient Greeks aging was a fate worse than death.[7]

The militaristic, sensual and grandiose Romans continued the Hellenic deprecation of the aged and aging. Their imitation of Greek traditions extended not only to language, religion and philosophy, but also to their wavering between an official posture of good will toward the aged and a more practical unconcern for those regarded as past their prime.[1] Retaining dignity by committing suicide was an honorable end for many Romans, a view that is periodically upheld to this day. The intolerable situation is resolved by removal of the sufferer.[32]

The vacuum of authority created by the decline of Rome was filled by the rise of two spheres of influence — the sacred and the secular — organized Christianity and the feudal landholding system. Of the two, The Roman Church assumed the lion's share of power and consolidated its strength throughout Europe. The aged received much more official recognition and consideration than they had under Greek and Roman traditions.

Medieval life was essentially agrarian, with certain securities guaranteed to cooperating classes. By far the greatest boon to the aged was the solicitude and compassion extended them by the growing body of canon law, backed by an obedient priesthood that commanded considerable wealth.[25] The sincere dedication of the Church to the salvation of souls did not exclude the humble, the poor, the ill, or the aged. Charity, hospitality and care were essential elements in parish life and comforted many of the aged in their time of need. If the land laws or the family circle could not sustain them, the aged could find solace through the three institutions of the church: the parish, the monastery, and the hospital. Finally, under the leadership and urging of the Church, homes for the aged, ill and handicapped were established. Hundreds of hospitals in Europe provided custodial as well as medical care for older persons.

To conclude this brief overview of the history of the social treatment of the aged a few observations should be made as Judeo-Christian traditions, supplemented by Greco-Roman ideas, left a post feudal Europe and were transplanted into the New World. The rigors of colonial life demanded strong, healthy adults and tended to exclude the very young, weak, overburdened, and elderly. Male domination continued unabated on the frontiers and farms, in the villages and towns. Women were subordinated by the mores of the times as well as by public declarations. Large families, the glorification of work (known as the Protestant Ethic) and patriarchy were characteristic of colonial life. Obedient, servile, God-fearing children were living assurance that the advanced years, if they were reached at all, would not be lonely and without material comforts.

The persistence of early American patterns concerning the aged may be observed in the unique customs of contemporary Amish.[11] These religious people have steadfastly held to principles, passed along intact from late seventeenth and early eighteenth century Europe and colonial America, that are rooted in ancient Hebraic traditions.

This comparative study of ancient Hebrews, Greeks, Romans, medieval Europeans, and colonial Americans does not reveal much progress toward greater respect and influence for the aged. Instead, it unveils a tendency to idealize and to honor, and a need to come to terms with the loss of power with the passage of a lifetime. Although there was considerable care for the aged, action was not forthcoming without community pressure. Fortuitous social structures either granted great power to the aged or left them vulnerable to suffering and neglect. The sketches drawn from the European-American historical record of social treatment of the aged provide a sobering picture of the reluctance to meet the needs of the elderly.

Ancient ideals provide impetus to be morally correct, but pragmatically, the interests of the aged may not be in the societal mainstream and so may be devalued. As America moved from a pre-industrial, or agrarian society, to an industrial society the social climate for the aged changed. With industrialization, specialization, urbanization and automation now well entrenched in this country, the aged are all too frequently placed in the difficult position of being dysfunctional or nonfunctional as members of their society. The multi-faceted problems of the aged in America which have risen and have become the concern of many will be the subject of the next section of this chapter.

SOCIAL TREATMENT OF THE AGED IN THE PRESENT

Probably no other group in America has been more thoroughly studied in the past fifteen years than the aged, in terms of health, housing and employment. More research is constantly being started, and still more will follow. Studies grew mainly out of the realization, shortly after World War II, that this country was developing a sizable population of older people, that they had unique problems and interests, and that very little was really known about them as a group. Their number, for example, had increased in the first half of the 20th century from approximately 3 million, representing 4 per cent of the population, to 12.3 million, representing more than 8 per cent. By 1980 it is estimated 24.5 per cent of the population will be 65 years or older, and by the year 2000 this proportion will have risen to 32.3 per cent.[49]

It was recognized by economists, social scientists, physicians, government officials and others that America was going to have a serious crisis on its hands if this growing group did not receive special attention. As a result, government agencies, universities and colleges, community and national organizations, employers, and private foundations began to probe and study. Rarely, if ever, have so many spotlights been trained so steadily on a social development.

Progress has been made through the establishment of the social security system, which provides a foundation of financial security on which the individual older person can build greater security through his own devices. By 1935, when the Social Security Act was passed, only about 1100 employers had pension plans and only about 2.2 million employees were covered. By 1965 there were 25,000 plans covering 23 million workers. However, despite the relatively early discovery of the need for the establishment of public and private systems of providing income in retirement, adequate income among the aged is still the exception rather than the rule. In fact, for all the interest and activity which has surrounded the aged in the past 15 years, one conclusion stands out. The older person has gained longer life — as a result of scientific, economic and social advances in this century — but is left without the financial means to solve satisfactorily many economic, social, and medical problems. This conclusion is one that we, as a nation, have not fully faced. It is one that millions of our elderly have to face daily. Many more are poorly housed and poorly fed. Many are forced to turn to their children or to the public for the medical care they need. Many have been shoved into a dull, meaningless existence because the opportunities to remain active and to use their skills and talents are not available.

What we need to keep constantly in mind is that the same society which has given Americans longer life has not developed enough ways for making additional years useful and meaningful. It must be recognized that a citizen's desire to live a purposeful life does not end with his retirement. It must be made clear that skills and talents do not suddenly end with retirement. There is a need to seek out new means to use these talents, which all too often go unused. Does the average American, supposedly blessed with longevity but faced with mandatory retirement at 65 years, make any preparation for retirement? A nationwide survey indicates that in preparing for retirement the overall picture for older people in the United States is one of gross negligence:[24,53]

Of those retired: 57.6% made no plans
                    27.4% made a few plans
                    14.5% claimed to make any plans.
Of those close to retirement:
                    23 % said they had made plans
                    76.7% said they had made no plans.
When asked if employers had assisted them in making plans:
                    83.7% denied receiving any help
                    15.4% could say they had received help.

The dilemma retirement presents for the American man in particular, arises from the fact that the leisurely life expected of the retired person contradicts the pervasive work orientation of our society. Our society does not yet accord to retirement the positive value it accords to work.

A second related problem arises from the fact that retirement has not yet been institutionalized. According to Thompson, retirement is what one makes of it.[48] The retiree must create for himself a pattern of activities which serves as an effective substitute for his work. Adjustment in retirement involves considerable personal *input*, over and above that required to assimilate new activities and patterns of interaction. Successful adjustment, then, means that the individual must find self-fulfillment through socially acceptable means. Society may have to define what is socially acceptable before the retired status is institutionalized.

THE MEANING OF INDEPENDENCE

To most of the elderly, a high degree of independence is almost as valuable as life itself. It is their touchstone for self-respect and dignity. It is the measure they use to decide their importance to others. And, it is their source of strength for helping those around them.[28]

Whether they enjoy the degree of independence they desire depends partly on the role they play in the community, partly on the conditions of their health, and partly on the adequacy of their incomes, housing, medical care and other essentials. Their importance will vary not only from person to person but from time to time depending on a given situation.

HEALTH PROBLEMS

Millions of older Americans enjoy relatively good health, and many of them can be almost as active as they were when they were years younger. Many of those with disabilities have learned to live with them and accept their limitations.

Most of the elderly, however, have become the prey of at least one disease that will remain with them as long as they live. The causes of and cures for the diseases that come with age still have to be discovered. It is dramatic proof of the health-care problems faced by our older Americans who are caught between rising medical and hospital costs and their relatively low, fixed incomes.

More than 12 million elderly persons in this country have at least one chronic condition such as high blood pressure, arthritis, diabetes, heart disease or a mental disorder. More than half of those with a chronic ailment have some limitation on their activities. More than 800,000 of our elderly are in institutions. About 1,250,000 elderly people are invalids who, though not in institutions, are unable to get along without help from others. Tragically, many of those with serious conditions would be in better health if known preventative and restorative services had been promptly used.

Accidents, many of them preventable, take a high toll among older people. They have nearly twice as many home accidents as the average adult and three times as many fatal accidents. Information gleaned from recent health surveys indicates that the average older person is incapacitated 5 weeks of the year by illness or injury, with two of these weeks spent in bed.[20] One out of every six of the elderly will go into a hospital during a year. The average hospital stay for an older person is 2 weeks, twice as long as for the average younger person.

Nursing homes and other long-term institutions are largely populated by older persons. The average age of patients in many nursing homes is as high as 80 years.[25] It has been estimated that older persons constitute roughly 33 per cent of the patients in mental hospitals, 20 per cent of those in tuberculosis hospitals, and about 50 per cent of those in long-term institutions.

Older persons are much more likely to require home care of some kind; fifteen times as likely as younger people. Ethel Shanas has estimated that 7 to 8 per cent of the elderly are either bedridden or housebound.[52] Of the ambulatory aged, she estimates that approximately 30 per cent have difficulty walking stairs, 10 per cent have difficulty bathing, and 8 per cent have difficulty dressing.

The significant economic fact about the health problems of older persons is that, whereas their medical costs run twice as high as those of younger people, their incomes are only half as large. Only a relatively small proportion of older persons have substantial incomes and are able to afford ordinary medical costs. The overwhelming majority of older persons do not have adequate financial resources to cover medical emergencies. Those with the most limited resources are also those with the highest rates of illness.

The Medicare Program, which became law in 1965, was an attempt to relieve some of the high cost of illness. This program is a part of the Social Security System. Though it promised to offer some needed help to older people in meeting the costs of their medical care, the Medicare plan is certainly not adequate to solve the health problems of the elderly. Significantly, about one third of those older persons who elected not to sign up for the supplementary part of the Medicare Program, designed to provide partial payment of doctors' bills and other expenses, said that they could not afford to pay even $3.00 a month for the added benefits.[56] Five years later, 1970, this fee had risen to $5.00 a month, which incurred even a greater burden.

Loether states that there is a definite relationship between the state of a person's health and his feelings of dignity and self-respect.[16] Older persons who feel rejected or neglected are more likely to see their health as being poor than those who are accepted. The problem is much deeper than the physical problems of health. It is a problem whose solution lies more properly in some basic changes in the American value system. Recognition of the fact that ever larger numbers of our citizens will be among the elderly and the assignment to them of a respected place in our social system, could do much to alleviate their health problems — particularly the problem of mental health.

IDENTIFICATION WITH THE COMMUNITY

Next in importance to the aged individual's state of health is his place in the community. Some sources would list it as his primary concern. Be that as it may, for many, nothing is quite so important or as difficult as maintaining a useful and congenial place in the community around them.

For the first time, perhaps since childhood, the aged have extra hours — hours with no demands. Too frequently, the consequence of excessive time available to the elderly is one of disillusioned persons suddenly being forced into a completely strange period of inactivity, with no place to go, nothing to do, no purpose. Inertia, boredom, and tentative withdrawal can quickly lead to isolation. This condition has been called "retirement shock." Burgess states that the aged upon formal completion of working for a living assume a "roleless role."[4] He concludes that this role is thrust by society upon the older person at retirement, and to a greater or lesser degree he has accepted it or become resigned to it. Certain stereotypes and myths have grown up in Western cultures particularly to sanction this roleless role. Burgess mentions the following:

1. *Passive behavior*, the expected pattern of the older person in retirement. He should now "take it easy, loaf, and fish."

2. *Dependence* on others for advice and assistance is the natural and inevitable consequence of advancing years.

3. *Custodial care* in institutions as the answer to chronic illness, invalidity and mental disturbances common in old age.

4. *Withdrawal* from social participation which tends to accompany departure from employment.

5. *No preparation* for retirement is required or expected, asserting older persons need only to relax, read and listen to radio and/or watch television.

6. *Circulation of myths* which have no basis in fact and are prejudicial to older persons. Typical of these are that the older workers are unable to learn new skills, have more accidents, are less productive than younger workers. When these stereotypes are prevalent in the public mind and often accepted by older workers they are the greatest obstacle to progress by society and by the older person himself.

Other researchers have proposed two theories about the aged person's inclination to withdraw from society after the formal period of his working life ceases. These are the engagement and disengagement theories. Though they emphasize different aspects of the adjustment problem, these theories supplement each other. Both focus on the individual's role complex and on the changes that take place in it as the person ages. The engagement theory has been proposed by Havighurst in what he calls *role flexibility** as the key to successful adjustment to aging.[32] In research he conducted in conjunction with Albrecht, Havighurst found that those individuals who were active in a wide variety of social roles or highly active in a given social role were more likely to be happy and to make a good social adjustment to old age than were those who were less active.[1]

The assumptions made in the engagement, or role flexibility, theory are that significant changes occur in an individual's role complex between the ages of 50 and 75 years. Some roles are reduced or discontinued, some are intensified, others are intensified with effort, and still others are assumed for the first time. Some older persons intensify their homemaker roles (e.g., by gardening, decorating, repairing or entertaining); others play more active roles in their community (e.g., in their churches, as citizens, members of friendship groups, and members of extended families). Participation in recreational activities may be increased. Creative activities may be undertaken. The roles which may be reduced or discontinued are the roles of worker, parent and spouse. Among the new roles that might be assumed are the grandparent role and the role of a member of a senior citizens' organization.

The disengagement theory, proposed by Cummings and Henry, is that as a person ages he begins to withdraw from society by surrendering some of his social roles.[6] These researchers conclude that disengagement is an inevitable process in which many of the relationships between a person and other members of society are severed, and those which remain are altered in quality. As a person grows older, he begins to acknowledge the inevitability of death and begins preparing for it by gradually withdrawing from active roles. In addition, the disengagement process is accelerated by declining health and motility. Because of differences among individuals the time in life at which the disengagement process begins and the rate at which it proceeds vary. Furthermore, the degree of qualitative change which occurs in interpersonal relationships differs from person to person; but once it has begun, the disengagement process becomes self-perpetuating.

Rose and Peterson have carefully examined the disengagement theory and they suggest that some persons in their later years, rather than being alienated from others and thus disengaged, tend to develop an "aging group consciousness," and an "aging subculture," which

---

*Role flexibility is defined in the above context to mean the ability of an individual to change roles easily and to increase or reduce activity as the social situation demands it.

provide a network of interrelationships and serve as a social and cultural milieu for the older person.[22] Such a group self-consciousness and participation system tends to develop as old persons come to share common interests based on common past experiences, and as a consequence of withdrawal or exclusion from other relationships. However, Rose further notes that those who have disengaged have been forced into such a position by such pressures as youth orientation, compulsory retirement, and minimal opportunities in self-employment.[21] None of these is irreversible.

Those who endorse the engagement theory have won strong support for action programs to provide for or prolong firm bonds between aging individuals and their society. Those who favor disengagement insist that the bonds between aging individuals and their social milieu must inevitably be reduced and finally severed. The latter perspective has not as many advocates as the former. The "adding life to the years" and "retirement to life" slogans make good sense in terms of socio-psychological well-being. Study after study reports positive results in terms of good health and continued services to the elderly. On the other hand, "growing old gracefully" implies to some a shifting to a new, rather threatening status of being shelved, sidelined, and side-stepped. Recognition of limitations imposed by the aging process, also well documented by numerous studies, leads to the "roleless role" of the aged which may be filled with attractions of its own. Research in these matters has hardly begun, but knowledge is accumulating.

The engagement or role flexibility theory and the disengagement theory are not incompatible, but rather, they supplement each other. The disengagement theory describes the process by which the individual's role complex is voluntarily or involuntarily altered as he grows old. The disjunctions, described by Cummings and Henry, occur between the expectations of society and those of the individual, which may account for the many cases of poor adjustment among aged individuals. The theory of engagement, or role flexibility, serves to explain why many persons who are involuntarily disengaged from their central life roles are still able to make successful adjustments to old age. These are the people, according to Havighurst, who have cultivated that personal quality called role flexibility. The aged person's place in the community might well be determined on the basis of these proposed theories.

A PROSPECTIVE VIEW OF THE FUTURE FOR THE AGED

The problems which the aged have had to face under present social conditions may not, from a pragmatic point of view, be problems of the future.

Persons retiring five, ten or more years from now will be accustomed to more free time in their active, earning years than are most older Americans today. Shorter work days, shorter work weeks, longer yearly vacations and earlier retirement will help prepare tomorrow's elderly for active later years. Retirement will more often be anticipated as an opportunity to embark on a second career. It will provide a chance to grow in new interests, to find new avenues of creativity and to continue to live fully, adventurously and generously, with the knowledge that activity itself is an essential part of successful living in later years.

Kastenbaum has enumerated the following aspects where future generations of the elderly in the United States might differ from today's elderly.[36]

1. *Better educated.* Many of today's elderly were "dropouts" at an early age. Education offers many opportunities for an adult to continue as part of his community. One of the less obvious, but important values of preretirement education is the reminder to persons approaching full retirement that education for education's sake can be stimulating and enjoyable. Some older people welcome the chance to learn a new language, to be guided into greater appreciation of music or art, or to experience for the first time the joy of painting, modeling, orchestration, or discussion.

Basic elementary education, when classes are offered in convenient neighborhood locations and in sheltered environments, such as homes for the aged and senior citizens' residences, is eagerly accepted by older adults who lacked educational opportunities when they were growing up. Colleges and universities, community colleges, and public school adult education agencies in several areas across this country are offering courses especially designed to meet these increased needs. Many libraries have developed special services and programs for their older patrons.

2. *Demographic changes.* Many of today's elderly were born in other lands. One source estimated there are more than 3 million people among today's aged who migrated from Europe to the United States.[20] This large group has suffered from changes the future elderly will not have to endure. Modern economic social trends have brought losses as well as gains to all age groups in the population. But the full adverse effects have been experienced by the aging. Rather than to forecast it might be more advantageous at this point to recapitulate the serious blows which will not be experienced in the future. First, they lost their economic independence. They were demoted from the status of employer to that of employee. Their place of work was no longer the home but the factory or office. Second, in increasing numbers they had to give up rural residences for urban living. Third, they were forced to

retire from work by the decision of the employer rather than of their own free will (as in the past). Fourth, they lost their former favored position in the extended family. No longer were the grandfather and grandmother the center of the absorbing life of their descendents but often became unwanted hangers on, taking part by sufferance in the activities of their children or grandchildren. And fifth, deprived of the society of their family and having lost associates on the job and other friends by death or departure to other communities, they found themselves cursed instead of blessed by leisure time in abundance and the inability to utilize it.

The extent to which older persons become visible (as enumerated in demographic studies) often determines whether they will be superficially treated or given appropriate status within a population. This being the case, that older persons are becoming and will continue to become more visible, the United States may be described now, in demographic terms, as a young nation shifting to a maturing nation. It is estimated that private enterprise will gear itself more to an aging market offering goods and services calculated to appeal to this aging populace in the future.

3. *Better health.* The future generations will more likely enjoy better health throughout life. Medical advances and the increasing availability of medical services to all members of society should reduce the numbers of infirmities and ailments that people carry with them in their later years. Prompt management of health problems as they arise will arrest many conditions that have been chronic with elders today; rehabilitative medicine should also be more effective and widespread.

4. *Adequate income.* The impoverished or near-impoverished status of many older persons today has been widely advertised, although still disputed by some. Recent legislation and other developments that are likely to follow probably will ease this financial situation. Additionally, many future elderly persons will enjoy relatively affluent careers. This circumstance will contrast with the life history of many of our present elderly who have lived through some very lean, if not destitute, times.

5. *Higher standard of living.* In the future, elderly persons will be accustomed to a relatively high standard of living. They will have greater independence, better education, improved health and will be more career oriented. Therefore, fewer older perons will have to satisfy themselves by "scraping by."

6. *Preparation for retirement.* They are more likely to have thought about aging and retirement. Part of the "lost" look that characterizes some of the elderly can be attributed to lack of preparation for their present condition. Aging and retirement, not especially popular topics today, were even less popular in past decades. Future generations of the elderly are likely to grow up with greater appreciation for the retirement years, with more plans, more provisions and greater expectations.

7. *Less guilt about retirement.* Many of the elderly feel uncomfortable, and some feel guilty about their post-occupational existence, particularly men. At the present time, even if there were no economic necessity for them to work, most men would work anyway. It is through the producing role that most men tie into society, and for this reason and others, most men find the producing role important for maintaining their sense of well-being. Morse and Weiss contend that not only is work central to the life of the average American male but increasingly so to the American woman.[42] However, as this society becomes less work oriented (with the advent of shorter work days and weeks, and earlier retirement), the use of leisure time will become more institutionalized and thus socially acceptable.

8. *Acceptance and expectations of programmed assistance.* Today some of the elderly are more attuned to patterns of mutual aid as delivered by family, neighborhood or close knit groups. These elderly have been reluctant and have thus resisted or avoided organized programs of assistance such as housing, medical care or financial aid. Future generations of the elderly may be more practiced both in giving and receiving assistance through governmental and other formalized operations.

9. *Continued intellectual growth.* Future generations of the elderly will be more interested in continued education and in creative, recreative and civic activities. These elderly will bring a variety of interests with them. Already well educated, they will be capable of and motivated toward, further intellectual stimulation. They will not have to be satisfied with busy work or amusement situations.

Many of the elderly now show resistance to geriatric environments that underestimate their resources. This trend should be even more pronounced in subsequent generations.

10. *Social force.* Future generations of elderly will be more aware of themselves as a social force. The elderly, conscious of their group potential, will become increasingly influential in political and social spheres. Instead of feeling isolated or powerless, they might well have a realistic sense of membership in a reasonably powerful group.

11. *Social expectancy.* The problems facing the elderly of the future will be anticipated. Much of the difficulty experienced today both by them and by the community is associated with time pressure. Today we are attempting to solve the social problems *ex post facto* simply because we did not prepare for the present generation of elderly. The urgency and the impulse to do *something,* and do it quickly will hopefully be over. A more appropriate tempo of events will facilitate transition and adjustment.

This discussion has included three time dimensions — past, present and future — in which the social treatment of the aged and aging has been considered. Although many inequities still exist, in some respects, conditions have improved. However, the proportion of elderly people in the population has increased so rapidly in comparison to other categories that their presence began to be felt because of the multi-faceted problems which arose needing public attention. Some progress has been made but courses of action still remain to be taken to improve present conditions which exist among the elderly.

To appreciate the areas in need of attention, Tibbitts succinctly lists the needs of the aged:[54]

To render some socially useful service.

To be considered a part of the community.

To occupy their increased leisure time in satisfying ways.

To enjoy normal companionships.

For recognition as an individual.

For the opportunity for self-expression and a sense of achievement.

For health protection and care.

For suitable mental stimulation.

For suitable living arrangements and family relationships.

For spiritual satisfaction.

Not only are they needs but they are rights. With these rights, however, each citizen must assume certain obligations:[54]

To prepare himself to become and resolve to remain active, alert, capable, self-supporting and useful so long as health and circumstances permit and to plan for ultimate retirement.

To learn and apply sound principles of physical and mental health.

To seek and develop potential avenues of service in the years after retirement.

To make available the benefits of his experience and knowledge.

To endeavor to make himself adaptable to the changes added years will bring.

To attempt to maintain such relationships with family, neighbors, and friends as will make him a respected and valued counselor throughout his later years.

Some of our existing problems can be solved if these rights and obligations become reality in the form of a workable program. Without such a plan of action they will remain platitudes. Much can be accomplished by making such a program a challenge to us now and in the future.

PART TWO

IMPLICATIONS FOR THE OCCUPATIONAL THERAPIST

At the time of incorporation, The American Occupational Therapy Foundation made a statement of position: " . . . we (the profession) identify as our unique contribution a concern for the developmental process of man during his entire life span: his relationship with his environment and his development toward assuming satisfying life tasks . . . total health needs . . . our evaluation of his capacity to relate to and master his environment provide the basis for a program design which speak to his age-specific role or task mastery needs. . . ."[23] These are some of the tenets on which occupational therapy as a profession rests. In the specialty area of geriatrics they (tenets) are put through one of their most rigorous tests.

Having given a brief overview of the scope of the multi-faceted problems of the elderly, those past, present and anticipated in the future, we will now look for the thread that weaves throughout and serves as implications for the occupational therapist. Nothing in life is ever isolated, and no generational phenomenon stands by itself. Everything is interrelated and some things are culturally transmitted as the society deems fitting.

The roles of the Patient and the Therapist

Into the treatment milieu the patient and the therapist, usually of different generations, come together. Each has preconceived ideas of what is expected, but these are seldom, if ever, clear to the other. Each has his own attitudes, his own experiences and thus, his own judgment of what is possible and not possible. Some of these are idealistic and some realistic, but nevertheless, they are present during therapy. As time passes, either favorable or unfavorable assessments of the situation will take place. The possible rationale of the approach to treatment, the evaluation and re-evaluation of progress made will be of major concern to both the patient and the therapist.

Emphasis in this section will be placed on the role of the therapist as he interacts directly with the elderly patient, and further as he interacts with other medical specialists and personnel concerned with the welfare of the elderly individual's progress. The role performances of the patient, the therapist, and everyone involved in the patient's welfare are assessed in terms of society's needs. These needs have a direct bearing on the outcome of the treatment.

Initially there was a moral obligation to take care of the aged. This moral obligation is a part of the mores which have been passed down in a culture—from one generation to another. Sometimes social conditions are such that this obligation is not practical and therefore not binding, but some remnant of it remains nevertheless in the conscience. It plays a part in the kind of respect shown to the aged.

In addition, there is a self-image which Cooley called the "looking-glass self."[5] He held that self and social are two sides of the same coin. Our ideas, loyalties, attitudes and points of view are derived from others. In interaction the individual infers how he is regarded by others, how others see his appearance and actions and how others interpret his verbal and nonverbal responses. Then, he imagines what others' judgment is of what he infers that others see. In brief, he derives his own self-concept from others.

Therapist's Attitude Toward the Elderly

Newton states that members of the health professions are frequently unaware of how or why they reject the elderly patient.[17] All around us in the social scheme we find that the aged are less wanted than the young. Shrinking from the reminder of aging in ourselves, she concludes, we may then identify ourselves with our elderly patient, and, in rejecting the image, we may reject the patient.

The Elderly Patient's Initial Reaction

The patients, generally speaking, seldom regard themselves as old; at least not as old as the younger person envisions them to be. With the knowledge of his rights, by being older than his therapist, and consequently, feeling more experienced in living, he has to be convinced of the therapist's integrity. Just these aspects alone will reveal the gap in communication in this dyad (therapist and patient). In addition to the complexity of the dyadic relationship, we must consider the setting for treatment.

Patient's Use of the Sick Role

If the patient is living in a protective environment, such as a hospital, nursing or rest home, convalerium, or geriaterium, the aged person is ascribed a "sick role" whether he wishes to fill his role or not. It is, therefore, arbitrary, and illness becomes institutionalized as a social role. According to Parsons there is an institutionalized expectation system relative to a sick role.[18] First, there is the expectation that the sick individual will be unable to fulfill his normal social responsibilities, and furthermore he should not try to fulfill them. Secondly, it is assumed that the individual cannot make himself well by an act of will; his condition is such that he must be taken care of. Thirdly, being ill is undesirable, and the individual has an obligation to cooperate with those concerned about his condition so that he will regain his health. From a therapeutic standpoint it would be more advantageous for the aged patient to stress the last two points, since they emphasize the active sick role. However, we must keep in mind the aged person's self-image prior to his admission.

The sick role of the aged person incorporates within it the economic and physical spheres of influence. The physical sick role may be discussed first. It is impossible for the older person to return to his former state of health, especially if his illness is a result of the degenerative aging process itself. Superimposed upon this physical sick role is the economic factor. Although mentioned in the first part of this chapter, it is worth repeating in this context that society, which has no need for the older person in the work force, drives him out of the occupational role into compulsory retirement, and removes his major source of income. Age-discriminatory hiring practices and Social Security regulations make it virtually impossible for the aged individual to return to full participation in the economic order. As his savings and/or pension plan become increasingly inadequate he becomes poor. Our society now "rescues" him through the terminal sick role of the aged. Recall in the time of the ancient Romans that the intolerable situation is resolved by removal of the sufferer (suicide). Now, the trend is to remove an intolerable situation rather than the sufferer. Dependence is thus condoned for the aged individual who must play the economic sick role; he is allowed legitimately to receive some support on the basis that he can no longer help himself, no matter how much he might want to do so. The existence of Social Security programs, Old Age Assistance, Medicare, subsidized housing, etc., indicates that the terminal sick role in the economic sphere has been institutionalized in our society. Thus in the therapeutic setting, the terminal sick role for the aged, in both the economic and physical sphere, lacks the temporary nature described as characteristic of the active sick role.

Numerous empirical studies indicate that the morale of the dependent aged is lowered by their uncomfortable, unpalatable, and anxiety producing role, and the values internalized by the elderly person himself degrades his role in his own eyes.[15,35] With entry into a new situation—in this instance the therapeutic one—the aged person tends to seek clues and signals (How am I defined here, and how does this relate to the way I am accustomed to define myself?). When the person brings with himself a self-definition that already is tentative or partially "spoiled"—by the attitudes of others—then he is even more at the mercy of his immediate environment.

The communication gap referred to earlier seems even wider in the light of the above discussion. As a professional person, the therapist in a therapeutic situation is placed in a position of "detached concern." He must remain sufficiently detached to be objective and exercise sound judgment yet concerned enough to give the aged patient sensitive, understanding care.

The Concept of What Makes a Good Therapist

Much has been written in terms of what makes a good therapist. Inskip states that in addition to being creative and energetic, the more effective therapists believe in what they do.[34] They have a purpose in living. They have an enthusiasm about their work and about life. This basic attitude is communicated non-verbally to the patient. It says, *I believe in you, I believe in myself, I believe that if we pull together you can be helped, I believe that the goals we set together can be accomplished.* Essential in a therapeutic environment is a therapist who possesses the basic attitude that he is a worthwhile person, a person who has a purpose he believes in and a job to do that he feels is important. When the therapist believes in himself, he believes in others. This attitude gives hope and without hope the goal to be reached might not seem worth the necessary energy expended to accomplish the task.

Mullan is one of several specialists in the field who has studied the factor of emotional response to the aged and to the individual's own aging process. He has listed a number of characteristics that are conducive to healthy relationships in working with the aged.[43] A partial list of the most favorable characteristics is:

In relationship to self

Those who accept the aging process, who do not feel that they have lost out in life, who are generally satisfied with their status and role. Those who do not conceal their own age, who are not overly concerned with their appearance, who do not require of themselves perfection, complete understanding and immediate results. Those who are patient.

In relationship to parents and/or grandparents

Those who are accepting of parents and/or grandparents, seeing them as reasonable and nonrestricting, who believe that they have lived productive lives and did not unduly sacrifice themselves, who feel free and satisfied, although separated from parents.

In relationship to the cosmos

Those who view sickness and death as another experience in life, neither denying it nor ignoring it, whose religious beliefs include a conviction that there is a hereafter and that life is but an aspect of the total experience.

ESTABLISHING RAPPORT

Intrinsic to the above discussion is the establishment of rapport. It involves the use of a common language (through shared frames of reference), so that each person, by what he says or the postures he takes, calls out in himself the response that his gestures, postures and symbols call out in others. Not only do differences in class spell differences in language, values and general perspective; so too, and often in greater degree, do differences in ethnic and national background, in age and in sex. The occupational therapist frequently must deal with all these differences in a single patient. Becker, Blanc, Leznoff, Vogt, Von Hoffman and Cassidy, as well as Paul, have called attention to special transcultural problems, and Benney, Riesman and Star have shown the importance of age and sex differences in eliciting information in interviews.[46,19] One would suppose that the initial interview would present a setting in which these differences would be likely to affect rapport and in a greater degree, especially when they are compounded by other cross-cultural and intra-class differences.

Rapport would appear to have much in common with transference. Frequently, we are accustomed to think of transference bilaterally, but to think of rapport only unilaterally. Goffman states that in any situation where interaction is involved, the patient and the therapist each put on a "performance" for the benefit of the other.[8] Each puts on his best "front," most calculated to impress the other; neither one will be "taken in by the routine."[9] The occupational therapist, in this case, while trying to maintain the professional prescription of tacit self-constraint, will probe for the "dark secrets" he presumes the other to have. If the patient is equally sophisticated he will either conceal these secrets or use them to negotiate for whatever it is that he thinks he can get out of the relationship. Each in his own way, but especially the occupational therapist, will engage in what Goffman calls certain acts of "mystification."[10] These will involve, on his part, the use of esoteric words or professional jargon, and the allusion to powers (e.g., the doctor would like. . . .) outside the interview situation. He justifies the use of mystification to himself in terms of the "professional role," but actually he uses it to create or maintain his authority to probe for secrets. He already holds two trump cards in this; frequently his class superiority and his role of functionary in the agency that employs him. However, though his use of mystification tends to enhance his authority, it also tends to diminish rapport.

This is the predicament in which class and other cultural differences, including the difference in age between the occupational therapist and the patient, place the former. Control and rapport are both necessary, though paradoxical, requisites if interaction is to go as the occupational therapist defines it. The interview he is having with the patient will fall apart without control and will be meaningless without rapport. But the social distance between the patient and the occupational therapist results in secrets on both sides, especially on the side of the patient. The enchancement of control through mystification at this point only results in lessening of rapport, whereas rapport is the needed tool with which to disengage the secrets. The occupational therapist's attempts to pry at this juncture, into what Goffman calls the "back regions" or back stage where the patient lives with those most intimate to him, only increase the difficulties weakening rapport, even if they divulge a few secrets. Berne refers to these as the "first and second degree games."[3]

If we regard the patient-therapist relationship in the interview in a positive and constructive way the individual discovers himself and establishes his own identity. This interview, then, is not a situation — as it is commonly taken to be — in which a film (in the form of the interviewer) is exposed to an already established self which will then be developed (the occupational therapist's evaluation in preparation for starting therapy), so that the image of the self can be studied and diagnosed. It is rather, at least ideally, a constructed situation in which an individual acts out in conversation, the essentials of what Faris calls the "retrospective act,"[30] Rose believes it should be called the "conspective act" for it has present and future reference as well as past reference.[21] It does not stem from the past frustrated acts alone, but also from anticipations and intentions. These latter acts are of particular significance in the occupational therapy environment. In the interview process the patient is led to rehearse his past actions and the evaluations which others who matter to him put upon them. He is led to consider alternatives, or redirective actions, to imagine the responses of significance of others, and to define, assess and reassess himself as an object with each rehearsal.

It would seem to be the prime requisite of the occupational therapist that he present himself in this dialogue in such a way and in such a light as will most facilitate this rehearsal and this self-definition. To do this he must have achieved a certain degree of clarity in his own self-definition. It involves a reasonable congruence between role ideal and role actuality. It involves his knowledge and understanding of the various cross-cultural and inter-class rhetorics involved in any patient relationships. And it involves his understanding of the paradox of control and rapport and the aspects of the interview process for which each is distinctly requisite.

The analysis of the interview in terms of its nature as a social act has received very little attention by most occupational therapists. Perhaps it is due to the fact that they have been much more interested in the interview as an information-getting tool than as a therapeutic instrument. The occupational therapist is not ordinarily in a position to exercise any significant degree of control, at least, over the patients assigned to him; for they are assigned to, rather than accepted by him. Yet this phenomenon, which is in the general realm of interpersonal attractions and avoidances, must play some kind of significant part in the initial interview and in the therapeutic environment once treatment starts. One does not have to be a devotee of extra-sensory perception to believe that affinity and avoidance can be and usually are subliminally communicated. They affect the nature, direction, and success of the interview as a social act, for both the patient and the therapist. If progress is to be made and goals attained it is essential that rapport be established beginning with the initial interview.

CONSIDERATIONS IN THE THERAPEUTIC SETTING

In Part I of this chapter, two theories of adjustment of the aged were discussed. In view of the tenets of occupational therapy it is assumed that members of this profession would be advocates of engagement, or flexibility role theory, rather than the disengagement role theory. However, we must keep in mind that both theories represent essentially "ideal types" and as such do not exist. Rather there will be gradations or degrees of difference; even a continuum from one to the other.

Looking again at the thread woven throughout the first part we are reminded that the aged person's status and power are in direct proportion to society's needs. Today's aged are the products of a work oriented society. The "Protestant Ethic" was in vogue at the turn of this century.[29] Work was glorified; idleness was sinful. This ethos is changing in our culture but very slowly and leisure is far from being institutionalized.

With the above as background several approaches in therapy will be presented, each for a different level of activity among the aged. Note how the change is occurring in the use of the media.

Kramer points to conflicts that therapists have in expecting from their patients—not just activity—but goal-motivated activity which sometimes takes the form of productivity.[13] The "democratic, self-growth therapeutic atmosphere" is not supposed to demand activity for its own sake. But inactivity is still seen as bad, regressive, etc. The result is often an alternation in the therapist's behavior between demand for activity and cessation of involvement. Kramer believes that when working with the aged in particular, we can be carried away with the idea of work as therapy. Rather, we must try to analyze the separate components of work to see which, for any particular individual, are of value.

It is not necessary to work to be creative, to have social contacts, or to have a regular structured day. Work permits social contacts, absorption and some psychological satisfaction. But work is activity, and according to some authorities, activity is a controversial issue.

Pearman and Newman would disagree in part with Kramer.[44] These former researchers stress that it is not work performance alone which is important, but the social interaction that takes place in a small group involved in planning their activities. They found significant differences in the geriatric patient's level of performance in areas of initiative, degree of effort, relationship with the therapist and social interaction.

Notice in this particular research that programming is inferred. The patients, as participants, begin to assume a more prominent place in their environment. It becomes less of a patient-therapist interaction, where the therapist assumes the role of teacher, model, and participant; now the therapist becomes a provider of resources and an interpreter of group responsibilities. The therapist still channels the program toward treatment objectives but the group becomes more autonomous. The program allows for patient-patient relationships. Increasing meaningful interpersonal relationships can be a tremendously rewarding experience. "High visibility media," such as arts, crafts, weaving and ceramics, are useful when the geriatric patient is able to perform such tasks, but the interpersonal relationship fostering socialization within the group permits involvement which increases motivation over a longer time sequence. Solomon notes there is a tendency for the aged to move away from task-oriented roles to emotionally supportive roles as a primary source of life satisfaction.[53] This is due in part to physiological and neurological changes occurring in the aging process which will be discussed later under characteristics of aging persons.

We have assumed that the aged of today are the products of a work oriented society but that the aged of the future will be more leisure oriented. Since the practicing occupational therapist will be in this latter group he is presently preparing his inputs for later utilization. To avoid the pitfalls that Kramer refers to above, he is in an advantageous position to foster the idea of leisure time pursuits in the therapeutic setting.

We are attempting now to recognize the beginning shift of emphasis from activity for activity's sake to kinds and levels of activity. Activity levels in the adult go down with increasing age, but at what rate and for what reasons at this time we can only surmise. Anderson implies from his research that the individual must be subjected to some minimal amount of general stimulation, and if this is not provided serious psychological dysfunction will occur.[2] His conceptualization suggests that lack of stimulation leads to diminution of activity, which circularly results in less stimulation, and ultimately in deterioration of behavior. Although this deterioration can happen at any age and to anyone, the aged are particularly vulnerable to it. Lessened sensory capacities, diminished energy, and frail physical condition predispose the aging individual to stimulus deprivation with its deleterious behavioral consequences. This predicament was referred to earlier as the disengagement role.

We must conclude from Anderson's findings that maintenance of activity, regardless of kind and regardless of the attitude of the person toward it, is highly important to forestall quick deterioration. Unquestionably, optimum activity levels vary between individuals and with differing physical conditions. Undoubtedly, excessive or stress-producing activities may also be deleterious. How such levels, that are beneficial to the individual, can be selected is more a matter of art than of science at this time. Probably, the optimum amount of activity is somewhat above the spontaneous level adopted by the person earlier in his life. Hoever, the answer to this question, remains speculative until more adequate research is directed toward this problem.

Characteristics of Leisure Activities

When the aged have become less task oriented, what might be said in favor of leisure-time activities?

Leisure may be characterized by activity, although not all activity is leisure. The very practical questions which concern us here are:

(1) What distinguishes leisure activities from other activities?

(2) Which leisure activities are most appropriate for older persons?

Max Kaplan has attempted the difficult job of distinguishing leisure from other activities by establishing a set of criteria.[12] The first of these is that leisure must not be considered work, particularly in the economic sense. By this Kaplan means the exclusion of activities done for pay rather than for the pure pleasure of doing them. The distinction, then, is in the *motivation* and not in the *kind* of activity.

In effect, leisure activity is not defined by what one does, but by why one does it. Leisure activities must be characterized by pleasant expectation and recollection. The participants should have freedom of choice of the available activities, and the activities should be acceptable in the social situation. From this kind of classification leisure may be considered a state of mind rather than a particular kind of activity.

Some occupational therapists would take exception to the above concept, in the belief that work substitutes, even for small remuneration, are beneficial. If the activities pursued help to maintain the individual at an optimum activity level, they are justified. In addition, if the person enjoys them, no further justification is required providing the therapeutic goals are met.

CHARACTERISTICS OF AGING PERSONS

Although few persons will admit to being old, they will confess to their decrements. The combinations of claims and denials emphasize that the problems of aged humans result from the onset of physical and psychic ailments and not from aging as a special developmental phase or process. The performance and fitness of the elderly are increasingly limited by a number of, presumably, physiological changes: muscle strength wanes, bones become fragile, skin becomes thin, translucent and wrinkled, joints may develop arthritic alterations, and connective tissues lose their elasticity.

The changes involving the central nervous system are the most handicapping of those which accompany advancing years. Changes in psychic activity which may occur are lessening of attention, decline in memory (particularly in the present as opposed to the past) and emotional instability. Alterations in neurological activity include diminished reflexes, as well as difficulty and inefficiency in initiating and maintaining movement.

The elderly tire more quickly and easily as age increases. Even the effort of intense concentration is often sufficient to exhaust them. Lawton states that their emotional states may be often seething ferments of hostility, sadness, competitiveness, knowledge of decline and fear.[38] Although hidden from the observer, these confused emotions may dominate the consciousness of the elderly so as to obliterate reason, care, training, and experience.

Sensory changes cause additional problems. Eye changes and loss of hearing are conspicuous with advancing years. Impairments in other areas of communicatory activity, diminution of vibratory sensitivity, and diminished taste and olfactory sensations closely follow increasing chronological age. Each change produces a series of induced problems ranging from limited communication to deleterious dietary habits.

While all these changes may be considered pathological alterations with senescence, all are common concomitants of the aging process as it is usually observed today. Each complicates and handicaps the activities of the aged individual who possesses it.

Reality Needs of the Aged

Of importance is the fact that the reality needs of many older people are uppermost in their minds. They are anxious about income security, health, family relationships, etc., and bring these concerns to the therapeutic setting. Perhaps one of the most difficult tasks, owing to the lack of attention that has been given to the matter, is the assessment of an older person's ego functioning. Which defense should be strengthened? What new defenses should be erected? What is the reality perception of the member? What is his "sense of autonomy" and when is he expected to be "dependent"?

The therapist's approach to evaluating individuals as individuals, and as group members, must be guided by two seemingly contradictory tendencies: (1) to take into account a member's total situation and his problems, keeping in mind that older people generally do not have available as many outside resources as younger people have (e.g., school, peers, homes, etc.); (2) to partialize a patient's problem or concern since he may be able to master only one segment of it and thereby get a sense of accomplishment. The patient may be a difficult member in the group one day because of a personal experience which he projects onto the rest of the group, including the therapist. The therapist's assessment skill requires ability to sort out the "data" in order to see their total interrelationship and relevance. At the same time the therapist has to attend to the smaller details which are part of the problems and which may assume tremendous importance for the older person.

Research done by the author indicates that the aged in protective environments initially reject the environment and themselves in the new surroundings.[28,55] Such a move is frequently not by choice. Independence has to be relinquished in favor of dependence. The approach in occupational therapy was to build self-esteem for each individual by encouraging respect for others. The goal was to gradually build in each person enough feeling of worth and acceptance of his living conditions that he would participate in some of the activities in the protective environment and begin to form interpersonal relationships. This approach requires a certain measure of input from the patient. It requires from the therapist the ability to discover, through adequate interviewing technics, assets which the patient may bring to the situation. Later in the group — patient to patient — situation each member's assets and strengths are stressed in an attempt to give each one a role that provides status and a new measure of independent functioning.

Encouraging Motivation in the Institutionalized Aged

The most difficult problem faced by the therapist in an institution for the aging is motivating those elderly patients who do not readily join groups of any size; in fact, they may even be threatened by others. For these types of patients, gradualism is recommended.

The individual who is reluctant to join a group situation may be persuaded to engage in a solitary creative activity. Once he has achieved a degree of excellence in that, sufficient ego strength may develop so that he is willing to take a chance in the more competitive environment of the small group.

Timidity may take another form. An individual might possess neither the social confidence necessary for group participation nor sufficient self regard to undertake a solitary task and pursue it to a successful goal. For the patient who does not wish to participate actively, Margulies recommends a peripheral (passive) membership.[40] Here he may feel a part of things yet the environment makes no demands on him beyond what he is willing to give. His participation may be as much or as little as he chooses.

Filer and O'Connell observe that some of the deterioration of behavior observed in aging seems to be fostered by the institutional climate and is not merely a result of the aging process.[31] The occupational therapist is only one of the many professionals represented who views his task as that of transforming the institutional setting into a climate that nourishes mental health and encourages social rehabilitation and personality growth.

Awareness of Factors Inhibiting Learning

Elderly persons do not learn as quickly or retain new information as long as younger subjects. This phenomenon has been explained in terms of **learning deficits** associated with old age. Recent research suggests other factors may be present which inhibit learning. These factors are of particular interest to the occupational therapist who must consider them in treating the geriatric patients. They are as follows:

1. A longer period of time may be needed for accomplishing tasks.
2. Stress should be kept to a minimum.
3. Incentives should be provided which the patient defines as being important, preferably related to life-long interests.
4. Tasks must be meaningful since the patient is concerned about his status and self image.[28]

In considering the importance of motivation and the environmental factors impinging on it, Pincus stresses the therapeutic value of the context in which the activity is performed.[45] He considers it as great as the therapeutic value of the activity itself.

Making Behavioral Deficits Less Debilitating

The suggestion has been made by Lindsey that "prosthetic environments" would permit less debilitating aspects of behavioral deficits.[14] By prosthetic environments he means the adapting of equipment to meet the needs of the geriatric patient who has deficits, predominantly sensory. Occupational therapists are in a unique position to offer leadership to the interdisciplinary team in designing and setting up prosthetic environments. The following is but a brief list of adaptations. The ingenious creative mind of the occupational therapist will undoubtedly think of many more adaptations as the situation warrants them.

Amplifiers — which increase the intensity of environmental stimuli (e.g., signs with large print).

Multiple sense displays — which appeal to more than 1 sense.

Expanded auditory and visual narrative stimuli — e.g., movie projectors adapted to slow down visual and audio tracks, enabling more elderly persons to understand a film presentation.

Response force amplifiers — e.g., automatic-opening doors, throat microphones for feeble voices.

Wide response topographies — e.g., telephones utilizing pushbuttons instead of dials.

Rate switches — safety devices which have to be continually pressed, or pressed repeatedly, at certain time intervals in order to operate a machine or pieces of equipment (e.g., such as on an electric iron to avoid being left on).

Response feed-back systems—for appropriate response such as an electric eye which acts as a warning signal of danger (e.g., when person places hand too close to the edge of a saw).

The problem of motivation pervades the whole field of occupational therapy, particularly when treating the geriatric patient. The encounter will be facilitated if adequate incentives are presented which meet the needs of the elderly person. It has been suggested, in the above discussion, that the occupational therapist, as part of the interdisciplinary team, be keenly aware of the geriatric patient's deficits. His perception and follow-through in approach, together with a conducive environment, may well make the difference between involvement or lack of involvement of the aged person.

THE FUTURE FOR OCCUPATIONAL THERAPY IN GERIATRICS

In the discussion so far the assumption has been that the therapist's concern is mainly with the aged patient in some kind of protective environment. There is presently beginning a change of emphasis from institutional care of the aged, except for short-term hospitalization, to care offered in their own homes.

The reasons for the gradual shift are many. One is the increasing high cost of medical care. Another reason is the growing knowledge that elderly persons are happier and remain active longer when they are encouraged to stay in, or return to, surroundings familiar to them and where care can be adequately rendered.

Under these circumstances occupational therapists will need to be more community oriented. The rationale and the approach to treatment will remain the same. The therapists will need to join forces with others in community programs. They can anticipate that they will be called upon by representatives of the health professions in the community to enter into planning, offering suggestions and making available skills unique to their profession.

There is, however, a shortage of registered occupational therapists. The supply available does not presently meet the demand. If this demand is to be met it might be that these highly trained professionals will have to be used less as staff therapists and more in supervisory positions or in the capacity of consultants.

The Role of the Occupational Therapist as a Consultant

Although very few occupational therapists have ventured into consultation, it seems both timely and appropriate to discuss this area of professionalism. Of those few therapists who consider themselves consultants, more are in the specialty area of geriatrics than any of the other fields of occupational therapy. Since the demand for occupational therapists in the field of geriatrics will be even greater in the future, especially in the national Medicare Program and its anticipated modifications, it behooves us to search for ways in which we may use our services more advantageously.

Traditionally the consultation process in any field enables the consultee to identify problems and work out solutions. The consultant gives advice when it is sought after by the consultee. The consultant's role lacks authority, thereby, leaving the consultee free to accept or decline the recommendations made by the former. According to Mazer, the power of the consultant's role lies only in his specialized knowledge, and sometimes in his position as an outsider who acts as a clarifier.[41]

Leopold states that the modern trend in consultation is in "spreading professional manpower."[39] Faced with a shortage of professionally trained personnel and, therefore, unable to hire a staff therapist an administrator might consider a consultant as an alternative. This is particularly the case in protective environments for the aged where there is a great demand for such a service.

The roles of the occupational therapy consultant and the staff member are quite different as the following points indicate:

1. Unless employed by an agency the consultant is usually self employed. As such he carries on his own practice with all its ramifications.
2. He may be a consultant to a patient, an institution or agency, usually the latter.
3. He may be an educator orienting the staff or the local community, influencing changes in attitudes and functioning.
4. He will be expected to define, analyze or diagnose needs and help develop programs according to the situation of the consultee.
5. He is task oriented not patient oriented or client oriented. The primary job of the consultant is to help other people to treat patients.
6. The consultant remains removed from treatment and deals with many other factors that influence all patients in any given social system rather than one patient.

Being a consultant has its advantages and disadvantages. Probably the one reason why there are so few consultants in occupational therapy is that the consultation relationship is relatively lacking in the deep personal gratifications offered by the patient-therapist relationship. However, consultation does merit our attention; particularly at a time in the history of our profession when the shortage of registered occupational therapists exceeds that of all the other representatives in the health professions.

SUMMARY AND CONCLUSIONS

In dealing with the aged, one is dealing with bodies and minds that cannot be returned to full health and vigor. The fact of residual defects must be accepted, but it is important to preserve remaining bodily functions and mental faculties. This not only requires the full pursuit of all scientific medical advances in their behalf, but necessitates the simultaneous preservation of the privileges, honor and integrity of personal independence for each elderly individual. While occupational therapists will be constantly concerned with the latest scientific discoveries as they apply to their particular area of interest, they will also be emphasizing tender loving care whenever possible as a part of rehabilitative and restorative procedures for the aged and aging.

Aging must be viewed as a developmental process, but when physical or social trauma occurs, a downward spiral of loss can produce psychopathology. This spiral can frequently be halted by intervention on the part of the therapist through differential use of programmed therapeutic activities to meet the specific needs of specific patients at specific times. The primary reason for the inclusion of a particular activity in a therapeutic program should always be its potential value for the intended recipient.

We addressed ourselves in this chapter to the needs of the aged and aging, within a framework of historical relevance and cultural derivations. The occupational therapist must be attuned to the significance of these overtones which have resulted in the multifaceted social problems of the aged. As part of his total experience the patient brings these problems to the therapeutic situation.

Within a frame of reference of the aged as a disadvantaged person in this society, and superimposed upon it the debilitations which come with aging, concepts have been presented which included the roles of participants in interaction and the expanding of roles to include significant others which assist in the adjustment of the aged person to his environment.

The therapist is a product also of this society. He is also in the process of aging, and the environment where he works serves as a microcosm of the larger society. Therefore, the attitude of the therapist requires a good deal of insight, development and coming to terms with his personal reaction toward aging if rapport is to be established and goals realized.

Theories on disengagement and engagement roles of the aged were presented with the proposition that these roles may be transitional on a continuum scale. If these theories have significance to the therapist emphasis in treatment may be placed on movement away from the former to the latter role.

Instead of accepting debilitating factors, emphasis has been placed on improving the environment to facilitate the learning process. Various approaches to treatment have been presented emphasizing the need to reduce dependency by restructuring treatment programs to permit ample opportunity for the geriatric patient to reconstruct a new self-image through finding in others an evaluation of himself, which he can internalize. It requires on the part of the aged patient an input of satisfactory assets, and on the part of others an appreciation for them which will enable the patient to have status which commands respect in his therapeutic environment.

Finally, and very briefly, the role of the therapist was discussed as a professional member of the community and the contribution he might make considering first, the trend toward providing care for the elderly patient in his own home and the reasons for this trend. Secondly, due to the increasing demand for, and the continual shortage of registered occupational therapists, particularly in the field of geriatrics, a proposal was made to consider consultation as a way of utilizing to better advantage, the available professional skills of these highly trained people.

REFERENCES

Books

1. Albrecht, R., and Havighurst, R. J.: Older People. New York, Longman, Green & Co., 1953.
2. Anderson, J. E.: The Use of Time and Energy, in J. E. Biren (ed.); the Handbook of Aging and the Individual. pp. 769-796, Chicago, The University of Chicago Press, 1959.
3. Berne, E.: Games People Play. New York, Grove Press, 1964.
4. Burgess, E. W. (ed.): Aging in Western Societies. pp. 383-384. Chicago, University of Chicago Press, 1960.
5. Cooley, C. H.: Human Nature and the Social Order. rev., New York, Scribner, 1922.
6. Cumming, E., and Henry, W.: Growing Old. New York, Basic Books, 1961.
7. Flaceliere, R.: Daily Life in Greece at the Time of Pericles. New York, Macmillan, 1965.
8. Goffman, E.: Encounters. New York, Bobb Merrill, 1961.
9. ———: Interaction Ritual. Garden City, N.Y., Doubleday, 1967.
10. ———: The Presentation of Self in Everyday Life. Garden City, N.Y., Doubleday, 1959.
11. Hostetler, J. A.: Amish Society. Baltimore, Johns Hopkins, 1963.

12. Kaplan, M.: Toward a Theory of Leisure for Social Gerontology. in R. W. Leimeier (ed.); Aging and Leisure: a Research Perspective into the Meaningful Use of Time. pp. 389-412, New York, Oxford University Press, 1961.

13. Kramer, C. H.: Day Hospital, New York, Grune and Stratton, 1962.

14. Lindsley, O. R.: Geriatric Behavioral Prosthetics, in R. Kastenbaum (ed.); New Thoughts on Old Age. pp. 41–60. New York, Springer, 1964.

15. Lipman, Aaron: Responsibility and Morale. Proceedings of the 7th International Congress of Gerontology. pp. 267–276. Vienna, Austria, June 26–July 2, 1966.

16. Loether, Herman J.: Problems of Aging; Sociological and Social Psychological Perspectives. p. 33. Belmont, California, Dickerson, 1967.

17. Newton, K.: Geriatric Nursing. ed. 3, St. Louis, C. V. Mosby, 1960.

18. Parsons, T.: The Social System. p. 436, Glencoe, Illinois, The Free Press, 1951.

19. Paul, B. D.: Interview Techniques and Field Relationships, in A. L. Kroeber (ed.); Anthropology Today. pp. 430–451, Chicago, The University Press, 1953.

20. President's Council on Aging: The Older American. pp. 1, 14, 15. Washington, D.C., U.S. Government Printing Office, 1963.

21. Rose, A. M.: Human Behavior and Social Processes; An Interactionist Approach. Boston, Houghton Mifflin, 1962.

22. Rose, A. M., and Peterson, W. A.: Older People and Their Social World. (eds.) p. 360. Philadelphia, F. A. Davis, 1965.

23. Snyder, N. V.: A Statement of Position. The American Occupational Therapy Foundation; Education and Research. p. 3. New York, The Amer. Occup. Therapy Foundation, Inc., 1965.

24. Tibbitts, C.: The Evolving Work-Life Pattern. Handbook of Social Gerontology. p. 386. Chicago, University of Chicago Press, 1960.

25. Tierney, B.: Medieval Poor Law; A Sketch of Canonical Theory and Its Implications in England. Berkeley, UCLA Press, 1959.

26. U.S. Department of Health, Education and Welfare: Health Care of the Aged. p. 25, Washington, D.C., U.S. Government Printing Office, 1962.

27. Walker, A. D.: Nursing Homes; A Metropolitan Survey. Dynamic Living for the Long Term Patient; Study Course III. p. 64. Third International Congress of World Federation of Occupational Therapists, New York, 1962.

28. ————: Occupational Therapy Potentialities in Homes for the Aged. Proceedings of the 1960 Annual Conference. p. 31. New York, The American Occupational Therapy Association, 1960.

29. Weber, M.: The Protestant Ethic and the Spirit of Capitalism. tr. by Talcott Parson. New York, Scribner, 1950.

Journals

30. Faris, E.: The restrospective act. J. Educ. Soc., 14:79–91, 1940.

31. Filer, R. N., and O'Connell, D. D.: Motivation of aging persons in an institutional setting. J. Geront., 19:15–22, 1964.

32. Havighurst, R. J.: Flexibility and the social roles of the retired. Am. J. Sociol. 59:309–311, 1954.

33. Haynes, M. S.: The supposedly golden age for the aged in Ancient Rome. Gerontologist, 3:26–35, 1963.
34. Inskip, W. M.: Development of personal integrity in the patient with chronic illness. Am. J. Occup. Therapy, 15:196, 1961.
35. Kalish, R. W.: Of children and grandchildren; a speculative essay on dependency. Gerontologist, 7:66, 1967.
36. Kastenbaum, R. J.: Projections. J. Geriatric Psychiat. 2:244–247, 1969.
37. Kutner, B.: Modes of treating the chronically ill. Gerontologist, 4 (Part 2): 44-48, 1964.
38. Lawton, A. H.: Characteristics of the geriatric person. Gerontologist, 8:120–123, 1968.
39. Leopold, R. L.: Consultant and consultee; an extraordinary human relationship, some thoughts for the occupational therapist. Am. J. Occup. Therapy, 22:72–81, 1968.
40. Margulies, M. S.: Classification of activities to meet the psycho-social needs of geriatric patients. Gerontologist, 6:210–211, 1966.
41. Mazer, J. L.: The occupational therapist as consultant. Am. J. Occup. Therapy, 23:417–421, 1969.
42. Morse, N. S., and Weiss, S.: The functions and meaning of work and the job. Am. Sociol. Rev., 20:198, 1955.
43. Mullan, H.: The personality of those who care for the aging. Gerontologist, 1:44–46, 1961.
44. Pearman, H. E. and Newman, N.: Work-oriented occupational therapy for the geriatric patient. Am. J. Occup. Therapy, 22:203–208, 1968.
45. Pincus, A.: New findings on learning in old age; implications for occupational therapy. Am. J. Occup. Therapy, 22:302, 1968.
46. Riesman, D., and Benny, M. (eds.): The interview in social research. Am. J. Sociol., Vol. 62, September, 1956.
47. Rosenblatt, D., and Taviss, I.: The home for the aged; theory and practice. Gerontologist, 6 (Part 1): 165–168, 1966.
48. Thompson, Wayne E.: Pre-retirement anticipation and Adjustment in retirement. The Journal of Social Issues, 14–35, 1958.
49. Walker, A. D.: Nationally speaking; report from the white house conference on aging. Am. J. Occup. Therapy, 15:167, 1961.
50. Wessen, A. F.: Some sociological characteristics of long term care. Gerontologist, 4, (Part 2): 7–14, 1964.
51. Willard, H. N.: Home care versus institutional care. Gerontologist, 4, (Part 2): 49–52, 1964.

Papers

52. Shanas, E.: Health Problems of the Aged. Paper presented at the annual meetings of the Western Gerontological Society, Los Angeles, California, November 13, 1965.
53. Solomon, B.: Social Functioning of the Economically Dependent Aged. Paper presented at the Western Gerontological Society's Twelfth Annual Conference on Aging on Social Behavior, San Francisco, California, September 19, 1966.

54. Walker, A. D.: Sociological Aspects of the Aged. Paper presented to the 1967 Convention of California Nurses Association, Los Angeles, California, March 8, 1967.

Thesis

55. Walker, A. D.: An Investigation Into Life Satisfactions of Geriatric Men and Women Living in Protective Environments. Los Angeles, University of Southern California, Unpublished Master's Thesis, January, 1959.

Newspaper Article

56 Medical Care is a Luxury. Los Angeles Herald Examiner, Los Angeles, California, December 20, 1965.

Index

Numerals in *italics* indicate tables or illustrations.

Trauma, and spinal cord injury, 292
Tumors, brain, factors affecting therapy, 159

Upper extremity. See *Extremity, upper.*

Vision, in cerebral palsy, 343
Visual deficiency, and patient instruction, 48
Visually handicapped. See *Blindness.*
Vocation. See *Job.*
Vocational counseling, relation of, to therapist, 9
Vocational evaluation, following stroke, 325
Vocational potential, following spinal cord injury, 305
Vocational problems, in stroke, 316
Vocational rehabilitation, for blind, 501
Voos, D., 375

Ward patients, supportive therapy for, 138
Watanabe, S., 90

Weaving, 173
  for restoration of function, analysis of, 179
Wheelchair, in cerebral palsy, *349, 351*
  in spinal cord injury, 300
  trays for, 351, *352, 355*
  with seatboard, 283
White, R. W., 123
Woodworking, 173
  for restoration of function, analysis of, 178
World Federation of Occupational Therapists, 3
Work, in occupational therapy, 124
Wrist, activities for, 176
  braid weaving as, 179, 181
  woodworking as, 178
  amputation involving, prostheses for, *269, 270*
  exercise of, 167
  joints, of, measurement of, 207, *207, 208*
  motion of, in daily living, *231*
  orthoses for, *238, 239*
  recovery of, in stroke, 320
Writing, dysfunctions associated with, 460
  motion used in, analysis of, 229
  orthoses for, *238, 239*